Trauma Assessments

TRAUMA
ASSESSMENTS

A Clinician's Guide

Eve B. Carlson

The Guilford Press
New York London

© 1997 The Guilford Press
A Division of Guilford Publications, Inc.
72 Spring Street, New York, NY 10012

Printed in the United States of America

This book is printed on acid-free paper.

Last digit is print number: 9 8 7 6 5 4 3 2 1

Library of Congress Cataloging-in-Publication Data

Carlson, Eve B.
    Trauma assessments : a clinician's guide / Eve B. Carlson.
        p. cm.
    Includes bibliographical references and index.
    ISBN 1-57230-251-8 (hard)
        1. Post-traumatic stress disorder—Diagnosis. 2. Psychic trauma.
    3. Dissociative disorders—Diagnosis. I. Title.
        [DNLM: 1. Stress Disorders, Post-Traumatic—diagnosis. 2. Stress, Psychological—psychology. WM 170 C284t 1997]
    RC552.P67C37 1997
    616.85'21—dc21
    DNLM/DLC
    for Library of Congress   97-17254
                                                              CIP

Acknowledgments

This book was made possible only by a considerable amount of kindness from strangers and more than a little help from my friends. I am grateful to work in a field in which generosity and a collaborative spirit are the norm.

I would like to acknowledge a number of people whose comments and suggestions greatly shaped the structure and contents of the book. Their insights and encouragement were invaluable to me. Thanks go to Judith Armstrong, John Briere, Mark Chaffin, James High, Steven Lynn, Elana Newman, Frank Putnam, and Lucy Quimby. I am also extremely grateful to the measure authors for their enthusiasm for the project and willingness to review the profiles. I appreciate the years of hard work they put into the development and validation of these innovative measures. Needless to say, these assessment tools provided the impetus to write the book.

I am particularly indebted to my friend Constance Dalenberg for her detailed comments and suggestions on the entire manuscript. Her ideas greatly enriched and enhanced the book. The best parts of the book are those that were refined as a result of her intellectual prodding.

At The Guilford Press, Rochelle Serwator and Seymour Weingarten were continual sources of enthusiasm and encouragement, renewing my energies at each stage of the long and sometimes tedious process of creating a book. Rochelle was a great help in my efforts to make this sometimes dense material more accessible.

I also thank the many trauma survivors who generously and patiently described their traumatic experiences and responses to me and my colleagues. Without their willingness to put into words the horror of their experiences and the disturbing and often difficult-to-describe consequences, we would not know what to ask or how to ask.

Finally, my husband, Kurt, deserves a great deal of credit for his patience and unflagging confidence in me. His constant support allowed me to enjoy the writing process and give it my best effort.

Preface

This book is intended for clinicians at all levels of experience with trauma and its effects. Those with little or no training in the trauma field will find a good deal of theoretical and practical information that will help them understand trauma and trauma responses and how best to assess them. Those who have some knowledge of trauma and assessment will find a broad review of theoretical issues and specific guidance on options for assessing trauma and trauma responses. Experienced trauma clinicians and researchers will find new theoretical formulations and innovations in measurement that can add to their stock of assessment tools.

Some fresh twists on venerable concepts that appear in this book include ideas about what makes an event traumatic and how dissociative symptoms fit into a conceptualization of posttraumatic responses. Innovations in measurement covered in the book include tools for assessing trauma that are broad in scope and provide for detailed inquiries and tools that can be used to assess responses to multiple traumatic events. Many of the measures profiled in the book have not previously been published or described in the literature. One of the primary goals of this book is make these assessment tools available to practicing clinicians.

Before treating traumatized clients, you must gather the information needed to plan treatment. This process is facilitated by access to assessment tools that are inexpensive and easy to obtain, use, score, and interpret. But in order to choose the most appropriate measures and interviews for a particular client in a particular setting and to interpret the results of your assessment, you need to have a good theoretical understanding of the effects of trauma.

This book begins with the theoretical foundation for understanding human responses to traumatic experiences. The first chapter addresses why mental health professionals need to understand and assess responses to traumatic experiences and how a better understanding of trauma theories and better assessment methods will foster appropriate, effective, and efficient treatment of traumatized persons. Chapters 2 through 5 describe a general, integrative theoretical framework for the effects of traumatic experiences. I believe that the most useful conceptual framework for practicing clinicians is one that encompasses the entire spectrum of traumatic responses and disorders. Accordingly, this framework applies to single-event traumas as well as to more chronic traumatic experiences. It specifies the most common core, secondary, and associated responses to trauma and the major factors that influence responses to trauma. These chapters also discuss the course of trauma responses and variations in responses seen across traumas that occur at different points in the life span.

The second part of the book addresses both conceptual and practical aspects of choosing and administering measures of trauma and trauma responses. Chapter 6 discusses the many challenges involved in accurately assessing trauma and trauma responses and offers suggestions for maximizing the accuracy of your assessments and minimizing the effects of client and interviewer expectations on your assessments. Chapter 7 provides information about the available options for assessment and about measure characteristics that should be considered when choosing measures for a particular client. Chapter 8 includes an explanation of what information is included in the profiles of measures and a discussion of the practical aspects of administering measures.

The third part of the text addresses how to proceed after the assessment is complete. Chapter 9 offers guidance in interpreting results of assessments and diagnosing trauma-related disorders. This chapter also includes discussion of a number of controversial issues relating to the diagnosis of posttraumatic stress disorder and dissociative disorders. Chapter 10 provides a brief introduction to the major forms of treatment of trauma-related disorders and cites sources of further information about these treatments. The final chapter offers some idea of developments you can expect in assessment of trauma and trauma responses in the coming years.

The final section of the book includes profiles of recommended measures of traumatic experiences and trauma responses. These include self-report and interview measures of trauma, self-report measures of trauma symptoms, structured interviews for posttraumatic and dissociative disorders, and measures for children and adolescents. Although it may be tempting to flip directly to the profiles, the information they contain is best understood in the context of the material covered in Part II.

Throughout the book, references are provided to support formulations, but these are not an exhaustive review of all relevant research or theory. Where possible, I have tried to include citations for sources of information that describe alternative conceptualizations or more detailed discussions of topics addressed.

Numerous examples are given to illustrate responses to a variety of traumatic stressors. Names of clients in examples are all fictitious, and details of the cases have all been altered so that the identity of the client cannot be recognized. Some examples are composites of different individuals, and some are fictional.

Contents

MEASURE PROFILES

Part I

UNDERSTANDING THE IMPACT OF TRAUMA

Chapter 1

The Importance of Understanding Responses to Trauma

Every new client presents something of a mystery. You and the client need to "solve the mystery" in order to develop an appropriate treatment plan or referral. Solving the mystery involves assessing the client's current symptoms and coming to an understanding of his or her psychological problems. For a number of reasons, it can be especially difficult for mental health professionals who have no special training in traumatic stress disorders to assess and understand the symptoms of a traumatized person. At the same time, studies of the prevalence of potentially traumatic events and of trauma-related psychological disorders such as posttraumatic stress disorder (PTSD), dissociative disorders, and acute stress disorder (ASD) have shown that traumatic events and related disorders are far from rare.

A review of studies of the prevalence of potentially traumatic events in the United States shows that rates of exposure vary from moderate to quite high, depending on the population sampled and the methods used to define and ask about the experiences (Green, 1994). For example, when a random sample of young adults from an urban area of the Midwest were asked whether they had experienced an event outside the range of normal human experience, about 40% of them said they had (Breslau, Davis, Andreski, & Peterson, 1991). When a random sample of women in South Carolina were interviewed, 34% of them reported at least one experience of sexual abuse before the age of 18 (Saunders, Villeponteaux, Lipovsky, Kilpatrick, & Veronen, 1992). A study of a women enrolled in colleges and universities across the United States found that 27% of them reported that they had been sexually assaulted or raped at least once since the age of 14 (Koss, Gidycz, & Wisniewski, 1987). Norris (1992) studied a community sample of men and women and asked them about their experience of a wide range of potentially traumatic events. She found that 69% of the subjects reported having been exposed to at least one potentially traumatic event. In another study of a community sample, lifetime exposure to potentially traumatic events was also found to be 69% (Resnick, Kilpatrick, Dansky, Saunders, & Best, 1993).

Rates of exposure to potentially traumatic events are also very high among people who seek treatment for psychological problems. When a sample of psychiatric outpatients was asked whether they had experienced an event outside the range of normal human experience, 81% of them reported having had one or more of these experiences (Davidson & Smith, 1990). Two studies of psychiatric outpatients found that between 64–68% of those sampled reported childhood experiences of physical or sexual assault when they were asked directly (Jacobson, 1989; Surrey, Swett, Michaels, & Levin, 1990). Similar studies of reported childhood physical or sexual assault in samples of psychiatric inpatients have found rates that vary from 63% to 81% (Bryer, Nelson, Miller, & Krol, 1987; Chu & Dill, 1990; Craine, Henson, Colliver, & MacLean, 1988; Jacobson & Richardson, 1987). It is clear, then, that a substantial proportion of people who come to mental health professionals for treatment have had an experience that may have been traumatizing.

Reviews of research on rates of traumatic stress responses have estimated that 25–30% of those exposed to extreme stressors develop PTSD (Green, 1994; Tomb, 1994). Research has not yet clearly established what proportion of those who experience a stressor develop other trauma-related disorders such as dissociative disorders or ASD. If rates of exposure to trauma are in the 60–80% range in psychiatric treatment settings, and 25–30% of those exposed develop PTSD, then clinicians can expect at least 15% of their clients to have current or past trauma-related symptoms. Although assessing trauma responses can be tricky, the task is one faced by virtually every clinician.

The difficulties of accurately assessing trauma responses have been exacerbated in the 1990s by increasing pressure on mental health professionals to assess and treat clients quickly and cost-effectively. In many clinical settings, it is no longer possible to conduct or order a full psychological evaluation or a complete battery of psychological tests on every client because the time and resources for this simply are not available. Similarly, most clinicians do not have the luxury of seeing a client five or six times before making a treatment or referral recommendation. The reality faced by many (perhaps most) mental health professionals today is that they must make a treatment plan or a referral decision after only one or two sessions and without using expensive assessment tools. In these circumstances, making sense of responses to trauma has become even more challenging, and the obstacles to understanding and assessing trauma responses have become more and more salient.

OBSTACLES TO UNDERSTANDING TRAUMA RESPONSES

One obstacle to understanding responses to traumatic experiences is the rich complexity of relationships among traumatic experiences, the moderating variables that influence the response to a traumatic experience, and the outcomes that the clinician observes in the form of symptoms. This is partly because the traumatic experiences a person might have can vary greatly in terms of their intensity, duration, frequency, meaning, and other factors. But even for a particular stressor, there is no clear and simple cause-and-effect relationship between a traumatic experience and subsequent psychological symptoms. Two people can have the same traumatic experience yet show very different responses. For example, suppose two people are in a convenience store when there is an armed robbery. Each of them might respond very differently to that event, depending on individual variables such as previous history of trauma, age, sex, cultural background, biological vulnerability (or resilience) to stress, perceptions about how much danger they were in, and the amount of social support they get following the experience. One person might largely have "gotten over" the experience a month later, whereas the other might have severe PTSD. In Chapter 4, I discuss the factors that influence responses to traumatic experiences in more detail.

Another obstacle to understanding traumatic stress responses is that most mental health professionals do not receive much (if any) training or experience with these disorders during their graduate training. Even though it may seem nonsensical that trauma-related disorders were not covered in courses or practicums taken by today's practicing therapists along with other psychological disorders, this situation probably results from the fact that this is a fairly new area of study in psychology and psychiatry. Traumatic stress reactions were described in rudimentary forms in the first and second editions of the *Diagnostic and Statistical Manual of Mental Disorders* (DSM) of the American Psychiatric Association, but PTSD was not recognized as a distinct diagnostic category until 1980 when the third edition of the DSM was published (Wilson,

1994a). Similarly, dissociative disorders, which research has linked to traumatic experiences (Classen, Koopman, & Spiegel, 1993), first appeared as a diagnostic category in DSM-III (American Psychiatric Association, 1987). Since diagnostic criteria (and measures of the relevant symptoms) are necessary for empirical research on a disorder, research on traumatic stress reactions did not begin in earnest until the 1980s. Trauma researchers and clinicians have had relatively little time to understand how traumatic events affect people, and the knowledge that the "first generation" of trauma researchers has acquired is just beginning to be incorporated into the curricula of graduate training programs. In short, most clinicians practicing today did not get training relating to trauma because most of their graduate faculty and clinical supervisors were not knowledgeable about trauma.

OBSTACLES TO ACCURATELY ASSESSING TRAUMA RESPONSES

There are several obstacles that make it especially difficult for clinicians to accurately assess traumatic stress responses and trauma-related disorders. One of these obstacles involves the more practical and technical aspects of assessment, while others result from the nature and complexities of the trauma responses themselves.

Using Psychological Tests to Assess Trauma Responses

In practical terms, in order to assess responses to traumatic experiences, it is necessary to ask about the relevant symptoms. Although I discuss the prominent responses to trauma in more detail later, it is safe to say here that measuring PTSD symptoms and dissociative symptoms is crucial to a good assessment of trauma response. Unfortunately, the most widely used psychological tests are not useful for assessing PTSD or dissociative symptoms. Worse yet, some of the results from these measures can be misleading for traumatized people.

Three of the most popular self-report symptom measures that are frequently given to people who seek treatment include the Minnesota Multiphasic Personality Inventory (current version is the MMPI-2), the Millon Clinical Multiaxial Inventory (current version is the MCMI-III), and the Symptom Checklist 90—Revised (SCL-90-R). Often, one of these global symptom measures is part of a routine intake assessment at outpatient clinics and psychiatric hospitals. All of these three measures yield subscale scores for various symptoms and characteristics, but two have no subscale for PTSD symptoms, and none of them has a subscale for dissociative symptoms. The MCMI-III has a PTSD subscale, but it has not been established as a valid measure of PTSD. Two of these inventories do have subscales for anxiety, which may be somewhat helpful in assessing trauma responses, but they will not help you with making a differential diagnosis between PTSD and another anxiety disorder.

For the MMPI, subscales have been developed to measure PTSD symptoms, but they may not be adequate clinical measures of these symptoms. For example, the Keane PTSD Scale (also known as the PK subscale) uses 46 MMPI-2 items to measure PTSD symptoms (Lyons & Keane, 1992). Unfortunately, since the items are drawn from MMPI-2 items, they do not fully represent the symptoms of PTSD. For example, there are no items about symptoms of intrusive images or emotional numbing that are commonly associated with posttraumatic responses. Also, studies of the subscale's ability to correctly identify those with PTSD have shown mixed results (Solomon, Keane, Kaloupek, & Newman, 1996). In some studies, the subscale did not do a very good job of picking out those with a PTSD diagnosis. Also, since norms are not yet available for various traumatized groups for the updated PK subscale that corresponds to the MMPI-2, it is difficult to make clinical interpretations of these scores. The PK subscale may be useful if you have access to MMPI results and no other options for measuring PTSD, but it is not optimal for that purpose.

Some results from general symptom inventories may even be misleading for those with trauma-related disorders. For example, the MMPI F scale is often elevated in those with posttraumatic or dissociative disorders (Carlson & Armstrong, 1994; Orr et al., 1990). The F scale was designed to be a validity scale to indicate carelessness in responding, gross eccentricity, or malingering (or "faking bad"), and it was originally made up of items that were thought to be rare psychiatric symptoms (Anastasi, 1988). It now appears that some of those symptoms are common to many with posttraumatic or dissociative disorders, particularly war veterans. For example, F-scale items include "I have nightmares every few nights" and "I believe my sins are unpardonable." Using the MMPI to assess a traumatized person might lead to the mistaken conclusion that the person is exaggerating his symptoms, when he is actually accurately reporting them. The danger of misinterpretation of an elevated F-scale score is very likely present in the MMPI-2 as well as the MMPI, as 60 of the 64 items that load onto the F scale were retained in the MMPI-2 (Butcher, Dahlstrom, Graham, Tellegen, & Kaemmer, 1989). It is possible that similar problems with other symptom measures might lead to misdiagnosis or misinterpretation of results, but too little research has been done on MCMI-III and SCL-90-R results in traumatized people to determine whether they might be misleading. Clearly, though, none of these major symptom inventories is optimal for assessing traumatic symptoms because these inventories do not directly assess the core symptoms of PTSD and dissociation.

In a standard psychological testing battery, other tests such as intelligence tests and projective tests are often used to gather clinical information. For example, those who use intelligence tests are familiar with the subscales known as the "anxiety triad" that indicates impairment of intellectual functioning due to anxiety. Theoretically, it might be possible to identify a similar "trauma triad" as a marker of impairment of intellectual functioning due to PTSD and/or dissociative symptoms, but to date, such a marker has not been identified.

Among projective tests, the Rorschach inkblot test is widely used in clinical assessments. In recent years, there has been increased interest in identifying Rorschach markers for trauma (Levin & Reis, 1996). Some very promising work has been done to develop a Traumatic Content Index (Armstrong & Loewenstein, 1990) that may provide information about how a person is responding to a known trauma. This index may one day be part of a Rorschach scoring system, but until then, a standard scoring and interpretation of the Rorschach will not be of much help in assessing trauma responses. Results from other projective tests such as the Thematic Apperception Test (TAT) or projective drawing tests (like the Draw-A-Person) may provide some interesting and useful clinical hypotheses, but since results from these tests tend to have questionable validity and are usually not objectively scored, they cannot provide clear and objective information about PTSD or dissociative symptoms. All in all, then, results from a standard psychological test battery are unlikely to yield the information you need for a systematic assessment of trauma responses.

Using Standard Intake Interviews to Assess Trauma History and Trauma Responses

Most clinicians use some type of assessment or intake interview to assess new patients and make initial treatment or referral plans. Most of us have some standard set of questions that we like to ask to find out about a client's life history and current problems. And most of the time, this standard interview provides us with enough information to give us confidence that we do know the important life events and that we understand the client's problems well enough to plan treatment. But there may be ways in which our standard intake interview may fail us without our realizing it. In particular, most intake interviews are likely to miss important traumatic experiences and to miss some of the symptoms most relevant to traumatic experiences.

For example, studies have found that routine assessments in psychiatric hospitals often fail to uncover potentially traumatic experiences of childhood abuse. This happens largely because most routine assessments simply do not ask people about these kinds of experiences. In one study, psychiatric inpatients were given detailed interviews about their experiences of physical or sexual assault as children and as adults. The researchers then checked the records of those who had had such experiences and found that 91% of the assaults reported in the interviews had not been noted in their records (Jacobson, Koehler, & Jones-Brown, 1987). Inadequate assessment of trauma and trauma responses may be especially prevalent in specialized treatment facilities where assessment and treatment are focused on a particular disorder. For example, clinicians working in a pain treatment center who do not systematically assess trauma and trauma responses may miss important information in those who have experienced traumatic injuries. Similarly, clinicians treating people with drug and alcohol dependency problems may miss important diagnostic information when drug and alcohol problems are comorbid with trauma symptoms.

It is worth noting that the lack of attention to trauma history (including childhood abuse experiences) predated the concern over the possibility of "false memories" that has troubled mental health professionals in the 1990s. I discuss the difficulties of asking about abuse in more detail in Chapter 6. For now, suffice it to say that epidemiological research on child abuse has unequivocally established that millions of children are abused every year in the United States (Panel on Research on Child Abuse and Neglect, 1993). Since it seems reasonable to expect that those experiences would have an impact on a person's psychological functioning, clinicians should ask about them.

Another problem that makes it hard to get an accurate assessment of a person's trauma history is that many people have partial or complete amnesia for traumatic events that occur to them (Loewenstein, 1996). Several studies have found that a substantial proportion of those who are physically or sexually assaulted as children have partial or complete amnesia for the experiences for some period after. In one particularly compelling study, a group of women, who had been examined and treated in a hospital emergency room after sexual assaults when they were children, were interviewed as adults (Williams, 1994). As adults, 17 years after their assaults, the women were asked if they could be interviewed for a study of women who had received hospital care as children. Despite detailed questions about past experiences of sexual assault, 38% of the women did not report the incident for which they had been treated at the hospital. Of those who did recall the incident, 16% reported that they had had amnesia for the event for some time following it (Williams, 1994).

Similar results were found in a study of a nationally representative random sample of adults. Of those who reported that they had experiences of sexual assault during childhood, 42% said that they had had some level of amnesia for the experience, and 20% said that they had

had complete amnesia for the experience for some time in the years following the event (Elliott & Briere, 1995). Another study found even higher rates of amnesia in a clinical sample of subjects. In a sample of people in outpatient treatment, 59% reported some level of past amnesia for childhood sexual assault experiences (Briere & Conte, 1993). I have found similar rates of amnesia in my own study of psychiatric inpatients (Carlson, Armstrong, Loewenstein, & Roth, 1997). Of those who reported sexual assault experiences in childhood, 61% reported having at some time experienced some level of amnesia, and 42% reported total amnesia for the event. A higher rate of amnesia for psychiatric patients compared to people who were not seeking treatment can probably be explained by the finding (from both studies) that people with more severe symptoms and more severe trauma are more likely to have amnesia for traumatic experiences (Carlson, Armstrong, Loewenstein, & Roth, 1997; Elliott & Briere, 1995).

Limited memory for traumatic events is also a problem for those who have traumatic experiences as adults. For example, in my own research on Cambodian refugees who experienced traumatic events as adults, 90% of the subjects reported having amnesia for important aspects of the events (Carlson & Rosser-Hogan, 1991). Partial or total amnesia has also been found in survivors of traumatic experiences such as combat, concentration camp incarceration, torture, and natural disasters (Loewenstein, 1996; van der Kolk, 1996d). In fact, lack of memory for important aspects of traumatic experiences is so common among traumatized persons that it constitutes one of the diagnostic criteria for PTSD.

It seems then that a substantial proportion of those who have traumatic experiences in childhood or adulthood will not remember part or all of their experiences later on. This means that it is likely that some people who come for treatment will not give complete reports of their trauma histories even when they are specifically asked about such experiences.

Another pitfall of intake interviews is that peoples' reports about their symptoms can be incomplete. Setting aside the possibility of intentional misreporting that may occur in a small minority of cases, many traumatized persons may unintentionally misreport their symptoms. In some cases, this might be because the client is not aware of what symptoms are relevant to her evaluation and treatment. At a time when a lot of therapists are not sure about the relationships between traumatic experiences and particular symptoms, we surely cannot expect the average person to have such knowledge. In some cases, a person might be reluctant to report symptoms that seem very unusual or "weird" to her. New clients might be especially unwilling to tell an unfamiliar therapist about "strange" phenomena such as flashbacks, intrusive images, or distorted perceptions of themselves or their surroundings—all common posttraumatic symptoms.

In still other cases, a client might not report an important symptom because she does not perceive it as a symptom. This might happen, for example, to a woman who has experienced chronic, severe, and traumatizing abuse as a child that resulted in the lifelong symptom of emotional numbing in the form of a restricted range of affect. This woman might not report "feeling numb" when she seeks treatment if she does not ever remember feeling differently. In other words, she may not perceive the restricted affect as a symptom of disorder because it is "normal" for her.

To summarize, a standard intake interview may sometimes fail to provide you with all of the information you need about a person's trauma history and symptoms. This can happen when an interview does not include specific questions about possible traumatic experiences, when a person has amnesia for part or all of his traumatic experience(s), or when a person's reports about his symptoms are incomplete.

Presenting Symptoms May Be Misleading

Another major obstacle to accurate assessment of trauma responses is the fact that presenting symptoms of traumatized people can be very misleading. Although assessing and diagnosing a new client is often a challenge, assessment of traumatized people can be especially perplexing and enigmatic because of the great overlap between trauma-related symptoms and symptoms of other disorders. There are many disorders that have symptoms in common with other disorders, but symptoms of trauma-related disorders such as PTSD, dissociative disorders, and ASD overlap or are similar to symptoms of dozens of DSM-IV disorders. This problem is compounded by the fact that many clinicians have little or no formal training in assessing and conceptualizing trauma-related disorders.

Because trauma-related disorders have a number of symptoms in common with other disorders, a therapist might interpret a posttraumatic symptom as part of some other, more familiar disorder and miss its significance as a response to trauma. The most common examples of this are trauma symptoms such as problems with sleep and concentration that may be mistaken for symptoms of other anxiety disorders or depression. Another example of a shared symptom is difficulty with reality testing. Although this may appear to indicate a psychotic disorder or borderline personality disorder, it may, in a traumatized person, simply be a temporary difficulty related to reexperiencing symptoms. Particular constellations of symptoms may also be mistakenly interpreted to indicate symptoms of other conditions. As mentioned earlier, although the constellation of symptoms measured by the F scale on the MMPI is usually interpreted to indicate malingering, this would be an inappropriate interpretation for a traumatized person.

Another reason why presenting symptoms of traumatized people are sometimes misleading is that trauma-related symptoms often occur simultaneously with other psychiatric disorders. Such comorbidity occurs frequently among trauma survivors, possibly because those with psychiatric disorders are more at risk for being traumatized. When a comorbid condition is present, symptoms of another disorder may confuse the presenting diagnostic picture. For example, a dramatic style of interpersonal interaction that is indicative of histrionic personality disorder may lead a clinician to believe that reports of trauma-related anxiety symptoms are exaggerated. This issue of comorbidity in the context of making a diagnosis is discussed in more detail in Chapter 9.

A third reason why presenting symptoms of traumatized people can be misleading is that symptoms may be present that are secondary to the trauma disorder. Here, new symptoms have developed as a result of symptoms related to the traumatic event. For example, trauma symptoms of loss of control over intrusive memories and emotions may lead to depression. In this case, a clinician might mistakenly believe that the client has an affective disorder rather than a trauma disorder.

Since, trauma-related disorders have symptoms in common with so many other disorders, it is not possible to go into detail regarding all of the commonalties. Here I limit the discussion to listing some disorders that seem particularly easy to confuse with trauma-related disorders and to giving some clinical examples to illustrate how such confusion might occur. There might be other disorders as well that can be added to this list. After reading Chapters 3 and 5, a reader with little familiarity with trauma-related disorders might find it useful to go through the list and identify the symptoms for each disorder that might be similar to those of PTSD, ASD, or dissociative disorders.

Below I have listed DSM-IV (American Psychiatric Association, 1994) categories of disorders and the names of any specific disorders within categories that might be particularly difficult to distinguish from a trauma-related disorder. Disorders seen in adults or children are listed separately from those usually first seen in children.

Anxiety disorders
    Panic disorder (with or without agoraphobia)
    Agoraphobia without panic disorder
    Generalized anxiety disorder
Mood disorders
    Major depressive disorder
    Dysthymic disorder
    Bipolar disorder (type I or II)
    Cyclothymic disorder

Somatoform disorders
  Somatization disorder
Eating disorders
  Anorexia nervosa
  Bulimia nervosa
Sleep disorders
  Primary insomnia
  Nightmare disorder
  Sleep terror disorder
Impulse control disorders
  Intermittent explosive disorder
Adjustment disorders
Amnestic disorders
Substance-related disorders
Schizophrenia and other psychotic disorders
  Schizophrenia
  Schizophreniform disorder
  Schizoaffective disorder
  Brief psychotic disorder
Personality disorders
  Antisocial personality disorder
  Borderline personality disorder
  Histrionic personality disorder
  Avoidant personality disorder
  Dependent personality disorder

Disorders usually first seen in infancy, childhood, or adolescence
  Attention-deficit and disruptive behavior disorders
    Attention-deficit/hyperactivity disorder
    Conduct disorder
    Oppositional defiant disorder
  Other disorders of infancy, childhood, or adolescence
    Separation anxiety disorder
    Reactive attachment disorder

Diagnostic Dilemma Cases

The diagnostic dilemmas presented below show how a trauma-related disorder might easily be mistaken for another disorder. Although a person may have more than one psychological disorder at a time, most mental health professionals do tend to make a primary diagnosis (or interpretation) and to focus on treating the client for that problem first. Similarly, although there may be more than one accurate interpretation of a person's symptoms, most therapists would agree that some interpretations (or diagnostic labels) are more accurate than others, and therapists try to make the most accurate interpretation they possibly can. As you read each case, consider what the consequences would be for the client if you went down the "wrong" diagnostic path.

Diagnostic Dilemma Case 1

Joan is a 42-year-old, divorced accountant with two teenaged children who comes to you for help with panic episodes that have been bothering her for about 6 months. She tells you that on five occasions over the past 6 months, she was suddenly seized with feelings of complete panic. Her heart would race, it became difficult for her to breathe, she began to sweat profusely, and her thoughts became confused and agitated. One of these panic attacks occurred when she was stopped at a traffic light while driving to work, one when she was at a PTA meeting, one when she was grocery shopping, and two when she was shopping at a mall. She reports no previous history of panic or anxiety. The panic attacks disturbed her greatly, and she was embarrassed about the attacks she had in public. Lately, she has found herself worrying more and more about the possibility of having another attack.

With this much information, you might naturally focus on the prominent symptoms of panic disorder and begin thinking about whether or not there is also agoraphobia. But suppose you assessed trauma-related symptoms and found that Joan is also hypervigilant, has been having nightmares about being attacked or in danger, has had trouble sleeping, and has been unusually irritable. Since Joan has so many posttraumatic symptoms, you might begin to wonder whether her panic attacks are related to some traumatic experience. You then assess for specific traumatic experiences and find that Joan was mugged by a man with a knife about 7 months before. Upon further discussion, you discover that Joan was terrified during the incident and feared for her life. She has been trying to "put the whole thing behind her" ever since by avoiding thinking about the incident. After further discussion and exploration of Joan's memories of the mugging, she suddenly realizes that just before each panic attack occurred, she saw a man resembling the mugger. The panic attacks turn out to be reexperiencing symptoms in the form of psychological distress and physiological reactivity in response to cues that remind Joan of a traumatic event.

Diagnostic Dilemma Case 2

Jim is a 38-year-old single man who works as an officer in an urban police department. He comes to you for help because he has been "feeling down" for the past 2 months. Jim says he feels sad and lonely, has trouble sleeping, and has not felt like going out with friends. His feelings have been affecting his work, and he is thinking of asking for a leave of absence so he can "get himself together," but he is not sure that he can afford to do that. He also tells you that Amy, his girlfriend of 5 years, moved out of their apartment 2 months ago. Amy isn't sure they should continue their relationship. When you ask Jim about problems in their relationship, he tells you that they fought a lot and he would lose his temper, which frightened Amy. Jim tells you that Amy complained that Jim's job had changed him and that he "was not the same gentle and kind man she had met 5 years ago." He does not know whether they will get back together, but he cannot stand being so miserable. He says that the only time he ever felt worse than this was when his mother died 12 years ago.

At this point in your assessment, it seems that Jim's major problem is depression over the loss of his relationship with Amy. You also wonder whether his current situation is bringing up feelings of loss relating to the death of his mother. When you give Jim a screening measure for PTSD symptoms, he reports sleeplessness, nightmares, and intrusive images. You then give him a trauma questionnaire, and he reports having witnessed a shooting 6 months ago. It turns out that during an arrest, Jim's partner had been shot and almost died. After some prodding, he tells you that he has been having intrusive thoughts and images and nightmares about the shooting. In the nightmares, sometimes his partner dies, and sometimes it is Jim who has gotten shot. He is also hypervigilant when on duty. Jim reports being somewhat ashamed of these feelings and has not mentioned them to anyone because "After all, I'm not the one who got shot, so why should I be a wimp about it."

Upon further exploration, you find that Jim's angry outbursts toward Amy all occurred in the evening on days when he had been in particularly threatening situations. He would lash out at Amy when she would ask him about what had happened that day or would suggest that his job was "too dangerous." It seems, then, that Jim's relationship problems and depression may have been secondary to his response to a traumatic event.

These case examples illustrate just a few of the ways that therapists can be misled by the complex presenting symptoms of traumatized persons. Such perplexing presentations make a formidable obstacle to accurate diagnosis and assessment. Since a standard psychological test battery and a standard intake are not likely to provide you with enough information about traumatic experiences or trauma-related symptoms to "solve" the diagnostic "mystery," you need additional clinical tools to make your best assessment.

HOW A BETTER UNDERSTANDING
WILL IMPROVE YOUR ASSESSMENTS

Although it is not hard to see how better assessment tools would help you evaluate traumatized people more effectively, it is less obvious how a better theoretical understanding of traumatic responses will enable you to make more accurate assessments and make them more rapidly. But a good working knowledge of the interconnections among aspects of traumatic experiences, individual characteristics, and responses to trauma will allow you to quickly choose your assessment tools and to make the most of the information they supply.

For instance, if you are knowledgeable about the core responses to traumatic stressors, and you know that a person has experienced a traumatic event, you can be alert to potential trauma-related symptoms. Such attentiveness can often help you to avoid focusing on comorbid symptoms to the exclusion of trauma-related symptoms. In other words, if you are knowledgeable about characteristic trauma responses, you are less likely to get distracted and waylaid by other symptoms that are present. You can see how such theoretical knowledge would be advantageous in the first diagnostic dilemma case. Suppose, at the beginning of your assessment, you gave Joan a brief self-report inventory of traumatic stressors and found that she had been in an armed robbery 6 months before. If you knew that the experience of that event was associated with a particular constellation of symptoms, and you knew that one of the prominent symptom groups was reexperiencing, then you would be more likely to understand her episodes of panic as reexperiencing symptoms and less likely to see them as "classic panic attacks." In this case, understanding the relationship between trauma and reexperiencing would improve your ability to assess Joan.

In the same way, awareness of the theoretical relationships between moderating factors and symptoms might lead to a more effective evaluation of a person's trauma response. Again, to use Joan's case as an example, if you were trying to understand why Joan's traumatic response to the mugging was persisting for so long, you might consider factors that are theoretically proposed to exacerbate or ameliorate a trauma response. For instance, if you were knowledgeable about the relationship between social support and severity of response to trauma, you might ask Joan some questions about how her family and friends have responded to the mugging. Since Joan was trying to forget about the experience, you might find that she minimized the event and gave people the impression that she did not need any help coping with her experience. Unintentionally, then, Joan cut off the social support that might have helped her recover. Here, again, in your effort to understand Joan's responses, a good conceptual appreciation of the trauma process could serve you well.

In other cases, if you were familiar with the theoretical relationships between aspects of traumatic experiences and later symptoms, particular presenting symptoms might cue you to ask about particular kinds of traumatic events and moderating factors. For example, suppose a new client reported long-standing problems with a wide range of posttraumatic stress and dissociative symptoms, including experiences of dissociated identity and amnesia for long periods of childhood. If you knew that this pattern of symptoms is thought to be related to early, severe, and chronic trauma, you could begin to investigate that possibility by choosing structured interviews for early experiences of abuse and neglect. The bottom line is that theoretical knowledge about trauma responses will help you to assess traumatized people more quickly and accurately.

HOW A BETTER UNDERSTANDING AND ASSESSMENT WILL LEAD TO BETTER TREATMENT

The ultimate goal of your efforts to understand and assess clients' psychological problems is to offer them treatment that is as effective and efficient as possible. There are countless ways in which understanding and assessing trauma and trauma responses well will help you to treat traumatized clients effectively and efficiently. A few of the most important benefits of understanding and assessing trauma and trauma responses are discussed here.

Familiarity with trauma theory is very valuable in the treatment planning process. Understanding the defining characteristics of traumatic events enables you to distinguish between events that have the potential to cause trauma responses and those that are simply distressing. Making this distinction allows you to choose the most appropriate treatment interventions for your client because different treatments would be optimal for a traumatic response and a distressing experience.

Familiarity with trauma theory can also foster your treatment efforts because understanding the psychological reasons for particular symptoms will help you decide how to address them. This is because the meaning of a symptom for a person in relation to his trauma is important to the process of resolution of the traumatic response. For example, in Diagnostic Dilemma Case 2, Jim's angry outbursts toward his girlfriend may have a very specific meaning and relation to his traumatic experience. For a person like Jim, his anger is really meant for the person who shot his partner and made him feel so helpless and fearful. Another man's outbursts might reflect a basic hostility toward women, an inability to control his angry impulses, or any number of other things. For Jim, understanding his anger as expression of his fear would lead to the most effective way to address that particular symptom.

Treatment can also be improved in a number of ways by a thorough assessment of trauma. A systematic assessment of trauma history will provide valuable information about early or multiple traumatic events in a client's life. As discussed in detail in Chapter 5, early childhood traumas and multiple traumas may call for different therapeutic approaches than single traumatic events in an adult.

Careful assessment of a client's trauma history will also provide valuable information about the role of traumatic experiences in a client's condition. The connection between current symptoms and past traumas often has important implications for treatment. For example, a client's chronic pain following a traumatic injury may be maintained or exacerbated by unresolved emotions relating to the trauma. In such a case, attention to resolving feelings relating to the trauma may be necessary before the pain symptoms can be addressed effectively. Another client's alcohol abuse problems might be a function of efforts at avoidance of intrusive trauma-related thoughts and feelings. Successful treatment of this client's alcohol problem may not be possible until intrusion symptoms are under control.

Detailed trauma history assessments can also help clarify connections between traumatic events and current problems by supplying important details that will aid prediction and control of symptoms and in implementing treatment interventions. For example, details about trauma history can help you identify cues that trigger traumatic reactions for a particular client. A woman who experienced traumatic abuse at the hands of her aggressive, dark-haired, Italian father might become anxious around her boss who is also an aggressive, dark-haired, Italian man. Although such a connection may seem obvious to the therapist, the link may be outside of the client's conscious awareness. In this way, identification of traumatic cues through knowledge of trauma history allows for greater prediction and control of trauma-related reactions. Identifying traumatic cues can also promote the implementation of treatment interventions. For example, trauma cues can provide content for developing anxiety hierarchies as part of behavioral techniques such as systematic desensitization.

Systematic assessment of trauma responses are also important to effective treatment. First, a good assessment of trauma responses enables you to identify traumatic stress responses rapidly and begin an appropriate treatment. Every therapist has had the experience of noticing and treating symptoms that seem prominent at first, only to realize later that the problem she has been working on is not really the most pressing problem. In Jim's case, if you had not investigated PTSD symptoms, it would have been very easy to become mired in a long, involved exploration of his loss of an important relationship and possible earlier emotional losses. The important issue for Jim, as is true for most clients, is what his most pressing psychological problem is. While work on emotional losses may be of benefit to Jim, it may not help relieve him of PTSD symptoms that interfere with his day-to-day activities. Addressing the trauma response might be all he needs to return to his previous high level of social and emotional functioning. If he chooses to continue treatment to work on emotional losses, he is likely to be more successful if he is comfortable at work.

In addition, careful assessment of trauma-related symptoms can help you identify the symptoms that are the most distressing and disabling for a particular client. Since different symptoms often require different treatment strategies, identification of the most pressing trauma symptoms is very important in your treatment planning.

SUMMARY

Traumatic experiences and trauma-related psychological symptoms are common enough among persons seeking help for psychological problems to warrant routine assessment, but understanding and assessing trauma symptoms can be especially difficult. It is hard to make sense of trauma responses because of the complex relationships among traumatic experiences, moderating variables that influence the response to a traumatic experience, and later symptoms. Most clinicians receive little if any formal training in the theory and assessment of trauma responses. Impediments to assessment of trauma responses include the inadequacy of standard intake interviews and global psychological measures for assessing posttraumatic and dissociative symptoms and trauma histories and the ambiguous presentation of many trauma-related symptoms. A good conceptual framework for trauma responses can improve your evaluations by allowing you to assess traumatized people more quickly and accurately and by affording you a better appreciation of the meaning of trauma-related symptoms. Effective assessments of trauma and trauma responses can save you and your client valuable time and energy as you pursue solutions to presenting problems.

Chapter 2

A Conceptual Framework
for Understanding Responses
to Trauma

As discussed in Chapter 1, a good conceptual framework for trauma responses can help you to conduct more accurate and efficient evaluations of traumatized people and to better understand the meaning of trauma-related symptoms. In this chapter, I present a framework for understanding responses to traumatic experiences. The next three chapters then expand upon aspects of the framework and show how the framework can be applied to particular kinds of traumatic experiences. To introduce this framework, I discuss why our understanding of the effects of traumatic experiences is still relatively limited to date. The framework attempts to address important questions about the effects of traumatic events. It is comprised of the defining features of traumatic events, the most common responses to trauma, the reasons for persistence of traumatic responses after the event, and the factors that influence responses to trauma.

WHY OUR UNDERSTANDING OF EFFECTS
OF TRAUMA IS LIMITED

The effects of traumatic experiences are still not well understood despite the great prevalence of these events and the magnitude of the distress they cause. Most of the knowledge about traumatic stress that has accumulated applies to the short-term effects of single-event traumas or combat trauma. Short-term effects and long-term effects of trauma have been explained separately by various theories, but no single theory has yet explained how both sets of effects can result from traumatic experiences.

If traumatic events cause substantial distress and are now and presumably always have been widely prevalent, why do we know so little about the short- and long-term effects of these kinds of experiences? The main reason for this is that the effects of traumatic events have only been studied systematically for a short period of time. As mentioned in Chapter 1, substantial research on responses to trauma did not begin until the 1980s when funding and interest in PTSD increased in response to the problems of Vietnam veterans. Arguably, traumatic stress researchers have made amazing progress in understanding trauma responses in only two decades of systematic research.

Progress in understanding trauma responses is hindered by several factors. First, it is very difficult to study trauma responses because researchers cannot control the circumstances surrounding the traumatic events. Since it is not possible to know who will experience a trauma, it is extremely difficult to pretest subjects to determine their pretrauma levels of psychological functioning. Obviously, it is impossible to manipulate aspects of traumatic events themselves in order to compare the effects of such variables on subjects' responses. Another hindrance to trauma research is that the treatment needs of trauma victims must always take precedence over the need to answer research questions. This means that research plans must be put aside if there is any possibility that participation in research would be distressing or would delay treatment for a traumatized person. Also, people are unlikely to be willing to participate in a research study soon after they have had a traumatic experience. Understandably, traumatized people feel the need to protect themselves and husband their psychological resources at such a stressful time.

Another impediment to trauma research is that it is sometimes difficult to get detailed information about the traumatic events themselves. This is because confusion frequently surrounds traumatic events, especially events such as disasters when there is disruption of whole communities. Trauma survivors themselves may be able to provide only limited information about what happened to them because of amnesia for aspects of the experience. Such gaps in memory are even more problematic when many years have gone by since the traumatic event because the normal processes of memory decay may exacerbate retrieval problems. Similarly, because objective records of events that occurred long ago are difficult and sometimes impossible to obtain, research on the long-term effects of traumatic experiences is hard to do.

Our understanding of the short-term and long-term effects of traumatic experiences in adults is considerably greater than our understanding of the long-term effects of early traumatic experiences such as child abuse. This is true, in part, because both knowledge and theory development are fostered by research and because much of the research on the effects of trauma has been done in Veterans Administration facilities. In such settings, it has been possible to study large samples of people who have had traumatic experiences in combat. Also, it is much easier to study the effects of traumatic events that are not personal in nature. For example, it would be relatively easy to identify subjects to study the short-term effects of a hurricane, earthquake, or flood, and we would expect most of these subjects to be willing to describe their traumatic experiences. On the other hand, it is much more difficult to do research on the long-term effects of childhood sexual abuse. These persons would be more difficult to identify and may be understandably reluctant to discuss their experiences. Additionally, the impetus to study childhood abuse experiences has only recently been spurred by a growing awareness among researchers and clinicians of the high prevalence of such experiences.

Theories of effects in adults have tended to be separate from theories of effects in children. This tendency for theories to be fairly specialized also results from the inclination of researchers to specialize in particular types of trauma in particular populations. Such inclinations are often driven by very practical considerations such as having clinical training that focuses either on adults or children or having access to a particular clinical population. Recently, enough research on the long-term effects of early trauma has begun to appear to allow progress in theory development in this area and integration of theories for short- and long-term trauma effects.

QUESTIONS A CONCEPTUAL FRAMEWORK FOR THE EFFECTS OF TRAUMA SHOULD ADDRESS

A useful conceptual framework for the effects of traumatic experiences should answer several key questions. Answering these questions is important to understanding clients' trauma responses and, ultimately, to assessing and treating them.

First, why do some individuals develop posttraumatic disorders following a traumatic event while others do not? As described in Chapter 1, not everyone who is exposed to a potentially traumatic event responds with symptoms that meet the criteria for a trauma-related disorder.

Estimates of the rate of PTSD in those exposed to extreme stressors range from 25% (Green, 1995) to 30% (Tomb, 1994). This means that following exposure to a potentially traumatic event, about one-quarter of those exposed will have enough of the DSM-IV PTSD symptoms to be given that diagnosis. The rate of PTSD following exposure appears to vary considerably depending on the type of traumatic event. For example, one study found that PTSD developed in 5% of those experiencing the sudden death of a loved one and 13% of those experiencing rape (Kilpatrick & Resnick, 1993). Another study found that 31% of Vietnam veterans exposed to combat later developed PTSD (Kulka et al., 1990d). What type of response occurs in the other 70–75% of people exposed is unclear because research has tended to focus on those who develop full-blown PTSD. Presumably, those not meeting criteria for a PTSD diagnosis respond to the events they experienced with fewer or less severe symptoms or with symptoms of shorter duration than 1 month. It is also possible that some who are exposed to severe stressors show no trauma-related symptoms at all.

To answer the question of why some people develop posttraumatic disorders while others do not, the framework addresses what makes an experience traumatic. Other important questions that a conceptual framework for the effects of trauma should address include: What are the core symptoms associated with being traumatized? What additional symptoms might be seen after the initial trauma response? What factors determine and influence the nature of trauma responses? Why do posttraumatic symptoms persist long after the trauma is over? This conceptual framework offers complex answers to these questions by explaining how aspects of stressful events and additional moderating variables affect the risk for developing various trauma-related disorders.

ORIGINS AND GOALS OF THE FRAMEWORK

This theoretical framework, like most others, is based on concepts that were developed and described by others. New frameworks are developed to answer questions that are not addressed or not fully answered by previous theories. A new framework might also improve upon previous conceptualizations by framing hypotheses so that they are open to empirical verification. As theory on a subject evolves, one can expect that some aspects of a framework will be confirmed while others will be disconfirmed and later replaced by more accurate conceptualizations.

This framework was developed drawing from the theoretical ideas of a variety of clinicians and researchers representing different theoretical orientations. It incorporates ideas introduced and elaborated upon by many, including van der Kolk and colleagues (van der Kolk, 1987b; van der Kolk, Boyd, Krystal, & Greenberg, 1984; van der Kolk & Kadish, 1987), Herman (1992), Janoff-Bulman (1992), McCann and Pearlman (1990), Foa and colleagues (Foa, Rothbaum, Riggs, & Murdock, 1991; Foa, Steketee, & Rothbaum, 1989; Foa, Zinbarg, & Rothbaum, 1992), Briere (1992), and many others. As I present my framework, I provide some citations for sources of previous discussions of concepts. These citations are meant to serve as examples of the foundations of concepts, not to be an exhaustive listing of sources. Because most of the ideas discussed have evolved gradually over time and are described in numerous theories, it is not always practical or possible to pinpoint the origin of an idea or to cite every source where an idea was discussed. Consequently, you should not assume that the authors cited in relation to a particular idea are the originators of the concept, the only authors to propose the concept, or the only influences on the development of the framework.

Alternative frameworks are also available to explain responses to traumatic experiences (Briere, 1996b; McCann & Pearlman, 1990). These differ from the framework I present in a variety of ways. Some are designed to explain responses to particular types of trauma, and some focus on particular theoretical models, such as cognitive or psychoanalytic models. Other frameworks such as those described by Wilson (1994b) and McFarlane and Yehuda (1996) overlap considerably with the framework presented here. Arguably, the differences among previous frameworks and that presented here are relatively minor compared to the similarities.

The present framework expands upon previous theories by addressing the effects of a wider variety of traumatic events, by addressing the causal connections between traumatic experiences and responses, and by incorporating constructs and hypotheses that can be empirically defined and tested.

One of the main goals in developing this framework is to expand on previous theoretical concepts so that they can be applied to a wider variety of traumatic events and be used to explain a wider variety of traumatic responses. There are two aspects of this framework that make it possible to apply it to a wider variety of traumatic events. First, the framework starts with different criteria for a traumatic experience than do most theories. These criteria make it possible to consider some events as traumatizing that would be excluded or poorly represented by criteria for traumatic events from other theories. For example, effects of traumatic events that are psychologically, but not physically, threatening are explained by this framework but not by many other theories.

Second, this framework includes factors that make it applicable to a very wide range of traumatic events, from early and chronic traumas to adult, single-event traumas. The framework can be used to explain a wider variety of traumatic responses than previous theories because it includes a wider variety of symptoms than many previous theories. For example, this theory discusses the role of dissociation in trauma responses in more depth than most previous theories.

This theory is also different from many others in that it specifically addresses the theoretical connection between the traumatic events and later symptoms. Although some theories provide explanations for what makes experiences traumatic and most describe symptoms that commonly follow traumatic experiences, many theories do not explain specific causal relationships between aspects of traumatic experiences and later symptoms. Causal relationships between traumatic experiences and anxiety symptoms have been explained fairly well, but relationships between trauma and other symptoms have not been clearly elucidated.

Another intended improvement of this framework is to define its constructs and hypotheses in ways that allow empirical testing. Some trauma theories are less appealing to many clinicians and researchers because they include concepts that are not readily measurable or hypotheses that are not easily tested. For example, if a psychoanalytic theory of trauma proposes that a weak ego increases one's vulnerability to trauma, it is very difficult to test this prediction because the concept of ego is not readily operationalized. There is no clear way to measure the strength of one's ego.

A strong theory must also include hypotheses that are amenable to empirical testing that can provide either clear support or a clear lack of support. Theories that are empirically testable are often referred to as falsifiable. Some theories, such as many psychoanalytic theories, are criticized because they are seen as "unfalsifiable." Theories are considered unfalsifiable when they do not allow clear, unambiguous predictions of relationships between causal factors and effects. For example, a psychoanalytic trauma theory might propose that traumatic experiences must be defended against by the ego because they are psychologically unacceptable to the individual. If a client shows frequent use of defenses (such as denying the importance of the traumatic experience), then the experience will be considered traumatic. If the client does not show defensive behavior, then the experience will not be considered traumatic. This formulation is circular and nonfalsifiable because the definitions of "traumatic" and "defenses" are not independent.

Theories from other orientations sometimes show similar problems. For example, traditional behavioral theory defines a reinforcer as a stimulus that results in an increase in a target behavior. A reduction in anxiety that results from avoiding a place that reminds a person of a trauma might be identified as a reinforcer because it results in an increase in avoidance behaviors. The causal explanation for the increase in the avoidance behavior is the process of reinforcement. But reinforcement is defined as an increase in the avoidance resulting from the presentation of the reinforcer! Here, the definitions of a "reinforcer" and "reinforcement" are circular. In the theory presented here, I have endeavored to define concepts in ways that are relatively easy to operationalize and measure and to propose hypotheses that can readily be tested.

THE CONCEPTUAL FRAMEWORK

This conceptual framework for the effects of trauma addresses what makes abuse traumatic, what psychological responses are expected following trauma, and why symptoms persist after the traumatic experience is over. Three elements are considered necessary for an event to be traumatizing: The event must be experienced as sudden, extremely negative, and uncontrollable. The initial responses to trauma include reexperiencing and avoidance in four modes of experience, and each of these symptoms is causally related to the traumatizing elements of the event. The framework proposes behavioral learning and cognitive processes that explain the persistence of the initial response to trauma. Five factors are proposed that influence the response to trauma including biological factors, developmental phase at the time of trauma, severity of the stressor, social context, and prior and subsequent life events.

What Makes an Experience Traumatic?

The first step in building a conceptual framework for the effects of traumatic experiences is to address some very basic questions about the nature of trauma. What is it about an experience that makes it traumatic? What makes an event cause sudden, severe emotional pain? To answer these questions, we need to determine the defining features of a traumatic experience. This turns out to be a somewhat daunting task because of the immense variety of experiences that have been known to traumatize people.

Green (1993) has described generic dimensions of traumatic experiences that can be used to define and categorize a wide variety of traumatic events. Green specifies seven dimensions including threats to life and limb, severe physical harm or injury, receipt of intentional injury or harm, exposure to the grotesque, violent or sudden loss of a loved one, witnessing or learning of violence to a loved one, learning of an exposure to a noxious agent, and causing death or severe harm to another. These dimensions account for most of the experiences that are considered potentially traumatic to humans such as disasters, both natural (e.g., floods, earthquakes, hurricanes, or tornadoes) and "unnatural" (e.g., technology-related events like the Chernobyl nuclear disaster); accidents (e.g., car accidents, fires, or explosions); human aggression (e.g., physical assault, some types of sexual assault, or terrorist acts); socially sanctioned aggression (e.g., war); traumatic deaths (e.g., the sudden death of a loved one); and witnessing death or violence.

While no theory may be able to explain the effect of every possible traumatic event, a theory that could explain all of those listed above would be very broadly applicable. It is also worth noting here that defining the features of potentially traumatic events will not provide an adequate explanation for their effects. Whereas some events may be so powerful that they would traumatize anyone, most potentially traumatic events are not so powerful. This means that the framework must also explain why a potentially traumatic event evokes a traumatic response in some people but not in others.

One way to develop an explanation of the effects of these traumatic events would be to determine what all of the events have in common. The predominant conceptualization of the defining features of traumatic events is reflected in DSM diagnostic Criterion A for PTSD (American Psychiatric Association, 1994). This criterion defines a traumatic event as one that involves "actual or threatened death or serious injury or a threat to the physical integrity of self or others" and a response of "intense fear, helplessness, or horror" (American Psychiatric Association, 1994, pp. 427–428). Using this definition, a theoretical explanation for how an event causes traumatic responses might be that the event is perceived as physically dangerous and that humans are naturally fearful of injury, death, and threats to physical integrity. This explanation works well for events involving the threat of injury or death to oneself, but it does not clearly explain why humans are fearful of the threat of injury or death to another person. The situation is complicated further by the observation that people are not necessarily fearful of the injury or death of any other person. In fact, in some instances, a person might intentionally injure or kill another person or witness such an injury or death and experience no fear or anxiety about the event.

The explanation that an event is traumatic when it is perceived as physically dangerous also does not apply well to potentially traumatic events such as acquaintance rape. It is very possible that a sexual assault by an acquaintance would be traumatic even if it were not perceived as physically injurious or life threatening. The fact that events that can clearly be traumatic do not meet DSM-IV Criterion A presents a problem in terms of assigning a PTSD or ASD diagnosis. Further discussion of problems with Criterion A is included in Chapter 9 (pp. 166–167). The inadequacy of a definition of traumatic events based on "dangerousness" highlights the need for a definition of traumatic events that take into account the interaction between the individual and the event. The importance of including this interaction in theories of trauma has been discussed in some detail by Wilson (1994b).

One solution to this theoretical difficulty is to propose that events are potentially traumatizing because they produce extreme fear. This conceptualization applies well to all of the potentially traumatizing events, regardless of whether they involve threat of injury or death, and it does take into account the interaction between the individual and the event. But it has the disadvantage of being somewhat circular. That is, events are designated as fear-producing occurrences when they produce fear. A definition of traumatic experiences that is applicable to a wide range of traumas, that incorporates the interaction between the individual and the event, and that is not circular would be more helpful in understanding why some events are particularly frightening to humans.

My colleagues and I have proposed three defining features of traumatic events (Carlson, Furby, Armstrong, & Shlaes, 1997). All three elements are considered necessary, though not sufficient, to make an event traumatic. The first element is the perception of the event as having a highly negative valence. The second critical element is the suddenness of the experience. The third element is the inability of the individual to control events and the subsequent threat to the individual's physical safety and psychic integrity.

Perception of the Event as Negative

The first critical element that makes an experience traumatic is that the event is perceived as having a severely negative valence. A traumatic event might have a severely negative valence because it is physically painful or injurious, because it is emotionally painful, or because it is perceived as likely to cause physical pain or injury, emotional pain, or death.

It is easy to understand why physically painful events would be traumatic: Humans and other animals have a natural desire to avoid physical pain. Avoidance of physical pain seems to be one of the few clear instincts that can be observed in humans. It makes sense for humans to possess an instinct to avoid severe physical pain because it is potentially damaging to the body and thus potentially life threatening. If a person is unable to control a sudden, severe physical pain, she may be traumatized: that is, she may experience sudden, overwhelming fear and may consequently by traumatized. The fear response functions to motivate the individual to avoid further injury or death.

Some events may be experienced as traumatizing because they involve a high likelihood of physical pain, injury, or death, even if none of these actually occurs. In other words, these experiences are negative because people experience the threat of physical pain, injury, or death. An example of this might be the experience of having a gun held to your head during a robbery. This experience might well be traumatizing even if no injury occurs and even if there was no real threat of injury because the gun was not loaded. It is your belief that pain, injury, or death is likely that triggers the fear instinct. Fear seems to be an emotion that has evolved to facilitate the avoidance of pain, injury, or death. It motivates you to act to control these negative outcomes. However, when you know that pain, injury, or death are highly likely no matter what you do, trauma is experienced due to the lack of ability to avoid the pain. In other words, not only failing to avoid these negative outcomes but also believing that you are highly likely to fail to protect yourself or be protected from negative outcomes results in psychological pain.

Some experiences are traumatic because they are emotionally painful or because they involve the threat of emotional pain. In this case, the negative valence is related to the psychological meaning of the event to the individual, not the physical consequences of the event. An example of an experience that might be traumatic because it is emotionally painful is witnessing the death of a loved one. The emotional loss associated with the death of someone you are close to would give a strong negative valence to the event.

In many cases, the psychological pain of a traumatic event involves damage or threat of damage to an individual's psychic integrity or sense of self. An example of this type of negative event would be an experience of sexual assault in which the victim did not expect to experience physical injury or pain. A woman might be raped by a man on a date and be traumatized by the experience even if she believed that she was not in physical danger during the experience. Such an experience might damage her sense of self because of the shame of being raped, guilt over any responsibility she feels for what happened, or anguish over her inability to protect herself from a very negative and unwanted experience. If such damage to a person's psychic integrity or sense of self were great enough, the experience might be traumatizing. The benefit of including emotional pain as a potential causal agent in traumatization is that the traumatic potential of events that do not involve threat of physical injury or death can also be understood. This is important because it is evident from research findings and clinical observations that sudden and uncontrollable emotionally painful events can also cause severe posttraumatic responses. A conceptual framework that can account for a wider variety of traumatizing events may be more useful than a less inclusive theory. One recent theoretical work that provides a detailed discussion of psychological pain as a traumatizing element is Freyd (1996).

It is possible for the negative valence of an experience to follow the experience in time and only become traumatizing when the negative valence is perceived. For example, a child might experience sexual assault but not understand the negative connotations of the events at the time they occurred. This person might become traumatized later when the negative meaning of the events was realized. Similarly, a soldier in combat might follow an order to burn a house where enemy soldiers were hiding and become traumatized some time later upon finding that the house sheltered innocent civilians.

A high likelihood of severe and uncontrollable psychological pain may also be experienced as traumatic. The perception that an extremely painful emotional experience is very likely may be traumatizing because the inability to control the anticipated event renders it negative, even if it does not occur. An example of such a traumatic experience might be having to leave your home during a firestorm and fearing that it will be destroyed. Even if no damage were done, the threat of psychological pain in this experience could be traumatizing.

In general, experiences with a negative valence because of actual or threatened pain, injury, or death are more universally traumatizing than experiences with a negative valence because of actual or threatened psychological pain. This is because there is little variation across individuals in what causes physical pain or damage, but there is a great deal of individual variation in what causes psychological pain. In other words, experiences involving no actual or threatened physical consequences involve a lesser risk of trauma. For example, it seems likely that almost anyone would be traumatized by the constant threat of death or injury involved in being a prisoner of war. On the other hand, the experience of witnessing another person being shot would be traumatizing only if it were experienced as psychologically painful. It might be psychologically painful if the person shot were a loved one, if one felt responsible for the person being shot, or if the shooting made one fear for one's own safety. It might not be psychologically painful if the person shot were considered an enemy or if the witness had little regard for human life.

The importance of the individual's perception of an event as negative can be seen by considering responses to negative events that were not perceived or were not perceived as negative. For example, suppose you were in a car accident but were knocked unconscious and did not remember anything about the accident. If you did not perceive the threat of injury or death, then you would not experience the fear that can precipitate a traumatic response. Results of a study of traffic accidents in Great Britain support this point. Mayou and colleagues (Mayou, Bryant, & Duthie, 1993) found that none of their subjects who were amnestic for the accident experience suffered from "horrific" intrusive memories about the accident.

It also seems clear that the perception of the event is more important than the actual danger associated with the event. For example, if a person pointed a gun at a child and the child was too young to understand the threat involved or believed the gun to be a toy, he would not be traumatized by the experience because no danger was perceived and no fear was generated. Such an event would only be traumatic if the danger of the situation were later conveyed to the child by an adult.

Clinical observations of traumatized persons lend support to the notion that the negative valence of an event is an important causal factor in the response to trauma. Traumatized persons often seem to be haunted by the fear and danger they have experienced. Many of the symptoms that follow traumatic experiences seem to reflect a preoccupation with the negative valence of the event. For example, the bus driver who killed a pedestrian might have intrusive negative thoughts about his child or wife being hit by a car. Here the negative valence of the event has become a focus for the client independently of the details of the actual event. His thoughts seem to be focused on the negative valence of the event rather than the event as it actually occurred. Similarly, he might have nightmares about hitting another pedestrian or about his bus driving off a cliff. The fact that some trauma victims become focused on the negative valence of their trauma supports the hypothesis that negative valence plays an important causal role in the development of symptoms.

Finally, it is important to note that the negative valence of an event must reach a certain threshold in order to cause traumatization. That threshold may differ across individuals and across types of trauma. Clearly, some events would not be negative enough to traumatize anyone, while others may be so negative that almost anyone would be traumatized by them. Empirical research is needed to clarify what factors influence the level of negative valence necessary for traumatization.

Suddenness

The suddenness of an event is also a key element in whether it is potentially traumatizing. Events that involve an immediate threat are more likely to cause overwhelming fear than experiences that involve danger or harm that occurs gradually. The critical factor here is the amount of a time between the person's awareness of a danger and the danger itself because that is the amount of time that a person has to act or to process the negative event. Janoff-Bulman (1992) has pointed out that some experiences are not traumatizing even if they are negative and frightening because they occur gradually and incrementally. These gradual changes can be adapted to cognitively and emotionally by gradual changes in a person's schemas about herself and the world. For example, if you gradually became ill with a fatal disease over a period of years, you would have time to accept the idea of your own death, and you might not be traumatized by the experience. This is not to say that you would not be fearful and depressed, but you might not be overwhelmed with fear to the degree that you had severe symptoms of anxiety. On the other hand, if you were trapped in a burning building, you would have no time to process the event cognitively or emotionally, and you might well become overwhelmed with fear and traumatized.

Similarly, actual or threatened psychological pain might not be traumatizing if it occurred gradually rather than suddenly. If your spouse were gradually to become ill and die of cancer over a period of years, there would be time to process the death cognitively and emotionally so that you might not be traumatized when your spouse did die. On the other hand, if your spouse died suddenly of a heart attack in front of you, you might easily be traumatized because you had no time to adapt to the emotional loss and change that such a death brings.

How much time is needed to process a frightening event is hard to say. Certainly, minutes, hours, days, and maybe even weeks would not be enough time to cognitively and emotionally process actual or threatened physical or psychological pain. Escaping a traumatic response is more likely if one has months or years to adjust to a negative event. It seems likely that PTSD would be a more likely response to an extremely negative experience that occurred over a period of minutes, days, or weeks, and depression would be a more likely response to an extremely negative event that occurred over a period of months or years.

Lack of Controllability

Lack of controllability of an experience is the third critical defining feature of traumatic events. There is considerable evidence to suggest that because protection from harm is a basic component of human (and animal) survival, people seek to control their environments so that they can protect themselves from harm. Research on both animals and humans has established that both are distressed by a lack of control over their immediate environment when that environment includes possible painful experiences (Abramson, Seligman, & Teasdale, 1978; Foa et al., 1989; Mineka & Kilhstrom, 1978). Building on this research, Foa and colleagues (1992) have argued that a lack of controllability of events is a defining element of trauma. The importance of the perceived controllability of an experience to its traumatic potential can be seen by contrasting the effects of an uncontrollable experience with one that was controllable. For example, if you came upon the scene of an accident and saw a person who was bleeding profusely and you felt that you had no control over the situation or ability to prevent the person's death, you might be traumatized by this sudden, very negative, and uncontrollable experience. On the other hand, if you were a trained paramedic who arrived at the accident and perceived yourself as having some control over the situation and some ability to prevent the person's death, you might not be traumatized by the experience.

Another illustration that shows the importance of perceived control in the traumatic potential of an experience would be the contrast between a physically painful event that was voluntary and one that was involuntary. If you chose to endure great physical pain to achieve some desired goal such as childbirth, the pain might be perceived as controllable, and you would be unlikely to be traumatized by the experience. This is true despite the fact that childbirth is somewhat dangerous, and you might be at risk of injury or death. On the other hand, the sudden onset of excruciating abdominal pains that were out of your control might well be frightening and traumatic.

Foa and colleagues (1992) propose that lack of predictability also plays a defining role in trauma. As they discuss in depth, predictability and controllability are not always independent of each other. The ability to control an event renders it more predictable, and the ability to predict an event may make control over it more possible. It seems, however, that predictability is not an essential element in the trauma process. Regardless of whether an event is predictable, it will be traumatizing if it is experienced as uncontrollable and sufficiently negative. If you are a victim of spousal abuse and can predict that you will be beaten every Friday night, the predictability of these events will only help you avoid traumatization to the extent that you are able to control the violence by ameliorating it or avoiding it. If you are unable to exert any control and find yourself suddenly faced with the threat of severe injury or death, you may still be traumatized by the experience. In some cases, it seems that predictability could even cause experiences to be more traumatic since the stress and tension of waiting for uncontrollable negative experiences could lengthen the period of distress.

Clinical observations of traumatized persons lend support to the notion that the controllability of an event is an important causal factor in the response to trauma. Traumatized persons often seem to be preoccupied with their own control over the traumatic event. This might be manifested in any number of different responses. For example, a bus driver who killed a pedestrian might have intrusive thoughts about what he might have done to prevent the accident. Trauma victims often report being bothered by frequent "if only" and "what if" thoughts following traumatic events. The bus driver might find himself thinking, "If only I had checked my side mirror a second time," "If only I hadn't been distracted by passengers getting on the bus," and "If only I had arrived at that intersection a few seconds later." Here the lack of controllability of the event has become a focus for the client. Similarly, he might have thoughts such as "What if I hit another pedestrian?" or "What if I hit another car?" Here his thoughts seem to be focused on his inability to control similar events rather than the event that actually occurred. The fact that some trauma victims become focused on the lack of controllability of the trauma supports the hypothesis that this factor plays an important causal role in the development of symptoms.

As with negative valence, the uncontrollability of an event must reach a certain threshold in order to cause traumatization. This threshold may vary across individuals and across events that carry valences of different degrees. Less control may be tolerable so long as the negative valence of an event is not too great. Research on the uncontrollability and valence of events that traumatize is needed to clarify where uncontrollability thresholds lie.

To summarize, the key defining features of a traumatic event are a negative valence, suddenness, and lack of controllability. All of these characteristics are necessary for an event to be traumatic, and all three are mediated by the individual's perceptions and understanding of the event. Remember, though, that while these features are all necessary for an event to be traumatic, they are not always sufficient to cause a posttraumatic disorder. Although an experience must be *sufficiently* negative, sudden, and uncontrollable to be potentially traumatizing, and even extremely negative, sudden, and uncontrollable events may not cause a posttraumatic response if the effects are moderated by favorable individual and situational factors.

Response at the Time of Trauma and Persistence

In the face of sudden danger, humans and other animals exhibit an innate "fight or flight" response that aids them in coping with or fleeing from danger (Lorenz, 1966). This reaction is characterized by high levels of physiological and affective arousal that are typically experienced as fear or anger. Cognitive distortions also frequently occur that seem to facilitate coping. Dissociative experiences such as depersonalization and derealization may help the individual continue to function by narrowing or distorting her experience of herself or the world around her. For example, a sexually abused child may experience depersonalization during an episode of abuse and may imagine that she is floating on the ceiling watching the events, but not experiencing them.

A complete conceptual framework for the impact of traumatic experiences must explain why responses to traumatic events persist once the event is over. If you are in a dangerous or frightening situation, why might you still be bothered by the experience weeks, months, or even years after you are out of danger? Several behavioral and cognitive theories can be applied to traumatic experiences to explain persistence of trauma responses. I mention these briefly here and provide a more detailed discussion of the concepts in Chapter 5.

Mowrer's two-factor theory has been applied to traumatic experiences by many trauma researchers (Foa et al., 1989; Keane, Zimering, & Caddell, 1985). This behavioral theory proposes that trauma symptoms result from both classical and operant conditioning. Through classical conditioning, new stimuli in the person's environment become associated with the traumatic event so that the new stimuli elicit the same fearful response as the original event. For example, the traumatized bus driver might be classically conditioned to associate driving his bus with the accident so that he becomes anxious whenever he drives his bus. The anxiety associated with driving is an affective reexperiencing of the trauma. This conditioned anxiety is not extinguished over time because of the accompanying avoidance of the conditioned stimuli (Mineka, 1979). Through operant conditioning, avoidance behaviors continue because they are negatively reinforced by relief from anxiety that they afford. For example, the bus driver might find driving his bus so aversive that he begins to call in sick to work so that he can avoid driving the bus.

Various cognitive theories are useful for explaining the persistence of trauma responses following multiple or chronic traumatic experiences. According to one theory, people develop general expectancy constructs to help them predict events (Mischel, 1973). If this theory were applied to fear and avoidance responses, their persistence might be understood as the result of the development of a general expectancy of danger and uncontrollability. Other theories propose that multiple traumas can lead to the development of highly individualized cognitive networks for processing cues for danger (Chemtob, Roitblat, Hamada, Carlson, & Twentyman, 1988; Foa & Kozak, 1986). Such networks might cause a person to interpret a very wide range of cues as threatening so that fear and avoidant behaviors become pervasive.

What Are the Most Common Responses to Trauma?

The next step in building a conceptual framework for the effects of traumatic experiences is to specify what responses tend to follow traumatic experiences. Although there is tremendous individual variation in how people respond to sudden, high-magnitude stressors, there are two basic categories of responses that are considered by many trauma researchers and clinicians to be common following a wide range of traumatic events. These are reexperiencing and avoidance symptoms (Horowitz, 1993; van der Kolk, 1987b). Both sets of responses can be manifested cognitively, affectively, behaviorally, and physiologically.

Although various authors may use somewhat different terms for the same symptoms, this conceptualization seems to have the advantages of being parsimonious while accounting for all of the major core symptoms associated with trauma. In Chapter 3, examples of symptoms that are manifestations of reexperiencing and avoidance across the four modes of experience are described in detail. These symptoms are considered core responses to trauma because they have been observed following a wide variety of traumatic events and because they seem to reflect the natural human response to sudden, negative, and uncontrollable events. We can see that these are natural human responses to traumatic events by examining theories and research findings relating to human and animal responses to danger.

Trauma clinicians and researchers have long noted that the symptoms associated with traumatic experiences seem to occur in particular patterns. Both van der Kolk (1987b) and Horowitz (1986) have described a two-phase model for the response to traumatic stress in which the individual alternates between phases of reliving and denial of the trauma. This model can also be used to describe alternating phases of reexperiencing and avoidance. For example, a train engineer who had been traumatized by accidentally killing a pedestrian might experience several weeks of intense feelings of anxiety, intrusive thoughts, sleeplessness, and irritability followed by a month of restlessness, emotional numbness, aversion to driving his route, and difficulty remembering the details of the event. Reexperiencing and avoidance symptoms can also cycle so rapidly that the person experiences both sets of symptoms in a brief period of time. The theoretical mechanisms that drive the alternating phases are discussed in detail in Chapter 3.

Secondary and Associated Responses to Trauma

Clinicians who have treated traumatized persons will no doubt have recognized symptoms in their clients other than those described as core symptoms. These seem to be related to traumatic experiences because they are seen following a wide range of traumatic events. My study of the literature on trauma has led me to believe that there are six responses to trauma that are either secondary to or closely associated with traumatic experiences. The responses that I describe as secondary are not directly caused by the traumatic experience, but occur later, as a result of the cognitive, affective, behavioral, or physiological manifestations of reexperiencing and avoidance. Associated responses, on the other hand, occur as a result of the social environment or other circumstances accompanying or following the trauma. Although there may be other secondary or associated responses that are common to trauma survivors, the six that seem the most prevalent are depression, aggression, low self-esteem, identity confusion, difficulties in interpersonal relationships, and guilt. These responses are discussed in detail in Chapter 3.

What Factors Influence the Response to Trauma?

The tremendous individual variation in responses to exposure to traumatic stressors raises the questions of why some persons develop posttraumatic disorders whereas some do not and why some responses predominate over others in a particular traumatized individual. Building on the formulations of van der Kolk (1987b) of factors that affect adjustment to trauma, this framework incorporates five basic factors to explain variations in responses to trauma. These five factors include individual biological factors, developmental level at the time of the trauma, severity of the trauma, the social context of the individual both before and after the trauma, and life events that occur prior and subsequent to the trauma. The severity factor, includes a number of variables such as the number of traumatic events experienced, the intensity of the event(s), the nature of the trauma, and the duration of the trauma.

All five factors affect an individual's response to trauma because they affect her perceptions of the valence, uncontrollability, and suddenness of the event. In this way, the basic theoretical model for what makes an experience traumatic can be related to factors that mediate the impact of trauma. These factors can either exacerbate or mitigate an individual's response to a potentially traumatic experience. In general, to the extent that the person is biologically vulnerable, the person is younger, the trauma is more severe (e.g., multiple, highly intense events of long duration), the social context is unsupportive, and previous or subsequent life events are very stressful, there would be a more pronounced and long-lasting traumatic response. On the other hand, to the extent that the person is biologically resilient, the person is older, the trauma was less severe (e.g., single, low-intensity events of short duration), the social context is very supportive, and previous or subsequent life events are very favorable, there would be a less pronounced response of shorter duration or perhaps no traumatization at all. A more detailed discussion of the effects of these factors is included in Chapter 4.

THE FUTURE OF THIS FRAMEWORK

The future of this framework depends upon the extent to which it is empirically supported. I offer this framework in the hope that others will consider whether these ideas can account for data from research better than previous theories or can account for more data than previous theories. Not surprisingly, the ideas presented are not all established or empirically tested to date. When research results are available that support particular concepts, that evidence is cited in Chapters 3, 4, and 5. It is possible that some aspects of the theory will not be supported by future research. There may be errors in thinking that come to light later or problems that arise when new data conflict with the framework's predictions. For this reason, I intend many of the ideas to be propositions that should be considered tentative until more evidence is available to support them.

SUMMARY

This chapter provided a framework for understanding responses to traumatic experiences. It began with a discussion of why our understanding of the effects of traumatic experiences is so limited to date. Next came a review of several key questions that the framework can help clinicians answer. The theoretical basis of the framework was described, and an explanation was given of how this framework expands upon previous theories. At the base of the framework is the specification of the defining features of traumatic events, including negative valence, lack of controllability, and suddenness. The most common responses to trauma were described, including cognitive, affective, behavioral, and physiological manifestations of reexperiencing and avoidance. Theories were briefly reviewed that explain the persistence of traumatic responses after the event is over. Secondary and associated responses to trauma were also described, including depression, aggression, low self-esteem, identity confusion, difficulties in interpersonal relationships, and guilt. Finally, the five most prominent factors that influence responses to trauma were described, including individual biological factors, developmental level at the time of the trauma, severity of the trauma, the social context of the individual both before and after the trauma, and life events that occur prior and subsequent to the trauma.

Chapter 3

Common Responses to Traumatic Experiences

This chapter focuses on the common responses to trauma that are part of the conceptual framework described in Chapter 2. When humans are exposed to extreme danger, they have a natural response of fear or anxiety. Under some conditions, behavioral and cognitive processes lead to the core symptoms of reexperiencing and avoidance and cause these responses to persist. Studies of human and animal responses to dangerous situations provide support for these formulations. During the initial trauma response, reexperiencing and avoidance symptoms are manifested cognitively, affectively, behaviorally, and physiologically. Although these core symptoms have been characterized as PTSD in the DSM diagnostic system, they can also be understood as forms of dissociation. Cognitive and psychodynamic theories are helpful in explaining why the initial responses to trauma tend to alternate between reexperiencing and avoidance. Secondary and associated symptoms can also be important aspects of the clinical picture. The former develop in response to core trauma symptoms, while the latter develop as a result of exposure to concomitant aspects of the individual's environment.

It is worth noting here that although all of the core, secondary, and associated trauma symptoms *can* occur as part of a posttraumatic disorder, all of these will not necessarily occur. Different symptoms may predominate in a client's symptom picture as a result of the influence of various individual and situational factors (reviewed in Chapter 4) and of the length of time that has passed since the trauma. Chapter 5 describes some of the distinctive symptom presentations that are observed following trauma along with research on core, secondary, and associated trauma symptoms.

RESPONSES AT THE TIME OF THE TRAUMA

To fully understand the function and process of symptoms that follow traumatic events, it is necessary to consider the experience at the time of a trauma. When faced with a sudden, uncontrollable, extremely negative event, a person is fearful and seeks to protect himself from danger. This "flight or fight" response observed in humans and animals facing danger (Lorenz, 1966) is characterized by high levels of physiological and behavioral arousal. In humans, high levels of cognitive and affective arousal have also been observed. High arousal when facing danger seems to be an unlearned, preparatory response of the body and the mind to danger. In other words, when you experience loss of control over your safety, your body and mind automatically go on "red alert" in an attempt to regain control. The "red alert" status might involve being hyperalert or hypervigilant to your surroundings and having an increase in physiological arousal to allow for flight or defense. Aggressive behaviors are also a natural response to danger (Lorenz, 1966). Such behaviors can be understood as an attempt to gain control over an unpredictable environment. This response to danger would seem to be an unlearned survival instinct.

Once a traumatic experience has ended, a number of symptoms appear that are related to the aroused state experienced in the midst of the traumatic event. These symptoms can be parsimoniously characterized as manifestations of reexperiencing and avoidance. Detailed examples of reexperiencing and avoidance symptoms are described later in this chapter. For now, I focus on the theoretical connection between the traumatic event and later symptoms.

PERSISTENCE OF TRAUMA RESPONSES

Mowrer's two-factor theory is a well-accepted behavioral model that explains the connection between an individual's aroused state during a trauma and the reexperiencing and avoidance symptoms that follow. As part of the two-factor model, classical conditioning principles can be used to explain conditioned arousal responses (Foa et al., 1989; Keane et al., 1985). According to classical conditioning principles, after repeated pairing of an aversive unconditioned stimulus (that evokes arousal as its unconditioned response) with situational cues, the situational cues become conditioned stimuli (CSs) that elicit conditioned responses (CRs) similar to the original unconditioned response (arousal). The CRs elicited take the form of reexperiencing in cognitive, affective, behavioral, and physiological modes.

Although classical conditioning of a response after only one event is not common, there is empirical evidence that fear responses can be strongly conditioned in only one trial (Kleinknecht, 1994; LeDoux, Romanski, & Xagorans, 1989; Rudy, 1993). Support for the concept of conditioned fear responses in traumatized persons has been found in studies in which severity of the trauma or fear during the trauma was related to the severity of later reexperiencing symptoms (Bryant & Harvey, 1996; Shalev, 1996).

To illustrate this process, the model could be applied to the experience of a traumatic car accident. The model predicts that the cues that are related to a traumatic event would become associated with previously neutral stimuli in the environment and that the neutral stimuli would then elicit arousal that was originally associated with the danger of the accident situation. For example, when driving a car following a traumatic accident, a person might experience racing thoughts, anxious feelings, and physiological arousal. Furthermore, stimulus generalization would result in stimuli similar to the original CSs also eliciting the CRs so that object, people, and situations even more distantly related to the accident, such as riding in a car, might also become associated with the aroused state at the time of the trauma.

According to operant conditioning principles (the second factor of Mowrer's model), behaviors aimed at escape and avoidance of stimuli associated with a trauma are negatively reinforced. That is, these behaviors increase because they are followed by a decrease in the arousal that was triggered by the conditioned stimuli. If this two-factor model is applied to traumatic experiences, we would expect cues associated with traumatic experiences to come to elicit arousal responses, and we would expect escape and avoidance behaviors in response to these cues to increase after the trauma. For example, following a car accident, a man might experience difficulty remembering details of the event and numbing of emotions and might go out of his way to avoid being in cars.

Application of this model to traumatic disorders is also supported by the success of behavioral techniques at reducing PTSD symptoms. These techniques are designed to break the connections between triggering stimuli and classically conditioned PTSD symptoms. In a study of veterans with substantial PTSD symptomatology, Bowen and Lambert (1986) found that systematic desensitization to combat imagery significantly reduced the symptom of physiological arousal that followed trauma reminders. In this study, counterconditioning of a relaxation response to combat imagery reduced the power of trauma-related thoughts (CSs similar to the combat images) to produce anxiety. Similarly, Keane and colleagues (Keane, Fairbank, Caddell, & Zimering, 1989) found that reexperiencing symptoms of veterans with PTSD were significantly reduced after implosion (flooding) therapy, and Cooper and Clum (1989) found that imaginal flooding was effective in reducing anxiety and sleep disturbances in Vietnam veterans with PTSD. In both of these studies, extinction of the conditioned association between combat images and anxiety resulted in a reduction of daily anxiety symptoms.

Mineka (1979) has pointed out that one weakness of the two-factor theory is that it cannot explain the fact that PTSD symptoms are often present for many years following a traumatic experience. The two-factor theory would predict the extinction of associations between neutral (conditioned) and trauma-related stimuli over time if the conditioned stimuli were no longer paired with aversive events. It may be that the expected extinction of associations does not occur for some because these individuals manage to cognitively, affectively, behaviorally, and physiologically avoid CS. Without adequate exposure to CSs in the absence of aversive consequences, extinction does not occur. This formulation is supported by the effectiveness of the flooding treatments described above and of other PTSD treatments involving exposure to trauma-related stimuli (Rothbaum & Foa, 1996). In all of these treatments, exposure to trauma-related stimuli (CSs) in the absence of aversive consequences did seem to foster extinction of the associations between CSs and CRs.

Cognitive theories of PTSD may also help explain the mechanisms for maintenance of reexperiencing and avoidance responses. After an uncontrollable and aversive experience, a person may develop a general expectancy of danger and uncontrollability. Mischel (1973) has argued that expectancies are personal constructs that individuals use to predict events and that expectancies are an important influence on behavior. General expectancies of danger and uncontrollability may persist for many years after trauma has ended if the individual does not have sufficient contradictory experiences of safety and controllability.

Another cognitive model that helps explain the persistence of posttraumatic symptoms was developed by Chemtob and associates to explain PTSD reactions of combat veterans (Chemtob et al., 1988). They proposed that the constant dangers of combat situations lead soldiers to develop cognitive networks that cause them to interpret cues as threatening and consequently dictate escape and avoidance responses to these stimuli. A bias toward interpreting ambiguous stimuli as dangerous might often be adaptive in a combat situation. One can easily imagine a soldier in combat being hypervigilant and shooting at an innocuous stimulus such as a moving branch. Once removed from danger, soldiers may continue to interpret ambiguous or neutral cues as threatening and consequently try to escape or avoid the danger (Chemtob et al., 1988). But these behaviors would be maladaptive once the person is out of danger. The misinterpretation of cues is thought to be maintained by a narrowing of attentional focus on potential threats that results in inattention to competing information and evidence of safety. This model could easily be applied to other types of trauma as well. For example, traumatically abused children may continue to be symptomatic long after they have escaped from abusive environments. They may continue to interpret ambiguous and neutral cues as threatening and therefore respond with reexperiencing and avoidance. Further discussion of cognitive processing of trauma can be found in Creamer, Burgess, and Pattison (1992) and Foa et al. (1989).

Psychodynamic theories have also been used to explain the development of posttraumatic symptoms. Although beyond the scope of this book, these theories propose that posttraumatic symptoms serve defensive functions for the trauma survivor, protecting her from emotional harm. Psychodynamic formulations of posttraumatic responses can be found in van der Kolk (1987b, 1996b), Brett (1993), and Herman (1992).

COMMON RESPONSES TO TRAUMA

As described in Chapter 2, there is great individual variation in response to traumatic events. Underlying this variation, however, there are a number of symptoms that seem to closely follow a wide range of traumatic events. Although different authors use different terms for some of the symptoms, reexperiencing and avoidance have long been considered to be the core responses to trauma (Horowitz, 1976; van der Kolk, 1987a). Reexperiencing and avoidance are manifested in the form of a variety of cognitive, affective, behavioral, and physiological experiences and symptoms. Examples of symptoms in each of these modes are shown in Table 3.1. Researchers and clinicians have come to see these symptoms as core responses to trauma for two reasons. First, studies have shown that various forms of reexperiencing and avoidance frequently occur in persons who have had traumatic experiences. Second, theory and research indicate that the symptoms are part of the natural human response to sudden, negative, and uncontrollable events.

TABLE 3.1. Manifestations of Reexperiencing and Avoidance across Modes of Experience

Mode	Reexperiencing	Avoidance
Cognitive	Intrusive thoughts Intrusive images	Amnesia for trauma Derealization/ depersonalization
Affective	Anxiety Anger	Emotional numbing Isolation of affect
Behavioral	Increased activity Aggression	Avoidance of trauma-related situations
Physiological	Physiological reactivity to trauma reminders	Sensory numbing
Multiple modes	Flashbacks Nightmares	Complex activities in dissociated states

As noted above, any particular traumatized individual may not appear to have all of these symptoms at all times. As discussed in Chapter 4, the factors that influence trauma responses may be largely responsible for variations in individual symptom patterns soon after a trauma. As discussed in detail in Chapter 5, multiple traumatic events and the passage of time may result in new symptoms and shifts in the initial symptom patterns. Another reason that all of these symptoms are not manifested following trauma is that the symptoms tend to alternate (as is described below). Also, particular symptoms may sometimes be masked or obscured by other behaviors that a person engages in. For example, a traumatized person who is initially anxious may drink heavily and effectively "self-medicate" so that he shows relatively few overt symptoms of anxiety (Stine & Kosten, 1995).

It is also possible that particular symptoms may predominate in a traumatized individual as a result of cultural influences. As with all psychological disorders, we should expect culture to greatly influence how symptoms are expressed. Although the bulk of research and clinical reports relating to trauma responses has focused on white, middle-, and upper-middle-class Americans, the research on trauma responses of persons from other cultures (and U.S. subcultures) that is available indicates that there may be considerable variation in the symptoms observed following trauma in different cultures (Marsella, Friedman, Gerrity, & Scurfield, 1996). At the same time, my own research on Cambodian refugees and research of others leads me to believe that, while the manifestations of symptoms may vary somewhat, the basic underlying responses to trauma are fairly consistent across cultures (Carlson & Rosser-Hogan, 1994). Consequently, you should keep in mind that clients from different cultures will have the same basic response to trauma, but they may express their symptoms somewhat differently from one another.

Reexperiencing

Trauma-related reexperiencing is reflected in a wide range of thoughts, feelings, behaviors, and physiological responses. This set of symptoms includes many of the DSM-IV symptoms for PTSD such as intrusive thoughts, anxious and angry feelings, physiological arousal and reactivity to trauma cues, and hypervigilance. For example, a client who has been robbed and threatened with a gun while walking alone at night might report that he can't get the incident out of his mind, that he feels anxious whenever he goes out at night, that his heart races and his palms sweat when he has thoughts about the robbery, and that he has felt on edge since the incident. Some reexperiencing responses might be observed in other forms as well, such as sleep problems or somatization resulting from chronic autonomic arousal. For example, the robbery victim might report that he has been having insomnia since the crime so that when he tries to go to sleep his thoughts are racing and he can't relax. Constant tension might also cause him to have headaches or stomachaches.

Cognitive reexperiencing symptoms often take the form of trauma-related intrusive images and thoughts (Horowitz, 1993). For example, a woman who has been raped may have flashes of the experience in her mind and be unable to stop thinking about the event. Other reexperiencing symptoms that involve a cognitive component include nightmares and flashbacks. Nightmares often involve thoughts about the trauma or being in danger, whereas a person having a flashback may believe that he is back in the traumatic situation again.

Affective reexperiencing symptoms that are most prominently associated with traumatic experiences are feelings of anxiety and anger or irritability. Following a traumatic flood experience, for example, a woman might feel constantly nervous and irritable. Traumatized persons may be troubled by unusually high levels of anxiety and anger as well as by the inability to modulate these feelings (van der Kolk, 1996a). They may be distressed and frustrated that they cannot control their extreme emotional reactions to relatively innocuous stimuli.

Behavioral reexperiencing might be manifested in several different ways, such as restlessness and increased activity levels. But the most notable and disruptive presentation of behavioral reexperiencing is physical aggression toward oneself or others. This type of aggression would reflect a reexperiencing of aggressive impulses experienced at the time of trauma. A traumatized prisoner of war, for example, might be more physically aggressive following his traumatic experiences. A child traumatized by a fire that destroyed her home might hit and kick her younger brother more after the event. Aggression might take many other forms as well. It could be expressed as verbal aggression toward others. For example, a woman who is traumatized by a serious earthquake might report finding herself yelling at her children and husband much more frequently than before the event.

In addition, some trauma victims may direct aggression toward themselves in the form of self-destructive behaviors. Self-destructive behaviors that seem to be related to traumatic experiences include suicidal behavior, self-harming behaviors such as cutting oneself, disordered and dangerous eating behaviors, sexual impulsiveness, and substance abuse. A woman who experienced traumatic sexual abuse as a child might report frequent suicide attempts in adulthood and problems with drugs and alcohol.

While behavioral reexperiencing in the form of aggression may be explained by the behavioral theories described above, other models for aggression toward others following trauma have also been proposed. Horowitz (1991) developed a model focused on children that may also apply to adults. He proposed that when children are traumatized by adults, they are made to feel extremely vulnerable. Some children may relieve their anxiety over this vulnerability by reversing roles to become the aggressor in imagination. Some abused children may act out their fantasies as children or when they are older and victimize others.

Differences in how aggression is expressed may be explained in part by biological and social aspects of sex and gender. Males seem to be more likely to express their aggression by violent or hostile behavior toward others. Aggression is one of the few behaviors that have been linked to sex and hormone levels in animals and humans (Bertilson, 1991). What is more, in many cultures, it is acceptable or even encouraged for males to express their anger physically.

Self-directed aggression, on the other hand, seems to be a more common response to trauma in females than it is in males. This may be because cultural norms often proscribe that aggression toward others is unacceptable in females. One way for a girl or woman to make sense of what happened to her is to believe that the event was her fault (Janoff-Bulman, 1992). Such self-blame may be accepted because it does not require a challenge to the cultural assumption that females are inferior and usually at fault in conflicts with males. Furthermore, aggression toward oneself can be understood as an attempt to gain mastery over painful experiences. Self-harming behaviors may effectively give the individual control over painful experiences, thus increasing the overall perception of controllability.

Reexperiencing in the form of physiological arousal is a prominent posttraumatic symptom. It is involved in many of the PTSD symptoms listed in DSM-IV, including physiological reactivity to reminders of trauma, sleeplessness, difficulty concentrating, and exaggerated startle (American Psychiatric Association, 1994). Chronic physiological arousal is also thought to contribute to the development of somatic problems such as headaches and gastrointestinal illnesses, which have been found to be elevated in many studies of trauma survivors (Green, Epstein, Krupnick, & Rowland, 1996).

As indicated in Table 3.1, some posttraumatic symptoms reflect reexperiencing in more than one mode. For example, hypervigilance involves reexperiencing in both cognitive and affective modes, such as thinking one is in constant danger and feeling "on edge." Similarly, nightmares may have cognitive, affective, and physiological components. A person could wake up from a nightmare sweating (the physiological component), be able to remember the details of the dream (the cognitive component), and still "feel" the emotions of the dream (the affective component). Flashback experiences may involve all four modes of experience. A combat veteran might suddenly find himself back in a combat, with all the accompanying sights and sounds, feelings, behaviors, and bodily sensations.

Avoidance

Avoidance following traumatic experiences can also be manifested cognitively, affectively, behaviorally, or physiologically. Several types of avoidance are listed as criteria for PTSD in DSM-IV, including avoidance of thoughts, feelings, conversations, activities, places, people, or memories associated with the trauma (American Psychiatric Association, 1994). All of these types of avoidance serve the purpose of protecting the individual from exposure to reminders of the traumatic event. Just as humans naturally try to avoid negatively valenced events to begin with, they also try to avoid reexposure to negatively valenced events. This means that after a person experiences a trauma, he will become particularly alert to any cues that remind him of the traumatic experience. Trauma cues can have dual meanings for traumatized people. First, the cue brings back the emotional pain of the traumatic event. Second, the cue tells them that they might in danger again.

Cognitive avoidance can involve putting the traumatic event or reminders out of a person's thoughts, or it can involve distortion of an individual's perceptions. For example, a person who survived a terrifying house fire might find that she remembers little of what happened that night. In addition to amnesia, many other avoidance symptoms involve a cognitive component. Distortions in perceptions of the environment (also known as derealization) and of oneself (also known as depersonalization) can also be means of avoiding "knowing" about a traumatic event through distortion of the meaning of an individual's experience. Volitional cognitive avoidance is also common in trauma victims. Intentionally trying not to think about a traumatic event is one of the DSM-IV criteria for PTSD (American Psychiatric Association, 1994).

Affective avoidance following trauma is commonly experienced as feelings of emotional numbness. Avoidance of all strong emotions protects the traumatized individual from the experience of emotional arousal that is associated with the trauma. A man who was unable to save his wife from drowning in a boat accident, for example, might report that he rarely has strong feelings of happiness since her death. He might avoid situations that involve any strong emotions, such as arguments or going to movies that are frightening. Affective avoidance might also take the form of isolation of affect. For example, a victim of a robbery might report the details of the event with no accompanying affect.

Behavioral avoidance typically involves avoiding reminders of the traumatic experience. This might involve avoiding situations, places, or people associated with the trauma. A common example of this would be how a traumatized paramedic might avoid watching TV shows that depict medical emergencies. Behavioral avoidance may sometimes be intentional, but sometimes the purpose of the avoidance behaviors is outside a person's awareness.

Physiological avoidance might be manifested as a numbing of sensations or analgesia. Traumatized individuals often report feeling no pain from an injury or feeling that their pain is somehow dulled or blunted. One example of this might be a man whose arm was torn off during a factory accident who reports that he felt no pain as he waited for the ambulance to come.

As indicated in Table 3.1, some posttraumatic symptoms reflect avoidance in more than one mode. For example, complex activities that occur when a person is in a dissociated state may involve cognitive, affective, behavioral, and physiological components. A person who has been in a severe car accident involving fatalities, for instance, might wander from the scene in a dissociated state that involves alterations in thinking, emotion, behavior, and physiology. Similarly, some depersonalization experiences may involve both cognitive and affective components. A person experiencing depersonalization, for example, might report disturbances in thought, such as perceiving that she is not "in charge" of her behavior, and disturbances in affect, such as feeling emotionally cut off from events happening around her.

Integrating Dissociation Symptoms into the Framework

Trauma clinicians and researchers have struggled to understand the role of dissociative experiences in the response to trauma. Dissociation is a confusing term because it has been used to describe such a wide range of experiences and symptoms. Dissociative experiences have been reported to occur both at the time of a trauma (Marmar, Weiss, Metzler, Ronfeldt, & Foreman, 1996) and following a trauma (Classen et al., 1993). Dissociative experiences are also observed as the predominant symptomatology of dissociative disorders, which are also thought to be trauma-related (Allen, 1995a). But experiences that are considered by some to be dissociative occur in other, nonclinical contexts as well. For example, subjects in normative samples commonly report dissociative experiences such as mild depersonalization and absorption (Putnam, Carlson, et al., 1996). Hypnosis researchers and practitioners have used the concept of dissociation to explain hypnotic phenomena such as hypnotic analgesia or posthypnotic amnesia (Frankel, 1994). Psychologists have also used the term dissociation to refer to phenomena of parallel streams of consciousness and divided attention (Hilgard, 1986). Research and theory relating to these nonclinical or normative forms of dissociation have sometimes made defining dissociation more confusing (Cardeña, 1994).

Some of the confusion surrounding the term dissociation may be reduced by making a distinction between pathological and nonpathological forms of dissociation. Such a distinction has been supported empirically by a study showing that some dissociative symptoms are experienced almost exclusively by subjects with posttraumatic and dissociative disorders (Waller, Putnam, & Carlson, 1996). Pathological forms of dissociation would include more severe experiences or symptoms that cause disruption in daily functioning or are experienced as subjectively distressing. Focusing attention on this more narrow range of dissociative experiences reveals that use of the term "dissociative" rather than "posttraumatic" to describe a symptom may simply be a matter of semantics. That is, we may simply be using different terms to describe the same phenomenon.

As it turns out, reexperiencing and avoidance symptoms in all four modes (cognition, affect, behavior, and physical sensations) have been labeled dissociative. For example, reexperiencing in the form of flashback experiences involves cognitions, affect, behavior, and physical

sensations and is considered to be dissociative (van der Kolk, van der
Hart, & Marmar, 1996). Reexperiencing phenomena are considered
dissociative because they are experienced "out of place" so that the
experience is disconnected from its original context.

Avoidance phenomena, on the other hand, are considered dissociative because they tend to cut the traumatized person off from aspects of
her own experience. For example, various manifestations of cognitive
avoidance are considered dissociative, including depersonalization (distortions in perceptions of the self), derealization (distortions in perceptions of objects or the environment), gaps in awareness, or dissociative
amnesia (unusually extensive lack of recall of autobiographical information). All of these forms of dissociation serve to distance an individual
from a traumatic event or from trauma-related stimuli. A woman who
survives a plane crash, for example, might experience depersonalization
and report that when faced with reminders of the crash, such as talking
to investigators, "It feels like I'm going through the motions, but I'm
not really there." She might also have gaps in her memory for the details
of the crash. By this use of cognitive avoidance, she keeps herself distant
from reminders of the traumatic experience. Experiences involving
affective and physiological avoidance have also been referred to as
dissociative. For example, both emotional numbing and lack of awareness of pain have been considered dissociative (American Psychiatric
Association, 1994; Giolas & Sanders, 1992; van der Kolk, van der Hart,
et al., 1996). Though all of these symptoms have been categorized and
studied as forms of dissociation, measurement of dissociation and
dissociation research of the past decade have largely focused on cognitive
avoidance symptoms including amnesia, depersonalization, derealization, absorption, and imaginative involvement (Carlson & Putnam,
1993).

It might help to clarify use of the term "dissociation" if pathological
dissociation were more clearly defined. Definitions of dissociation have
sometimes focused on symptoms or outcomes of trauma and sometimes
focused on the psychological function of the phenomena. Although there
is no single, accepted definition of dissociation, some representative
definitions include: "the lack of the normal integration of thoughts,
feelings, and experiences into the stream of consciousness and memory"
(Bernstein & Putnam, 1986, p. 727); "a compartmentalization of experience" (van der Kolk, van der Hart, et al., 1996, p. 306); and the
"disruption in the usually integrated functions of consciousness, memory,
identity, or perception of the environment" (American Psychiatric Association, 1994, p. 477).

Arguably, these definitions focus on the outcome or symptoms
observed following trauma and would be useful clinically as a way of

describing the effects of trauma. Characterizing dissociation as forms of reexperiencing and avoidance emphasizes the psychological process or function of trauma responses. Such a functional definition is useful because it helps to clarify the relationship between traumatic experiences and dissociative symptoms. This conceptualization is also very useful clinically because it focuses on connecting traumatic experiences to symptoms and would foster use of interventions to sever these connections.

A definition of pathological dissociation that combines these two conceptualizations might be optimal both theoretically and clinically. Pathological dissociation could be defined, then, as cognitive, affective, behavioral, and physiological reexperiencing and avoidance that results in a lack of integration of thoughts, feelings, behaviors, and sensations into the stream of consciousness. An advantage of a definition of pathological dissociation that incorporates both function and outcomes is that it allows integration of theory, clinical observations, and research related to PTSD with that related to dissociative disorders. It is worth noting that the definition does not imply a particular theoretical perspective or mechanism for dissociation. The definition could be compatible with behavioral, cognitive, or psychodynamic theories of reexperiencing and avoidance. This more comprehensive definition may also lead to more complete operationalization and measurement of trauma-related dissociative symptoms. Given that dissociative symptoms cover such a broad scope, and encompass numerous reexperiencing and avoidance phenomena, it is increasingly necessary for clinicians and researchers to be more specific in the future about exactly what form of dissociation they are focused on.

CYCLING OF PHASES

As mentioned in Chapter 2, trauma clinicians and researchers have long noted that the symptoms associated with traumatic experiences seem to occur in particular patterns. After a trauma, a phase of reexperiencing (or reliving or intrusion) is seen to alternate with a phase of avoidance (or numbing or denial) (Horowitz, 1986; van der Kolk, 1987a). Horowitz (1986) has explained these alternating phases using both psychodynamic and cognitive models.

According to Horowitz's (1986) psychodynamic model, when an event occurs that is traumatic, the individual experiences a great deal of anxiety. Later on, when faced with trauma-relevant information, he becomes anxious again because he fears the trauma will recur. When this anxiety threatens to overwhelm the individual and impair his or her functioning, defensive inhibitions begin to reduce the amount of incoming information relevant to the traumatic event. Trauma-relevant information can be controlled in two ways. One is the inhibition of memories of the trauma; the other is the inhibition of perceptions that are associated with the trauma. Once defensive inhibitions have successfully lowered the anxiety level, the motivation for the defenses decreases, and the individual begins to be more aware of trauma-relevant information. With the increase of awareness of the trauma, anxiety increases again, thus continuing the cycle.

A clinical example of this psychodynamic model of alternating phases might be the experience of a woman who has been traumatized by a rape. When she is exposed to a cue that reminds her of the rape, such as seeing a man who resembles the man who raped her, she becomes extremely anxious. She might even become so anxious that she cannot go on with the activity she is engaged in. If a man resembling the man who raped her works in her office, she might begin to be so overwhelmed by her anxiety when she sees him that she cannot perform her job. In order to protect her functioning, she might defend against the anxiety. For instance, she might arrange her work activities to avoid the man who reminds her of the rapist. This would allow her to avoid being reminded of the rape and thus would reduce her anxiety. She might also avoid going to work and feel more inclined to call in sick. If she used these defenses and succeeded in lowering her anxiety level, she would no longer need to defend. At that point, she might start having more interactions with the man at work and begin to be anxious again.

Herman (1992) proposes a somewhat different mechanism for alternating states of reexperiencing and avoidance. Herman applies her model to childhood abuse trauma and proposes that the avoidance phase is manifested as dissociative states that children use to protect themselves from emotional and physical pain. She hypothesizes that this dissociation can go "too far," leading to feelings of disconnection and detachment that are themselves profoundly disturbing. Self-injurious behaviors such as self-mutilation are then used in an effort to "jolt" the abuse survivor out of detached dissociative states. Herman's formulations reflect clinical observations that persons who inflict harm on themselves often intentionally engage in the behavior in order to interrupt their emotional numbness and to "feel something."

According to the cognitive model described by Horowitz (1986), there is a tendency for traumatic events to occupy conscious awareness. Horowitz attributes this tendency to a motivation to "process" the event, which he defines as cognitive/emotional work toward making one's interpretation of events consistent with one's self and world schemas. The tendency might also be explained as the result of conditioned stimuli evoking memory of the experience. In any case, evidence that traumatic events continually reappear in consciousness is suggested by the prominence of reexperiencing symptoms typical of trauma survivors. The resurfacing of cognitions related to traumatic events provokes negative emotion because the events were emotionally painful. Awareness of trauma is often interrupted when other pressing cognitive demands take precedence or when cognitive controls are activated to reduce emotional responses that threaten to impair functioning. Whenever the emotional response is controlled enough to allow normal functioning, thinking about the traumatic event will begin again. In this way, the individual alternates between thinking about the traumatic event and avoiding thinking about the event.

A clinical example of this cognitive model of alternating phases might be the experience of a bus driver who has hit a pedestrian. When he drives his bus along the route where the accident occurred, he finds himself thinking about the accident and seeing images of the scene. This becomes so distracting and agitating that he is in danger of having another accident. Because of his need to maintain awareness to avoid danger and decrease his agitation, he begins to employ cognitive avoidance strategies. He becomes increasingly interested in controlling his speed and timing his route very precisely so that he can avoid stopping at traffic lights. Soon, he becomes so absorbed in this mental task that he is not aware of when he reaches the scene of the accident. His absorption and lack of awareness of the accident site is a form of dissociation that results in a reduction of his anxiety and an increased ability to function normally. Eventually, though, when his anxiety level has decreased sufficiently, he will begin to process the trauma again, launching him into another phase of reliving.

Support for the concept of cycling of reexperiencing and avoidance has been demonstrated in at least one study of psychiatric inpatients. Spurrell and McFarlane (1995) found that cognitive avoidance symptoms following adverse life events were dependent on the level of the individual's cognitive intrusion symptoms. In other words, avoidance seemed to be a reaction to reexperiencing symptoms in these patients.

SECONDARY AND ASSOCIATED RESPONSES

In addition to the core responses to trauma, there are a number of important responses that are either secondary to the core trauma responses or associated with the trauma situation. Secondary symptoms develop in response to the core trauma symptoms. Associated symptoms develop as a result of exposure to concomitant elements of the traumatic environment. One way to think of secondary responses is as the "second wave" of symptoms that follows the initial trauma response. For example, a traumatized combat veteran having an initial response of reexperiencing might be angry and assaultive when reminded of the trauma. These behaviors are very likely to evoke social disapproval and rejection, which could lead to a secondary response of low self-esteem. Categorizing responses into initial, secondary, and associated responses is meant to reflect the causal and temporal progression of behaviors, rather than the clinical significance of the responses as effects of trauma. For some individuals, secondary or associated responses to trauma may well be their most troublesome symptoms. This seems to be particularly the case for those who experience severe and chronic traumas and who are still symptomatic for years after the trauma. Understanding some responses as secondary to trauma symptoms or associated with the trauma situation may enable clinicians to address these symptoms more effectively in treatment. For example, low self-esteem experienced by a combat veteran as a secondary response related to his aggressive behavior would be addressed in treatment differently than would low self-esteem from another source.

The most prominent secondary and associated responses include depression, aggression, decreased self-esteem, disturbances in identity, difficulties in interpersonal relationships, and guilt and shame. These responses have all been identified and discussed in much detail in the trauma literature (Briere, 1992; Gil, 1988; Herman, 1992; McCann & Pearlman, 1990).

Depression

Depression might be expressed in a number of different ways following a traumatic experience. Traumatized persons might demonstrate their depression cognitively, emotionally, behaviorally, or physiologically. Typically, traumatized persons show depression in several or all of these realms. For example, it could take the form of inactivity or lethargy, negative thinking, problems concentrating, depressed mood, feelings of hopelessness or apathy, sleep problems, or loss of appetite. Negative thinking and feelings of hopelessness can also be manifested in suicidal thinking or behavior. A child who witnesses a friend die in a bike accident might appear listless and sad, and his mother might report that he has not been eating or sleeping well since his friend died. A college student who has been raped by an acquaintance might report that she finds herself sleeping late and missing classes, doesn't have enough energy to continue playing on the softball team, and feels depressed most of the time.

Both secondary and associated forms of depression seem to be related to the perception of a loss of control. As a secondary symptom, depression might reflect the perception of a loss of control over one's ability to modulate or control one's own feelings of anxiety or anger. As an associated symptom, depression might relate to aspects of the trauma situation. For example, depression might reflect the perception of a loss of control resulting from loss of one's home or possessions. Trauma situations may also alter one's ideas about safety and protection from harm causing a perception of little control over safety.

The belief that you have no control over what happens to you can lead to despair, especially when the events that you cannot control are very negative. This idea is consistent with a learned helplessness model of depression described by Seligman (1975). According to this model, people (and animals) become depressed when they find that they are helpless to control or prevent negative events. In essence, when people are exposed to negative and painful events that they cannot control, they learn that their attempts to protect themselves from harm are to no avail, and they stop trying to help themselves. Lethargy, negative thinking, and negative emotions are all observable responses of people who have learned that they are helpless to prevent harm to themselves. Evidence of a connection between lack of control over negative events and depression has been found in numerous animal studies in which uncontrollable painful events were found to cause depressed behaviors (Maier, 1984).

The cognitive elements of learned helplessness are critical factors in creating and maintaining depression because trauma victims may often perceive themselves as powerless long after they might have regained some control. For example, the college student who had been raped became depressed when she perceived herself as powerless to protect herself from harm. She remains depressed because she continues to believe that she cannot protect herself. Even if she would, in fact, be able to prevent a similar experience and not be in any danger, her depression may continue because of her perception of continued helplessness.

Aggression

In addition to being a core response to trauma, aggression may be a secondary or an associated response. Although it may often be difficult to know whether aggressive thoughts, feelings, or behaviors are part of an initial, secondary, or associated response to trauma, it may sometimes be helpful to make these distinctions because they may have implications for treatment. For example, you are likely to take different treatment approaches to aggressive behaviors that seem to be reexperiencing symptoms than to aggressive behaviors that are the result of anger over inability to modulate anxiety or to aggressive behaviors that are socially learned through living in a violent home environment.

Aggression toward others that is a secondary symptom may result from frustration over the experience of core trauma symptoms. For example, a man who is traumatized by a terrorist bombing, might be frustrated at his own lack of control over his feelings of anxiety following the event and might lash out in anger at those around him. One way that aggressive behaviors toward others could be an associated response to trauma is that they could result from social learning of behaviors that are concomitant with the trauma. For example, a child who is traumatized by physical abuse by a violent parent may learn an aggressive coping style from his parent. In this way, the child might develop aggressive behaviors because he is imitating his parent's aggressive response to frustration or anger. Similarly, a teenager who is traumatized by witnessing urban violence may have a secondary response of aggression because he sees that aggressive behaviors are most adaptive in his environment. In this case, fear, social learning, and operant conditioning reinforcement may combine to make aggression likely. Fear would motivate the teenager to protect himself, and social learning would lead him to imitate the violent behavior of his peers. At the same time, violent behavior could be negatively reinforced if it were followed by relief from anxiety because the teenager believed that the aggression protected him from harm.

Self-directed aggression may also be a secondary response to trauma. One possible mechanism for such aggression would be that it is an attempt to interrupt the initial response of emotional numbing. As described above, emotional numbing is part of the core trauma response of avoidance. Some clinicians believe that self-harming behaviors may constitute an attempt at affect regulation. Herman (1992) has discussed how some abuse survivors may engage in self-injurious behaviors (such as self-cutting, vomiting, compulsive sexual arousal behavior, risk taking or exposure to danger, and use of psychoactive drugs) to alter and improve their affective states. Although it seems counterintuitive that self-harming behaviors would improve one's affective state, abuse survivors frequently report that self-inflicted physical pain is preferable to the emotional numbness they typically experience in the months and years following trauma.

Self-injurious behavior may also be associated with other aspects of abuse experiences. For example, it may result from feelings of self-hatred and disgust that represent trauma survivors' internalizations of the attitudes of others. For example, a father who sexually abuses his daughter may call her names and express revulsion and disgust with her. He might call her a "slut" and tell her that she deserves to be molested. Over a period of time, the daughter might incorporate this view into her self-concept and grow up to feel great self-loathing as an adult. Her adult suicidal behaviors may reflect a very negative self-concept and her belief that she is not worthy of living.

Self-Esteem

Many traumatic experiences indirectly impair self-esteem or interfere with its healthy development in children. Low self-esteem would be experienced subjectively as a lack of self-confidence, poor self-image, or negative evaluations of oneself and one's accomplishments. It might also be observed in a trauma survivor's behavior in the form of lack of initiative, a tendency to give up easily on endeavors, or self-defeating behavior. Impaired self-esteem might be a secondary response to trauma for those whose trauma responses impair or interfere with the development of their cognitive and social skills. For these people, preoccupation with self-protection during or following trauma hinders activities that would enhance cognitive and social skills. For example, a child whose home is destroyed in an earthquake might be anxious and distracted at school and feel emotionally numb. These initial responses to the trauma are likely to hamper the child's ability to do school work and to further develop her cognitive skills. As she falls further behind, academically, she may lose interest in trying to succeed at school, concluding that she is "just too dumb" to do well. At the same time, her emotional numbness and avoidance might cause her to become socially isolated and to fall behind in social development. Here, too, she may become discouraged about her ability to succeed socially, concluding that she will never be well liked by her peers, and gradually make fewer and fewer attempts to develop friendships.

To make matters worse, the initial aggressive responses to the trauma might be expressed by the child as antisocial behaviors at school and at home. Such negative behaviors might lead to rejection by teachers, peers, and family members, reinforcing the girl's perception of inadequacy. The downward spiral of self-esteem resulting from deficits in cognitive and social skills are likely to be further compounded for those whose traumas are intentionally and maliciously inflicted. For example, a child who is traumatized by sexual abuse may suffer the combined effects of poor performance in school, poor social skills, negative feedback from teachers and peers, negative feedback from an abuser, and negative self-evaluations (Putnam, 1990). In children, low self-esteem may well continue into adulthood in the absence of experiences that promote high self-esteem.

Impaired self-esteem might also be the result of concomitant aspects of the traumatic situation. For example, in addition to causing a trauma response through violent acts, an abusive parent might externalize her anger in other ways. Such a parent may blame a child for things that are not her fault and may fail to recognize any of her child's positive qualities or achievements. These concomitant aspects of the abusive situation are very likely to contribute to problems with self-esteem.

Identity

Disturbance in identity might be manifested by identity confusion, confusion over one's desires, tastes, or personal goals, or feelings of passive influence. Passive influence experiences are those in which a person does not feel in control or "in charge of" her own behavior so that behaviors are not experienced as volitional. Identity disturbance could be a secondary response to trauma symptoms such as avoidance symptoms. For example, a police officer who is traumatized in a shooting incident and is unable to do his regular work because of fear would experience disruption of his normal activities and relationships. He might also be avoidant of reminders of his work such as "cop" shows on TV or news coverage involving crimes. These disruptions and his avoidance might result in identity confusion, particularly if his work as a police officer were a major part of his identity. Unable to join his fellow officers when they responded to calls, he might begin to question his own courage, his loyalty to his friends and his profession, or his general "fitness" to do the work of a police officer.

Dissociative symptoms of depersonalization and amnesia might also lead to identity problems. Traumatized persons often experience depersonalization experiences such as feeling unreal, feeling detached from oneself, or feeling a lack of control over one's behavior. Similarly, they may experience amnesia for personal information and for aspects of their traumatic experiences. If experienced over a prolonged period of time, these kinds of disturbances in the perceptions of oneself and of biographical memory could lead to disruptions in one's identity. Further discussion of the impact of depersonalization and amnesia on identity is included in Chapter 5 (pp. 92–93).

Identity disturbance could also be an associated symptom when aspects of the trauma situation affect a person's identity. For example, aside from the immediately traumatizing effects of traumatic combat situations, a soldier might experience identity confusion because of acts he committed in combat. A man who sees himself as humane may not be able to reconcile having killed another person, and this conflict may threaten his sense of self.

Interpersonal Relationships

Difficulties in interpersonal relationships may also be a secondary or associated symptom following traumatic experiences. In adults, these difficulties might be manifested as problems in intimate relationships, conflict with family members, or trouble establishing or maintaining friendships. Interpersonal difficulties in adults can be secondary to the initial trauma responses of fear, aggressive behaviors, emotional numbing, behavioral avoidance of people, and depression (Young, 1988). Such difficulties will be most pronounced for people whose traumatic experiences were interpersonal in nature. For example, a college student who has been raped by an acquaintance may be fearful of other men. She might behave in a hostile way or avoid men altogether in an effort to protect herself. She might also be depressed and have little energy for pursuing or maintaining friendships with women. All of these initial responses to trauma would tend to damage her current relationships and impede development of new relationships.

Difficulties in interpersonal relationships can also be the result of concomitant aspects of a trauma such as when children are traumatized by physical abuse by their caretakers. In many cases physical abuse of a child is accompanied by emotional and physical neglect. Abuse and neglect may make children particularly vulnerable to developing difficulties in their interpersonal relationships because they may have no experience of healthy interpersonal relationships. Further discussion of the impact of childhood abuse on an individual's lifelong interpersonal relationships is included in Chapter 5 (p. 90).

Guilt and Shame

Guilt and shame are closely related emotions that can be powerful secondary or associated responses to traumatic experiences. Guilt reflects a person's sense of self-blame or responsibility for events, whereas shame reflects a sense of responsibility accompanied by embarrassment or disgrace. These may be manifested as remorse over surviving when others did not, as the belief that one is to blame for harm to others or oneself, or as shame over having behaved badly during or after the traumatic situation. As secondary symptoms, guilt and shame may be consequences of core trauma responses. For example, a firefighter might be traumatized in a fire and later be unable to function because of conditioned reexperiencing of fear when he sees fire. He might feel guilty and ashamed of endangering his coworkers and fire victims by not doing his job effectively. Another firefighter might feel guilty after a fellow firefighter dies in a fire if he felt that he should have acted to prevent the death. Clearly, guilt and shame are powerfully influenced by the person's perceptions about the traumatic event and its surrounding circumstances. Feelings of guilt may or may not be realistically related to any actual behaviors of the traumatized person, but they can be extremely disabling nonetheless.

Guilt that develops as an associated response to trauma seems to be a result of the traumatized person's ambivalence over the controllability of the traumatic event. On one hand, at the time of the trauma, the individual feels unable to exert control over the immediate and negative threat to his safety. On the other hand, the idea that he cannot protect himself or others from harm may be so intolerable that it is preferable to believe that he could have controlled the events, but did not.

There may be other mechanisms for the development of guilt and shame following traumatic experiences (Stone, 1992). For example, abused children may experience guilt because of a need to protect the image of their parents as blameless (Dalenberg & Jacobs, 1994; Herman, 1992). Because the child is dependent on the same people who abuse her (or fail to protect her), she must deny their guilt and blame herself in order to preserve her attachment to them. This self-blame results in shame and guilt because of negative social mores about children engaging in sexual activities.

SUMMARY

This chapter described core, secondary, and associated responses to traumatic experiences and the forms that they might take. First, the core responses to trauma were defined and explained, and examples of responses to particular traumas were provided. Explanations of how each response is theoretically linked to trauma were offered that explained how the responses reflect the natural human response to uncontrollable, negative, and sudden events. Research findings relating to human and animal responses to danger were described to provide support for these explanations. To better understand the complex patterns of responses that traumatized people present clinically, the alternating phases of posttraumatic responses were described. Cognitive and psychodynamic theories were presented that explain why these alternating phases occur. Finally, secondary and associated responses to trauma were described that are common across many types of traumatic experience. These include depression, aggression, guilt and shame, and disturbances in self-esteem, identity, and interpersonal relationships.

Chapter 4

Factors That Influence Responses to Traumatic Experiences

As discussed in Chapter 2, exposure to a potentially traumatic event will not necessarily cause a posttraumatic reaction in every individual. For some persons, no doubt, this is because the event was not perceived as sufficiently negative or uncontrollable. Others, however, seem to emerge from experiences that are extremely negative, uncontrollable, and sudden with relatively few and mild posttraumatic symptoms. There are several factors that seem to influence responses to trauma and that seem to account for much of the individual variation in trauma responses. As you consider the influence of these factors, keep in mind that there may well be additional factors that also influence responses. Some of the additional factors may be idiosyncratic to the individual or the circumstances of the traumatic event. Other factors may play a role in shaping responses of particular populations of people. For example, relationships between aspects of traumatic experiences and symptoms may vary depending on cultural background. As with other psychological disorders, we can expect culture to influence the process and presentation of the disorder greatly. Because most of the research and clinical work on traumatic stress has focused on white, middle- and upper-middle-class Americans, it may not generalize well to people from other cultures or to those from distinctive American subcultures. To the extent that a client's cultural background differs from the "mainstream," relationships between his experience and symptoms may also differ.

Building on the work of van der Kolk (1987b), I have identified five general categories of factors that influence responses to sudden, uncontrollable, negative experiences. These include biological factors, developmental phase at the time of trauma, the severity of the stressor, social context, and previous and subsequent life events. In general, these factors affect the trauma response because they affect either the perception of uncontrollability or the degree to which an event is experienced as negative. For example, a biological predisposition to psychopathology or biological effects of earlier trauma might decrease a person's perception of controllability of experiences. Earlier phases of development are associated with high levels of uncontrollability, since young children are very dependent and have relatively little control over what happens to them. Traumas involving more severe stressors such as those that are life threatening have a very negative valence. Little or no social support might make trauma experiences seem more negative and uncontrollable. Previous or subsequent life events that are negative might decrease perceptions of controllability.

Conversely, these factors might all help mitigate responses to trauma if they resulted in increased perceptions of controllability or reduced the degree to which experiences were perceived as negative. For example, a biological tendency toward resilience might moderate the perceived negative valence of an event and might increase a person's perception of controllability of the experience. Traumas that occur at a later period in development might be perceived as more controllable since adults have more capacities and thus more control over their environments than do children. Less severe or threatening traumas would be perceived as less negative. Strong social support might make trauma experiences seem less negative and uncontrollable. Positive previous or subsequent life events might moderate effects of early traumatic experiences by increasing perceptions of controllability. For each of the five factors identified, I discuss the theoretical basis for the effect of the factor and the empirical evidence that supports its influence.

BIOLOGICAL FACTORS

Two biological factors may influence responses to trauma. The first is a biological or genetic predisposition to vulnerability or resilience to trauma. The second is biological change(s) that may occur in response to traumatic experiences. At this time, the role of biological or genetic predisposition to mental illness or mental health is still unclear. Because theories that propose links between neurotransmitter function abnormalities and predispositions to mental illness are based largely on studies of animal brain tissue preparations, both the generalizability of the findings and the causal direction of the processes are left in question. In other words, we do not know whether findings from studies of animal brain tissue apply to humans, and we do not know if the neurotransmitter changes observed are the cause or the result of a particular mental illness. Also, although most theories assume a genetic predisposition model, biological abnormalities need not be genetically based. It is also possible that early environmental factors or experiences cause biological abnormalities in some individuals.

Studies have shown that there are individual differences among both children and animals in their reactions to the same stressful event under controlled circumstances (van der Kolk, 1987b; van der Kolk et al., 1984). These findings are of interest because they may have implications for human responses to high-magnitude stressors. Some have interpreted the findings to mean that genetically based temperamental differences cause some individuals to be more vulnerable to traumatic experiences than others. Personality researchers have only recently begun to explore the possibility that innate, biological tendencies in brain function are associated with temperament and affective responses to stressful, negative events (Davidson, 1992a, 1992b). If such innate biological tendencies are found, they may constitute a predisposition for vulnerability or resilience to negative life experiences.

But other factors may also be influencing biological temperament, which might then influence responses to stress. Temperament may be shaped through biological, cognitive, and behavioral mechanisms. Environmental or experiential factors may make contributions to temperament in humans, beyond those of genetic predisposition. A wide range of environmental factors (such as exposure to toxins or hormones in utero or early in development) and experiences (such as traumatic stress) can cause long-lasting biological changes in humans (van der Kolk, 1996b). It is also possible that the different responses to stressors result from differences in behavior and cognitive patterns learned from previous experience. With so many interacting causal agents and mechanisms involved, it is extremely difficult (and may be ultimately impossible) to sort out their respective influences completely. Studies are most informative if they are prospective and follow children from birth, but the practical aspects of conducting such studies make them extremely difficult to accomplish.

If biological changes occur as a result of traumatic experiences, they are likely to affect responses to later traumatic experiences. Some PTSD researchers have developed models that specify neurological changes following traumatic experiences (Lewis, 1992; van der Kolk, 1987a, 1996b; van der Kolk et al., 1984; van der Kolk, Greenberg, Orr, & Pitman, 1989; Yehuda, Giller, & Mason, 1993; Yehuda, Giller, Southwick, Lowy, & Mason, 1991; Yehuda, Resnick, Kahana, & Giller, 1993). Because these models focus on changes in neurotransmitter functions, they are as difficult to study as theories of biological predisposition described above. Consequently, theories of neurological changes following trauma have only been tested indirectly in humans, leaving open questions about their validity. Moreover, no clear picture of the biological response to trauma has emerged from research to date.

Despite the problems inherent in studying vulnerability to trauma, it seems likely that humans have emotional strengths and weaknesses that make them more or less vulnerable to mental illness, just as they have physiological strengths and weaknesses that make them more or less vulnerable to physical illnesses and injuries. In general, we can expect that those with biological predispositions to anxiety, aggression, or depression will develop more severe reactions when exposed to trauma. Childhood trauma might also play a role in precipitating mental disorder in a person who is biologically predisposed. This conceptualization is consistent with stress-diathesis models proposed for many mental disorders and has been raised as a possibility in regard to traumatic events in general.

Along these lines, Yehuda and McFarlane (1995) have proposed that PTSD may not be a normative response to a traumatic event but a disordered response that is related to some number of preexisting biological or psychological vulnerabilities. These authors have reviewed a number biological and psychological mechanisms that may account for differences in the development of PTSD across similar stressors (McFarlane & Yehuda, 1996). True and colleagues (1993) have found strong evidence of a genetic component to PTSD in their twin study of Vietnam era veterans. It does seem likely that a person's biological and psychological strengths and weaknesses contribute to his response to exposure to a traumatic event. But whereas biological factors are usually conceptualized as producing vulnerability to mental disturbances, it might be that these factors can also produce invulnerability or resilience. For example, findings of at least one recent study of abused children were consistent with the hypothesis that some children are relatively resilient to abuse experiences (Cicchetti, Rogosch, Lynch, & Holt, 1993). If such a resilience trait does exist, it may well be normally distributed so that biological factors produce extreme vulnerability to mental illnesses in some individuals, extreme invulnerability or resilience in others, and a moderate level of vulnerability in the vast majority of individuals.

These possibilities could be explored in relation to the effects of trauma by studying whether the majority of those who experience sudden, uncontrollable, and highly negative events are symptomatic or not. To date, most studies have focused on exposure to a potentially traumatic stressor without specifically assessing the individuals' perceptions of the event's uncontrollability and negative valence. Better assessment of these factors may shed light on the question of what is a "normative" response to trauma. For example, if most of those who perceive a sudden event as highly negative and uncontrollable show moderate posttraumatic symptoms, then it may be "normal" to be vulnerable to trauma and "abnormal" to be invulnerable or extremely vulnerable. Still, the picture is clouded by the impact of environmental and experiential variables (such as developmental level, social context, and previous and subsequent life events), and it remains possible that the contribution of initial biological factors to trauma responses is swamped by the effects of life experiences and social context variables. We should be able to discover whether this last possibility is probable by determining how much of the variance in response to trauma can be accounted for by experiential and environmental factors alone.

Finally, we agree with Wilson and his colleagues that some extreme stressors will produce symptoms in almost everyone, regardless of predisposing factors (Wilson, Smith, & Johnson, 1985). Evidence for this possibility was provided by my own findings from a study of a random sample of a group of Cambodian refugees living in the United States who had all experienced many years of severe trauma (Carlson & Rosser-Hogan, 1993). Fully 90% of the subjects reported high levels of two or more trauma symptoms (anxiety, PTSD symptoms, dissociation, and depression) when interviewed after 5 years in the United States.

The role of biological factors in the response to trauma is further complicated by the fact that biological and emotional factors are continually interacting. These interactions are particularly pertinent to understanding the responses of traumatized children because of the continuous changes in a child's underlying biology as he develops. For example, a child might experience somatic changes because of anxiety and depression following traumatic abuse. Any further traumatic abuse might then have a different impact because of the child's altered physiology. Another example of the interaction between biological and emotional factors involves children's hormonal systems. There is some evidence that experiences of chronic sexual abuse in children may alter hormonal mechanisms (Putnam & Trickett, 1993). These alterations may, in turn, have some effect on sexual behavior.

A close link between biological and psychological aspects of the trauma response can also be inferred from evidence that physiological and psychological responses to trauma seem to vary together. In a study of behavioral treatment of Vietnam veterans with PTSD, only those subjects who showed decreased physiological responding at 3 months following treatment also showed improvement in psychological symptoms (Boudewyns & Hyer, 1990).

DEVELOPMENTAL LEVEL AT THE TIME OF TRAUMA

The effects of the developmental level of the child at the time of trauma are extremely complex and difficult to study. In its simplest form, developmental level is often equated with age. In general, the age at the time of trauma is expected to be negatively related to severity of symptoms. In other words, if other variables are held constant, the younger the person is at the time the trauma occurs, the more severe her symptoms will be. This should be the case as children are forced to rely on emotional and cognitive methods of avoidance (such as emotional numbing and dissociation) because they typically do not have the option of behavioral avoidance. In other words, since children often cannot physically escape from trauma, they must rely on emotional and cognitive forms of escape. This conceptualization is supported by the finding of Kirby and colleagues of a negative relationship between age of onset of childhood abuse and level of dissociation in psychiatric inpatients (Kirby, Chu, & Dill, 1993). Also, Wolfe and colleagues found that age was negatively related to a range of posttraumatic symptoms in groups of sexually abused children (Wolfe, Sas, & Wekerle, 1994; Wolfe, Gentile, & Wolfe, 1989).

If the essential elements of trauma are uncontrollability and a negative valence, it would seem that the effects of trauma would be most severe during the period when sense of control and self are developing. This means that trauma should have its greatest impact on development between the ages of 2 and 7 years when the major tasks of regulation of self-esteem and control of environment and self are central (Cicchetti, 1989; Erikson, 1963).

Although an earlier age at time of trauma would generally be expected to result in increased posttraumatic symptoms, further predictions are complicated because variables such as psychological vulnerability to mental illness and pretrauma coping abilities are likely to vary greatly across children of the same age. Furthermore, for some types of trauma, more advanced development may make a child more vulnerable to trauma. For example, an older child who has a more sophisicated understanding of sexuality may experience sexual contact with her father as more negative (hence more traumatizing) than would a younger child who doesn't fully appreciate the meaning of the behavior. On the other hand, it is possible that younger children can be sensitized to later trauma. For children who experience repeated traumas, it seems certain that earlier traumas will alter their psychological disposition at the time of later trauma and influence their coping with any later traumatic events. Briere (1996b) notes that early abuse can be globally devastating to a child because it alters the child's sense of self.

Children's responses to trauma will depend on their emotional, social, and cognitive development. A child's emotional development will no doubt affect the response to trauma. For example, a child who had a secure attachment (or emotional bond with a caretaker) would be expected to show a more positive long-term adjustment to trauma than a child who had an insecure attachment. This issue can be complicated by the interaction between the abuse and the attachment when trauma occurs before or during attachment formation, particularly when the trauma takes the form of abuse inflicted by a caretaker. Detailed discussions of the relationship between child abuse and attachment are available elsewhere (Aber & Allen, 1987; Alexander, 1992; Cicchetti & Barnett, 1991; Cicchetti & Howes, 1991; Cicchetti & Rizley, 1981; Crittenden & Ainsworth, 1989; Lynch & Cicchetti, 1991). The potential impact of abuse on later interpersonal relationships is discussed further in Chapter 5 (p. 90).

A child's level of cognitive development and social development at the time of trauma will also be important to her adjustment. Higher levels of cognitive and social skills might enable the child to exert more control over her environment, thus reducing her anxiety and possibly avoiding further stress or traumatic experiences. These skills might also make it possible for a child to obtain social support that would have beneficial effects. Higher cognitive capacities would also make it more likely that a child could develop an intellectual understanding of events that could ameliorate effects of some types of trauma events. For example, a young child with limited cognitive development might perceive traumatic abuse to be the result of his being bad, whereas an older child with more capacity for logic and reasoning might perceive the abuse to be the result of a parent's alcoholism. The different conceptualizations would be expected to have different ramifications for the child's self-esteem. On the other hand, as mentioned above, a higher level of cognitive development may make children more vulnerable to some types of trauma when more advanced cognitive abilities result in greater perceptions of uncontrollability or a higher negative valence for the event.

Developmental level may also play a role in determining the nature of the trauma response. For example, severe and chronic trauma that occurs early in development before identity consolidation has occurred may lead to a predominantly dissociative response. This possibility is discussed in detail in Chapter 5 (pp. 92–93). More in-depth discussions of the role of developmental level in responses to traumatic stressors can be found in work by Pynoos and colleagues (Pynoos, 1993; Pynoos, Steinberg, & Goenjian, 1996), Ruskin and Talbott (1995), and Perry (1997).

SEVERITY OF TRAUMA

Severity of the stressor has been found to be related to later symptoms in a variety of traumatized populations (Shalev, 1996). For example, studies have found relationships between severity of traumatic experiences and later posttraumatic symptoms in samples of crime victims (Kilpatrick et al., 1989), combat veterans (Sutker, Allain, Albert, & Winstead, 1993), burn victims (Perry, Difede, Musngi, Frances, & Jacobsberg, 1992), refugees (Carlson & Rosser-Hogan, 1991), and sexually abused children (Wolfe et al., 1989). In these studies, severity of traumatic stressors has been defined in various ways. Several characteristics of an event can contribute to the severity of trauma including the intensity, nature, and duration of the traumatic experience.

The intensity, nature, and duration of the trauma would all affect an individual's perceptions of the controllability and negative valence of the event. Traumas that are more intense are thought to be more likely to provoke overwhelming fear and helplessness because of their more negative valence. For example, since more intense forced sexual experiences (such as intercourse) will have a more negative valence than less intense experiences (such as fondling), they will tend to result in more severe symptoms. Several studies have found more advanced forms of sexual activity to result in more severe short- and long-term mental health problems (Browne & Finkelhor, 1986; Hartman, Finn, & Leon, 1987; Herman, Russell, & Trocki, 1986; Kendall-Tackett, Williams, & Finkelhor, 1993; Wolfe et al., 1994). Similarly, intensity of combat experiences has been related to severity of later symptoms in veterans (Breslau & Davis, 1987; Buydens-Branchey, Noumair, & Branchey, 1990; Green, Grace, Lindy, Glese, & Leonard, 1990). These findings support the notion that the intensity of trauma is an important factor influencing later symptoms.

The nature of a traumatic experience might also affect an individual's response. For example, sexual abuse experiences seem to be related to particular kinds of later symptoms that do not seem related to other types of trauma. Several studies have found higher levels of suicidality in children, adolescents, and adults with histories of sexual abuse (Briere, 1988; Briere & Runtz, 1987, 1988; Briere & Zaidi, 1989; Browne & Finkelhor, 1986; Shaunesey, Cohen, Plummer, & Berman, 1993). In contrast, studies have shown higher rates of violent criminality in those who experienced physical abuse during childhood compared to those who experienced sexual abuse or neglect (e.g., Widom, 1989).

It is worth noting that an individual's subjective impressions and perceptions can greatly affect the perceived intensity and nature of a traumatic experience. This happens because subjective impressions and perceptions influence the valence and perceived controllability of an experience. For example, a woman who is threatened with a knife and believes that she may be injured, but not killed, may experience the event as less intense than a woman who is threatened with a knife and believes that she may be killed. Similarly, physical or sexual abuse by a parent may be perceived as more intense than abuse by a stranger because the parent is an expected source of safety (Janoff-Bulman, 1992).

Traumatic experiences that last longer would necessarily be associated with longer periods when the person would feel unable to control the aversive events. The greater perception of events as uncontrollable tends to result in higher levels of anxiety. Traumas of very long duration may also lead to despair and depression because of the ongoing inability to control aversive events. This is consistent with the learned helplessness model of depression (Seligman, 1975). Similarly, Horowitz (1986) has noted that traumas of longer duration lead to despair and depression that inhibit the adaptation to trauma. Unfortunately, although many studies have examined the length of time spent in chronically traumatic situations (such as combat or incest), I know of no studies that have measured the effects of the duration of a single traumatic event.

It is worth noting, however, that a long duration alone will not necessarily lead to a more severe posttraumatic response. Very intense traumas of shorter duration may be more traumatizing than less intense traumas of longer duration. But if intensity is held constant, longer duration will generally be related to greater symptomatology. An example of this might be the experience of being held hostage at gunpoint in a bank robbery. If that experience were to last for 10 hours, it would more likely be traumatizing than if it were to last for 10 minutes.

SOCIAL CONTEXT

An individual's social context includes his socioeconomic environment and family context as well as his individual and societal social support. Important aspects of socioeconomic environment and family include stresses of the socioeconomic environment and family dysfunction. Living in a stressful environment is likely to exacerbate posttraumatic responses. Examples of stressful environments would include living in poverty and living in a violent neighborhood. Although environmental stress probably exerts an important influence on recovery following traumatic stress, this variable has not yet been studied in trauma victims. Familial variables that might negatively affect adjustment following trauma include: neglect; psychological maltreatment; caretaker alcohol or drug abuse, mental disorders, suicidality, and disciplinary methods; poverty; and violence in the home (such as marital violence or abuse of other children in the household).

The influence of family dysfunction on responses to trauma has been of particular interest to those studying the effect of traumatic child abuse. Wolfe and colleagues make the point that since most child abuse occurs in the context of a family that is otherwise disturbed, it may be impossible to determine the unique contributions of abuse and distinguish them from the effects of other social and emotional deprivations (Wolfe et al., 1989). Several studies have investigated the influences of a wide range of family variables on long-term adaptation to abuse (Briere, 1988; Briere & Elliott, 1993; Justice & Calvert, 1990; Nash, Hulsey, Sexton, Harralson, & Lambert, 1993; Pollock et al., 1990; Wind & Silvern, 1994; Yama, Fogas, Teegarden, & Hastings, 1993; Yama, Tovey, & Fogas, 1993). In general, results of these studies show poorer outcomes for abused children who were also exposed to severe family dysfunction such as parental alcoholism, mental disorders in caretakers, and family violence.

Social support is also an important part of social context that would influence responses to trauma. Social support might occur in the immediate familial or social environment or it might be present on a broader level in community or school settings. The first type of social support would be provided by individuals such as a friend, family member, or by a therapist. Familial social support is an important factor in responses to trauma to the extent that the individual interacts with family members. An adult with close family ties may obtain considerable social support from parents, siblings, spouse, or children. In the case of childhood traumas, individual social support is even more important because children are so dependent on others for emotional support.

The second type of social support might be provided by community or societal institutions. For example, a traumatically abused child might have a lesson at school, read a book, or view a television program that addresses abuse and assures children that they are not to blame for its occurrence. Domestic violence victims might obtain community support through a domestic violence hotline or shelter.

Those who have social support available to them at the time of their trauma are expected to show lower levels of symptoms than those who have no one available to give them emotional support. In other words, the availability of social support is expected to act as a mitigating factor in the response to trauma. This is anticipated because those who do have support are expected to feel more hopeful of achieving control over the aversive experiences than those who do not have social support. In addition, those with social support may be less likely to develop secondary symptoms. For example, a child who suffers traumatic abuse but is told that he or she was not to blame for the abuse would be helped to maintain a positive self-concept.

There is considerable empirical evidence that social support is an important factor in the response to adult traumatic experiences. For adult trauma victims, social support has been found to be related to lower levels of later psychological symptoms in combat veterans (Green et al., 1990; Keane, Scott, Chavoya, Lamparski, & Fairbank, 1985; Perry et al., 1992; Solkoff, Gray, & Keill, 1986; Solomon & Mikulincer, 1990; Solomon, Mikulincer, & Hobfoll, 1987), flood victims (Solomon & Smith, 1994), burn victims (Perry et al., 1992), bereaved persons (Bunch, 1972), rape victims (Kilpatrick, Veronen, & Best, 1985; Moss, Frank, & Anderson, 1990), and women who had abortions (Belsey, Greer, Lal, Lewis, & Beard, 1977). Interestingly, in the study of burn victims by Perry and colleagues, social support at the time of the trauma was found to be a more powerful predictor of PTSD symptomatology than the severity of the injury.

Several studies have found that social context affects responses to abuse in children. Conte and Schuerman (1987) found a significant relationship between the availability of a supportive parent or sibling and a rating of the child's distress following sexual abuse. Conversely, a review of research on resilience in children has found that more stable families are associated with resilience to psychological symptoms in general (Luthar & Zigler, 1991). Similarly, a meta-analysis of studies of sexually abused children has found that children who had maternal support at the time of reporting abuse showed fewer symptoms overall (Kendall-Tackett et al., 1993).

Relatively little research has examined the relationship between social support and long-term posttraumatic symptoms, and most of that research has focused on social support provided by individuals. In a study of the effects of social support on psychological health in women who had been abused as children, Parker and Parker (1991) found that women exposed to both abuse and poor parenting showed lower self-esteem and confidence in social situations than abused females who reported positive parenting. Another study found that women who had been physically or sexually abused as children and who had a supportive relationship with a nonabusive adult were less likely to abuse their own children than women who had been abused but did not experience this type of positive relationship (Egeland, Jacobvitz, & Sroufe, 1988).

PRIOR AND SUBSEQUENT LIFE EVENTS

Just as family and environmental contexts are expected to affect adjustment to trauma, prior and subsequent life events could exacerbate or mitigate the long-term response to traumatic events. Only nontraumatic life events are discussed here as the effects of multiple traumatic events are covered in Chapter 5 (pp. 85–94).

There are two major perspectives on the effects of prior stressful life experiences on a person's ability to cope with a traumatic experience. The first is that stressful events may "innoculate" people so that they are more resistant to subsequent stressful events. Some authors have proposed that intermittent, moderate stressors can produce a "toughening" effect so that the individual is not as sensitive to later stressors (Dienstbier, 1989; Eysenck, 1983). Some evidence has supported this formulation, including Norris and Murrell's (1988) findings showing that flood victims with prior flood experience were less symptomatic than those with no prior flood experience.

On the other hand, stressful events prior to trauma may reduce a person's psychological resources and impede that individual's ability to cope with trauma. This formulation is supported by studies of higher PTSD rates among African Americans in the United States (Neal & Turner, 1991) and of higher rates of childhood abuse among veterans who developed PTSD following combat (Bremner, Southwick, Johnson, Yehuda, & Charney, 1993). Research has also found that psychiatric and personality disorders may increase vulnerability to traumatic experiences (McFarlane, 1990). More research is needed to clarify further the relationship between prior stressful events and trauma response. It seems possible, though, that both moderating and sensitizing effects could be explained by the conceptual framework described in Chapter 2. Prior events that make a trauma seem more controllable and less negative would have a moderating effect, while prior events that make a trauma seem less controllable and more negative would have a sensitizing effect.

Stressful or negative events occurring after a trauma, however, seem certain to exacerbate a trauma response. Having to cope with negative life experiences such as living in poverty, marital discord, a stressful work life, and difficulties raising children would be expected to impair the individual's recovery from trauma. With the exception of research on the effects of social support, I know of no published studies on the influence of negative life experiences subsequent to trauma.

Even less attention has been paid to the possible mitigating effects of positive life experiences. Undoubtedly this is a result of an inherent bias in clinical psychology and psychiatry toward study of "what is wrong" rather than "what is right." Nevertheless, it seems intuitively obvious that positive life events could mitigate the long-term effects of trauma by reducing perceptions of uncontrollability. Financial independence in adulthood, for example, might increase perceptions of control and decrease the perceived importance of earlier negative experiences. Apart from research on social support and family dysfunction variables cited above, I know of no research on the effects of positive life events in persons with trauma histories.

CASE EXAMPLES ILLUSTRATING THE INFLUENCE OF THE FIVE FACTORS

Contrasting responses of two men to traumatic experiences in combat provide a clear illustration of the effects of characteristics of the trauma and other mediating factors. John was 28 when he enlisted in the Navy at the beginning of World War II. During his tour of duty, there were two occasions when he felt that his life was in danger. Both of these events occurred when his ship was under fire for a period of about an hour. He was greatly frightened by these experiences, but he received considerable emotional support from his buddies on the ship after the battles were over. When he returned home from his tour of duty, his wife, family, and community received him as something of a "hero" as he had been decorated for his role in sinking a German submarine. After a period of adjustment, John returned to his former job with few residual psychological problems relating to his war experiences.

Jeff was 19 when he was drafted into the Army and sent to Vietnam. During his tour of duty, there were several periods lasting for weeks when he felt that his life was in danger. He witnessed horrors such as the killing and burning of children, the gruesome death of a buddy who stepped on a land mine, and the bombing of civilian villages. Since many of his buddies from his unit were killed, sent home, or transferred to other units, he received little emotional support following his combat experiences. When he returned home from his tour of duty, protests against the war in Vietnam were at their height. He was unable to find work because of employers' negative feelings about Vietnam veterans. After numerous experiences of people verbally abusing him for having fought in Vietnam, he withdrew from social contacts and tried to keep people from finding out that he was a veteran. Jeff suffered numerous PTSD symptoms following the war including nightmares, intrusive images of combat and atrocities, exaggerated startle, hypervigilance, physiological arousal to trauma reminders, and cognitive and behavioral avoidance.

The contrasting experiences and responses of these two men show the powerful effects of developmental level, severity of the stressor, and social support on traumatization and recovery following traumatic events. Jeff was relatively young when he experienced combat trauma and had not yet developed an adult identity or self-confidence in his work or interpersonal skills. Jeff's lower levels of social and emotional development made it more difficult for him to cope with the traumas he faced. John, on the other hand, had begun a family and a successful career and felt self-confident as a husband, father, and employee. The severity of Jeff's combat experiences was clearly greater than John's. Jeff's experiences were arguably more intense and had a greater duration than John's. These differences in severity would be expected to produce a more severe posttraumatic response. Perhaps most striking are the contrasting levels of social support received by the two men. While John's social support probably played a positive role in his recovery from war experiences, the lack of social support and hostility that Jeff experienced probably exacerbated his symptoms.

SUMMARY

This chapter described five factors that affect responses to trauma, including biological factors, developmental phase at the time of abuse, the severity of the stressor, social context, and previous and subsequent life events. For each factor, the theoretical basis and empirical findings relating to the factor's influence were reviewed. Case examples were provided to illustrate the differential effects of the various factors on responses to traumatic events.

Chapter 5

Understanding Responses to Discrete and Chronic Traumatic Experiences

The symptom picture of a traumatized person varies depending on characteristics of the trauma and of the individual. The trauma and individual characteristics that are most influential were discussed in Chapter 4. Some of these can be considered pretrauma variables (the individual's biological characteristics, developmental level, social context, and previous life events), one represents trauma characteristics (severity of the stressor), and some are posttrauma variables (social support following trauma and subsequent life events). As you assess a client, try to understand his symptoms, and perhaps assign a diagnosis; it will also be important to pay attention to the length of time since the trauma and the chronicity of the individual's traumatic experiences. These two factors will interact with one another (as the pretrauma factors do) so that the long-term course of a trauma response depends, in part, on whether a person experienced a relatively discrete or circumscribed traumatic event or a continuous series of traumatic events.

Categorizing traumatic experiences as discrete or chronic is useful because these types of histories seem to be associated with differing clinical pictures. Terr (1991) has proposed that traumas be categorized in this way and suggests that one-time-event traumas ("Type I traumas") are likely to have different effects on an individual than repeated, long-standing, or chronic traumas ("Type II traumas"). Examples of discrete traumatic events are those that are circumscribed in time such the experience of a tornado or a car accident. In contrast, chronic traumas are those that occur continuously over a relatively long period of time such as repeated assaults over years as a part of incest or spousal abuse. Other examples of chronic traumas include combat, war, and refugee experiences. In addition, Terr (1991) notes that discrete traumas followed by periods of extreme, ongoing stress may create a posttraumatic response with features of responses to both discrete and chronic traumas. Although some experiences fall into a gray area between discrete and chronic, this distinction still seems important to make because prototypical patterns of posttraumatic symptoms have been observed for responses to single or relatively circumscribed traumatic events and for responses to chronic trauma.

Unfortunately, in the past, researchers have not always distinguished between discrete and chronic traumas in studying their effects. Studies have tended to focus on the nature of the trauma without regard to chronicity. For example, studies of combat veterans sometimes do not specifically measure or study the chronicity of combat traumas, and studies of child abuse victims often do not distinguish between those who experience a single assault and those who experience repeated assaults or chronic abuse. It is also important to avoid confusing the chronicity of trauma (defined as the length of time a person was in a situation experiencing repeated traumatic events) with the duration of a trauma (defined as the length of time a single traumatic event lasts and discussed in Chapter 4). Studies of individuals with discrete traumas and those of individuals with chronic traumas seem to indicate that chronicity is a critical determinant of trauma responses.

This chapter briefly reviews research findings of core, secondary, and associated symptoms following discrete and chronic traumas. Diagnostic categories that are associated with particular trauma patterns are also described. Though an in-depth discussion of children's responses to discrete and chronic traumas is beyond the scope of this book, some distinctive aspects of children's responses are noted. Prototypical long-term responses to discrete and chronic traumas are also described. Familiarity with short- and long-term trauma response patterns will be helpful to you during your assessments because they may give you some indication of the current stage of the client's posttraumatic response and of whether the symptom picture is more consistent with a discrete traumatic experience or a series of traumas over an extended period of time.

RESPONSES TO DISCRETE TRAUMAS

In the weeks and months following a variety of discrete traumatic experiences, high levels of the core, secondary, and associated symptoms described in Chapter 3 are commonly observed. As discussed previously, these symptoms are closely tied to the experience of an uncontrollable, very negative, and sudden event through various behavioral and cognitive processes. According to McFarlane and de Girolamo (1996), among those who do develop diagnosable posttraumatic responses, circumscribed traumatic experiences seem to result in a relatively "uncomplicated" PTSD response.

Most of the studies that have examined reexperiencing and avoidance responses have focused on the DSM symptoms of PTSD in adult victims of single traumatic events. Table 5.1 shows the DSM-IV criteria for PTSD (American Psychiatric Association, 1994), and a comparison of Table 5.1 and Table 3.1 (p. 44) shows that all of these symptom criteria can be conceptualized as forms of reexperiencing and avoidance. Although many studies measured PTSD criteria from DSM-III-R, the results would be very similar as the symptom criteria of the two versions are virtually identical (American Psychiatric Association, 1987). PTSD symptoms have been reported in victims of discrete traumas such as natural and technological disasters (Smith & North, 1993; Ursano, Fullerton, & McCaughey, 1994; Weisaeth, 1994); accidents (Malt, 1994), rape (Foa & Riggs, 1993), and criminal victimization (Kilpatrick & Resnick, 1993). Findings and discussions of PTSD in response to a wide range of discrete traumatic events are available in Wilson and Raphael (1993).

In addition to findings of PTSD symptoms, high levels of reexperiencing and avoidance symptoms in particular modes of experience have also been found following discrete traumatic experiences. High levels of cognitive reexperiencing in the form of intrusive thoughts have been reported by survivors of diverse traumas including earthquakes (Anderson & Manuel, 1994; Weiss & Marmar, 1996), bushfires (McFarlane, 1992), railway accidents (Andersen, Christensen, & Petersen, 1994), and by victims of terrorist attack (Shalev, 1992), ship disasters (Joseph, Yule, & Williams, 1994, 1995), and motor vehicle accidents (Bryant & Harvey, 1996).

Affective reexperiencing in the form of high levels of anger has been reported in studies of those who experienced discrete traumas such as crimes (Riggs, Dancu, Gershuny, Greenberg, & Foa, 1992). Affective reexperiencing in the form of high levels of anxiety has also been found following a wide range of discrete traumas such as rape (Steketee & Foa, 1987), accidents (Malt, 1994), disasters (Koopman, Classen, Cardeña, & Spiegel, 1995), as well as countless other types of discrete traumas (Horowitz, 1993; Keane, Litz, & Blake, 1990; Pynoos, 1993).

Behavioral reexperiencing following discrete traumatic experiences has not yet been the focus of systematic research. Although instances of verbal and physical aggression toward others and self-harming behaviors

TABLE 5.1. DSM-IV Diagnostic Criteria for 309.81 Posttraumatic Stress Disorder

A. The person has been exposed to a traumatic event in which both of the following were present:

   (1) the person experienced, witnessed, or was confronted with an event or events that involved actual or threatened death or serious injury or a threat to the physical integrity of self or others
   (2) the person's response involved intense fear, helplessness, or horror. **Note:** In children, this may be expressed instead by disorganized or agitated behavior

B. The traumatic event is persistently reexperienced in one (or more) of the following ways:

   (1) recurrent and intrusive distressing recollections of the event, including images, thoughts, or perceptions. **Note:** In young children, repetitive play may occur in which themes or aspects of the trauma are expressed.
   (2) recurrent distressing dreams of the event. **Note:** In children, there may be frightening dreams without recognizable content.
   (3) acting or feeling as if the traumatic event were recurring (includes a sense of reliving the experience, illusions, hallucinations, and dissociative flashback episodes, including those that occur on awakening or when intoxicated). **Note:** In young children, trauma-specific reenactment may occur.
   (4) intense psychological distress at exposure to internal or external cues that symbolize or resemble an aspect of the traumatic event
   (5) physiological reactivity on exposure to internal or external cues that symbolize or resemble an aspect of the traumatic event

C. Persistent avoidance of stimuli associated with the trauma and numbing of general responsiveness (not present before the trauma), as indicated by three (or more) of the following:

   (1) efforts to avoid thoughts, feelings, or conversations associated with the trauma
   (2) efforts to avoid activities, places, or people that arouse recollections of the trauma
   (3) inability to recall an important aspect of the trauma
   (4) markedly diminished interest or participation in significant activities
   (5) feeling of detachment or estrangement from others
   (6) restricted range of affect (e.g., unable to have loving feelings)
   (7) sense of a foreshortened future (e.g., does not expect to have a career, marriage, children, or a normal life span)

D. Persistent symptoms of increased arousal (not present before the trauma), as indicated by two (or more) of the following:

   (1) difficulty falling or staying asleep
   (2) irritability or outbursts of anger
   (3) difficulty concentrating
   (4) hypervigilance
   (5) exaggerated startle response

E. Duration of the disturbance (symptoms in Criteria B, C, and D) is more than 1 month.

(continued)

F. The disturbance causes clinically significant distress or impairment in social, occupational, or other important areas of functioning.
Specify if:
    Acute: if duration of symptoms is less than 3 months
    Chronic: if duration of symptoms is 3 months or more
Specify if:
    With Delayed Onset: if onset of symptoms is at least 6 months after the stressor

Note. From American Psychiatric Association (1994, pp. 427–429). Copyright 1994 by the American Psychiatric Association. Reprinted by permission.

have been observed and reported in the clinical literature, I know of no empirical studies of victims of discrete traumas that have specifically assessed behavioral reexperiencing.

Physiological reexperiencing in the form of elevated levels of physiological arousal has been found following discrete traumatic experiences and in response to trauma cues in traumatized persons (Prins, Kaloupek, & Keane, 1995). Indirect evidence of physiological hyperarousal following discrete traumas is provided by findings of high levels of somatization (Friedman & Schnurr, 1995; McFarlane, Atchison, Rafalowicz, & Papay, 1994) and sleep disturbances (Woodward, 1995) in trauma victims.

Research on cognitive avoidance has largely taken the form of studies of dissociation, including experiences of amnesia, depersonalization, and derealization. Experiences of these forms of cognitive avoidance have been reported following a wide range of discrete traumatic events such as disasters (Cardeña & Speigel, 1993; Koopman, Classen, & Spiegel, 1994; Marmar et al., 1996), rape (Dancu, Riggs, Hearst-Ikeda, Shoyer, & Foa, 1996), and murder of a family member (Rynearson & McCreery, 1993).

Affective avoidance in the form of emotional numbing has been reported following many different kinds of trauma but has only recently been the focus of more extensive theoretical and empirical work (Litz, 1992). Recent work on development of a measure of affective numbing may stimulate further research in this area (Glover et al., 1994). Another means of achieving affective avoidance may be through the use of alcohol or drugs to achieve emotional numbness. Studies have found high rates of substance abuse in those who survived various discrete traumas (Saladin, Brady, Dansky, & Kilpatrick, 1995; Stine & Kosten, 1995).

Behavioral avoidance of trauma-related stimuli comprises one of the diagnostic criteria for PTSD, but it has not specifically been the subject of research. Behavioral avoidance is very difficult to measure, partly because much behavioral avoidance may occur without conscious intention or awareness. Similarly, physiological avoidance has not been empirically studied following discrete traumas, although physiological numbing in the form of analgesia has been reported by individuals who sustain traumatic injuries.

Evidence of most of the secondary and associated symptoms described in Chapter 3 has also been found in studies of victims of discrete traumas. High levels of depression have been found in virtually all traumatized populations including victims of rape (Resick, 1993), torture (Basoglu et al., 1994), motor vehicle accidents (Blanchard, Hickling, Taylor, & Loos, 1995), earthquakes (Goenjian et al., 1995), and hurricanes (Daniella et al., 1996). Although there has been relatively little empirical study of self-esteem in victims of discrete traumas to date, low self-esteem has been identified as a problem in victims of spousal violence (Frisch & MacKenzie, 1991; Orava, McLeod, & Sharpe, 1996) and in rape victims (Murphy, Anick-McMullen, et al., 1988). Similarly, little empirical work has been done linking discrete traumatic experiences with identity disturbances or disturbances in interpersonal relationships, although several authors have proposed that such links may exist (McNally, Eells, Fridhandler, Stinson, & Horowitz, 1993; Solomon, 1989; Young, 1988).

Researchers have found elevated levels of guilt in survivors of discrete traumas such as rape (Layman, Gidycz, & Lynn, 1996) and disasters (Joseph, Hodgkinson, Yule, & Williams, 1993). Elevated levels of shame have been reported in survivors of discrete traumas such as kidnapping (Terr, 1983), sexual assault (Ruch, Gartrell, Amedeo, & Coyne, 1991), rape (Dahl, 1989), and disaster (Joseph, Brewin, Yule, & Williams, 1993).

In addition to specific studies of these initial, secondary, and associated symptoms, various studies have focused on diagnoses associated with traumatic experiences. As discussed above, PTSD is the diagnosis most commonly associated with the experience of discrete traumatic events. Although few studies to date have assessed criteria for acute stress disorder (ASD), this set of symptoms has also been observed in some individuals following discrete traumatic experiences such as disasters (Koopman et al., 1995). As you can see, the DSM-IV criteria for ASD (shown in Table 5.2) are basically the same as those for PTSD, with the exception that more emphasis is placed on the presence of symptoms of dissociation (American Psychiatric Association, 1994).

As noted in DSM-IV, discrete traumatic events may also precipitate any of three dissociative disorders, including dissociative amnesia, dissociative fugue, and depersonalization disorder (American Psychiatric Association, 1994). Dissociative amnesia (formerly called psychogenic amnesia) is characterized by "the inability to recall important personal information that is usually of a traumatic or stressful nature and that is too extensive to be explained by ordinary forgetfulness" (American

TABLE 5.2. DSM-IV Diagnostic Criteria for 308.3 Acute Stress Disorder

A. The person has been exposed to a traumatic event in which both of the following were present:

    (1) the person experienced, witnessed, or was confronted with an event or events that involved actual or threatened death or serious injury, or a threat to the physical integrity of self or others

    (2) the person's response involved intense fear, helplessness, or horror

B. Either while experiencing or after experiencing the distressing event, the individual has three (or more) of the following dissociative symptoms:

    (1) a subjective sense of numbing, detachment, or absence of emotional responsiveness

    (2) a reduction in awareness of his or her surroundings (e.g., being in a daze)

    (3) derealization

    (4) depersonalization

    (5) dissociative amnesia (i.e., inability to recall an important aspect of the trauma)

C. The traumatic event is persistently reexperienced in at least one of the following ways: recurrent images, thoughts, dreams, illusions, flashback episodes, or a sense of reliving the experience; or distress on exposure to reminders of the traumatic event.

D. Marked avoidance of stimuli that arouse recollections of the trauma (e.g., thoughts, feelings, conversations, activities, places, people).

E. Marked symptoms of anxiety or increased arousal (e.g., difficulty sleeping, irritability, poor concentration, hypervigilance, exaggerated startle response, motor restlessness).

F. The disturbance causes clinically significant distress or impairment in social, occupational, or other important areas of functioning or impairs the individual's ability to pursue some necessary task, such as obtaining necessary assistance or mobilizing personal resources by telling family members about the traumatic experience.

G. The disturbance lasts for a minimum of 2 days and a maximum of 4 weeks and occurs within 4 weeks of the traumatic event.

H. The disturbance is not due to the direct physiological effects of a substance (e.g., a drug of abuse, a medication) or a general medical condition, is not better accounted for by Brief Psychotic Disorder, and is not merely an exacerbation of a preexisting Axis I or Axis II disorder.

Note. From American Psychiatric Association (1994, pp. 431–432). Copyright 1994 by the American Psychiatric Association. Reprinted by permission.

Psychiatric Association, 1994, p. 481). A person might experience dissociative amnesia following a trauma such as a terrorist bombing or a train wreck. In the "classic" presentation, such a person would be found wandering near the scene of the trauma and would have no memory of his identity or details of his life (Loewenstein, 1991). In dissociative fugue (formerly called psychogenic fugue), amnesia is also present, along with sudden travel and identity confusion or assumption of a new identity (American Psychiatric Association, 1994). Although there is little research on the prevalence or presentation of either disorder, both are thought to be relatively rare in their pure forms (Loewenstein, 1991). Systematic epidemiological studies are needed to determine the prevalence of these disorders.

Episodes of partial or complete amnesia are commonly observed as symptoms in those who meet diagnostic criteria for PTSD, ASD, or dissociative disorders. For example, in my study of psychiatric inpatients, I found rates of partial or complete amnesia that varied from 40 to 60% across different types of traumatic events (Carlson, Armstrong, & Loewenstein, 1997). Amnesia has also been reported following natural disasters, accidents, war-related traumas, kidnapping, torture, concentration camp experiences, physical and sexual abuse, and commission of murder (van der Kolk, 1996b). Amnesia is also found in all of those with dissociative identity disorder and many with dissociative disorder not otherwise specified as it is one of the criteria for diagnosis of the disorders (American Psychiatric Association, 1994).

Depersonalization symptoms have also been associated with the experience of discrete traumas (Shilony & Grossman, 1991). Depersonalization disorder is characterized by severe distortions in perceptions of oneself or one's body (American Psychiatric Association, 1994). For example, during or after a life-threatening car accident, a person might have the experience of feeling as though he is removed from his body, watching himself from a distance. He may feel that he is "going through the motions" of escaping from the wreck and helping others, but he does not feel as though he is actively directing his behavior. Like dissociative amnesia and dissociative fugue, symptoms of depersonalization disorder are probably more common as part of other trauma-related disorders than they are as a sole disorder.

It is also very important to remember that the majority of those exposed to discrete traumatic stressors have posttraumatic symptoms that are not severe enough to warrant any trauma-related diagnosis (Blank, 1993). Some of these individuals may not develop a more severe response because they did not experience the necessary traumatizing elements of lack of controllability and negative valence. Those who did experience a full-fledged trauma may have been protected from a more severe response by biological or characterological resilience or by the ameliorating effects of intervening social support.

Responses to Discrete Traumas in Children

Although a detailed discussion of children's responses to trauma is beyond the scope of this book, research has established that children often experience reexperiencing and avoidance symptoms following discrete traumatic events (Fletcher, 1996a; Nader, 1996; Putnam, 1996a). Because less research has been done on trauma responses in children, there is less certainty about their patterns of responses to discrete traumatic events. Pynoos and colleagues have noted the extreme complexity of posttraumatic reactions in children and suggest a developmental approach to understanding children's trauma responses (Pynoos et al., 1996). While PTSD is observed in some children following some types of traumatic events, research has indicated that full-blown PTSD responses are less likely in children following traumas such as disasters (McNally, 1993; Ribbe, Lipovsky, & Freedy, 1995).

The finding of less severe PTSD in children after some traumas may reflect underdiagnosis due to differences in presentation of PTSD in children. Posttraumatic symptoms following both discrete and chronic traumas are often expressed differently in children than in adults and are highly dependent on the developmental level of the child (Pynoos et al., 1996). Some distinctive responses to discrete traumas in children include regressive behavior, separation anxiety, fears related to the trauma, generalized fears or anxiety, omen formation, eating problems, repetitive drawing and play related to the traumatic event, and reenactments of aspects of traumatic events (Fletcher, 1996a; Terr, 1991; Vogel & Vernberg, 1993; Yule, 1994). While some of these responses are included as notes in the DSM criteria for PTSD (repetitive play and reenactments), the others are also important to note and are measured by some of the self-report and structured interview measures reviewed in the Measure Profiles section of this book.

On the other hand, as mentioned in Chapter 4, children's incomplete cognitive development may contribute to lower rates of PTSD among children exposed to trauma. Younger children, in particular, may be somewhat protected from traumatization because they do not fully understand the nature of the traumatic event. It seems likely that younger children may mistakenly believe that adults who are with them have some control over the traumatic situation, and they consequently may not understand that they are in great danger. In some situations, adults may suggest or foster these ideas by giving assurances of safety to children during a traumatic event.

Although there has been a great deal of research on the effects of the stressor of sexual abuse on children, these studies show mixed results, with some indicating high levels of PTSD responses and others indicating very low levels (McNally, 1993). This apparent inconsistency may be due to the fact that the nature and chronicity of sexual abuse experiences vary greatly across children. Those experiencing a discrete sexual assault would be expected to have very different responses from those experiencing chronic sexual abuse. Similarly, those experiencing sexual assaults that produce overwhelming fear (such as rape) would be expected to have different responses than those experiencing less frightening molestations (such as fondling). Unfortunately, because most of the research on sexual abuse of children does not distinguish among these different types of sexual abuse experiences, the nature of children's responses to sexual abuse is not yet clear.

Long-Term Course of Responses to Discrete Traumas

Studies of the long-term course of symptoms in those who do develop PTSD responses to discrete traumas indicate that there is great variability in the persistence of symptoms after the traumatic experience. For example, of a group of persons traumatized when fighting bushfires in Australia, about half still had PTSD symptoms 3½ years later, and 4% still had PTSD symptoms 8 years later (McFarlane & Yehuda, 1996). Similarly, of a sample of women who were physically assaulted, almost 8% met criteria for PTSD 15 years after the event. It seems, then, that while some traumatized persons experience a gradual reduction in their posttraumatic symptoms in the months following discrete traumas, others do not.

In Chapter 4, I discussed in detail many factors that influence initial responses to trauma. These factors are also likely to account for differences in long-term adjustment to trauma across individuals. For example, biological vulnerabilities may affect both the initial response to a stressor as well as the process of recovery. Biological changes that result from traumatic experiences may also affect recovery (McFarlane & Yehuda, 1996). Posttrauma variables such as social support, social environment, and subsequent life events are also likely to greatly influence the course of posttraumatic symptoms.

Although some authors have noted that a PTSD response to a discrete traumatic event can have a delayed onset (Blank, 1993), others have noted that it is uncommon and that symptoms typically begin immediately following discrete traumas such as disasters and accidents (McFarlane & Yehuda, 1996). McFarlane and Yehuda (1996) note that the appearance of a delayed onset may sometimes result from a client's failure to recall or report her acute posttraumatic symptoms.

There can be considerable variability in the relative prominence of various symptoms over the course of a posttraumatic response. Those with the most severe PTSD responses are more likely to have persistent intrusion and avoidance symptoms over time (McFarlane & Yehuda, 1996). In those whose symptoms do decline over time, there seems to be a gradual decrease in intrusion symptoms. Levels of physiological arousal may remain elevated, however, long after the intrusive thoughts and memories have faded (McFarlane & Yehuda, 1996). Secondary symptoms such as somatic problems (De Loos, 1990; Kulka et al., 1990c; Leserman, Toomey, & Drossman, 1995) and depression (Carlson & Rosser-Hogan, 1993; Goenjian et al., 1995; Hubbard, Realmuto, Northwood, & Masten, 1995; Orsillo, Weathers, et al., 1996; Yehuda, Kahana, Southwick, & Giller, 1994) may also become prominent long-term symptoms following trauma. Because of these fluctuations in symptomatology over the course of posttraumatic disorders, a trauma-tized client who is 1 or 2 years posttrauma might meet criteria for disorders such as depression, dysthymia, somatization disorder, or generalized anxiety disorder and not meet criteria for PTSD.

RESPONSES TO CHRONIC TRAUMA

Repeated, long-standing, or chronic traumas have been found to result in all of the same posttraumatic symptoms observed in those experiencing discrete traumas. The core, secondary, and associated symptoms discussed in Chapter 3 have all been found the be prevalent among survivors of chronic trauma. I first discuss responses to chronic trauma observed in adults and then address responses to chronic trauma in children. Reexperiencing and avoidance symptoms in particular modes of experience have also been studied following chronic traumatic experiences. High levels of intrusive thoughts have been reported in those with experiences of repeated combat trauma (Hendrix, Jurich, & Schumm, 1994), other chronic war-related traumas (Carlson & Rosser-Hogan, 1993), and repeated sexual abuse (Alexander, 1993; Murphy, Kilpatrick, Amick-McMullan, & Veronen, 1988).

Affective reexperiencing in the form of high levels of anger has been reported in studies of those who experienced chronic traumas such as World War II veterans (Hovens et al., 1992) and Vietnam veterans (Chemtob & Roitblat, 1994; Kulka et al., 1990d). Affective reexperiencing in the form of high levels of anxiety has also been found following a wide range of chronic traumas such as sexual abuse (Beitchman et al., 1992; Koverola, Pound, Heger, & Lytle, 1993; Mennen & Meadow, 1994), combat (Scurfield, 1993a), refugee camp experiences (Kinzie, 1993), as well as numerous other chronic trauma survivor groups (Horowitz, 1993; Keane et al., 1990; Pynoos, 1993).

The form of behavioral reexperiencing following chronic trauma that has been studied the most is aggression. Researchers have found elevated levels of aggression toward others in studies of survivors of chronic trauma including war veterans (Beckham et al., 1996; Lasko, Gurvits, Kuhne, Orr, & Pitman, 1994), refugees (Hauff & Vaglum, 1994), and physically abused children (Scerbo & Kolko, 1995). Aggression toward the self, in the form of suicidality and self-harming behaviors has also been found in samples of Vietnam veterans (Everly, 1990; Kramer, Lindy, Green, Grace, & Leonard, 1994) and in adolescents and adults with histories of sexual abuse (Boudewyn & Liem, 1995; Brand, King, Olson, Ghaziuddin, & Naylor, 1996; Romans, Martin, Anderson, Herbison, & Mullen, 1995; van der Kolk, Perry, & Herman, 1991).

Symptoms of physiological arousal have been found to be elevated following a wide range of chronic traumatic experiences (Prins et al., 1995). In addition, increased physiological arousal in response to trauma cues has been found in several studies of veterans of combat trauma with PTSD (McFall, Murburg, Ko, & Veith, 1990; Orr, Pitman, Lasko, & Herz, 1993; Pitman, Orr, et al., 1990). These findings support the connection between trauma cues and physiological arousal in those with PTSD. In addition, findings of high levels of somatization (Friedman & Schnurr, 1995; Kulka et al., 1990c; Leserman et al., 1995) and sleep disturbances (Mellman, Kulick-Bell, Ashlock, & Nolan, 1995; Woodward, 1995) following chronic trauma provide indirect evidence of physiological hyperarousal.

Research on cognitive avoidance following chronic trauma has largely taken the form of studies of dissociation, including experiences of amnesia, depersonalization, and derealization. Experiences of these forms of cognitive avoidance have been reported following a wide range of chronic traumas (Loewenstein, 1996) including combat (Branscomb, 1991; Bremner et al., 1992; Hyer, Albrecht, Boudewyns, Woods, & Brandsma, 1993), refugee experiences (Carlson & Rosser-Hogan, 1991), and physical and sexual abuse (Carlson, Armstrong, Loewenstein, & Roth, 1997; Kirby et al., 1993; Nash et al., 1993; Waldinger, Swett, Frank, & Miller, 1994).

Clinical reports have noted affective avoidance in the form of emotional numbing in victims of chronic traumas such as sexual abuse and combat trauma (Herman, 1992). Unfortunately, as mentioned above, affective avoidance symptoms have only recently become the subject of theoretical and empirical work (Litz, 1992). High levels of substance abuse that may reflect intentional efforts to achieve emotional numbness have also been found in chronically traumatized populations (Stine & Kosten, 1995).

As mentioned above, behavioral avoidance of trauma-related stimuli comprises one of the diagnostic criteria for PTSD, but it has not specifically been studied in victims of chronic trauma. Such behavioral avoidance is difficult to measure and may occur without conscious intention or awareness.

Physiological avoidance has been observed in the form of numbing of sensations and has been associated with the experience of chronic trauma (Herman, 1992). Numbing of pain or analgesia has been reported in studies of veterans who survived chronic combat trauma

(Pitman, van der Kolk, Orr, & Greenberg, 1990; van der Kolk et al., 1989).

Evidence of the secondary and associated symptoms described in Chapter 3 has also been found in studies of victims of chronic traumas. High levels of depression have been found in chronically traumatized populations including war veterans (Orsillo, Weathers, et al., 1996), refugees (Carlson & Rosser-Hogan, 1993), and victims of the Holocaust (Yehuda et al., 1994). Some evidence of aggression as a socially learned, associated response to chronic trauma has been found in studies of aggression in children of aggressive parents (Herrenkohl & Herrenkohl, 1981; Kobayashi, Sales, Beckers, & Figueredo, 1995).

Although relatively little empirical work has focused on levels of self-esteem in chronic trauma victims to date, low self-esteem has been identified as a problem in victims of spousal violence (Frisch & MacKenzie, 1991; Orava et al., 1996), combat veterans (Wong & Cook, 1992), and child abuse survivors (Gil, 1988; Herman, 1992). Similarly, little empirical work has been done linking traumatic experiences with identity disturbances, although identity problems have been described in association with combat trauma (Silverstein, 1994) and traumatic childhood abuse (Herman, 1992). Further discussion of the long-term identity disturbances following early and chronic trauma can be found below (pp. 92–93).

Disturbances in interpersonal relationships have been found in survivors of a variety of chronic traumas including combat (Kulka et al., 1990b; Nezu & Carnevale, 1987; Solomon, 1989; Solomon & Mikulincer, 1987) and child abuse (Herman, 1992; Kaufman & Zigler, 1987; Mullen, Martin, Anderson, Romans, & Herbison, 1994). Researchers have also found elevated levels of guilt in survivors of traumas such as combat (Kubany et al., 1995) and elevated levels of shame in combat veterans (Orsillo, Heimberg, Juster, & Garrett, 1996; Wong & Cook, 1992) and refugees (Boehnlein, 1987). Further discussion of long-term effects of chronic childhood trauma on interpersonal relationships can be found below (p. 90).

Chronic traumas seem to have even greater potential than discrete traumas for producing responses that are severe and chronic. While moderate, intermittent stress may foster resilience to later trauma (as discussed in Chapter 4, p. 72), traumatic stressors seem always to exacerbate trauma responses. For example, studies have shown chronicity of abuse to be related to severity of posttraumatic symptoms in sexually abused children (Kendall-Tackett et al., 1993). In terms of chronicity of posttraumatic responses, the relationship between chronicity of trauma and severity of symptoms has been found to persist for years and sometimes decades after the trauma in combat veterans (Buydens-Branchey et al., 1990; McFall, Mackay, & Donovan, 1991) and in adult survivors of chronic sexual abuse (Briere & Zaidi, 1989;

Herman et al., 1986). In other words, many years after the trauma, posttraumatic symptomatology is greater in those who had longer periods of repeated traumatic experiences.

Furthermore, some recent studies have begun to indicate that the effects of early, chronic trauma and later traumas may be cumulative. For example, Bremner and colleagues found higher levels of PTSD in combat veterans with histories of childhood physical abuse than in those with no such history (Bremner et al., 1992). Similarly, Dancu and colleagues found higher levels of dissociation in rape victims who reported childhood rape or attempted rape than in rape victims with no such early assault experiences (Dancu et al., 1996). Follette and colleagues studied childhood abuse and adult physical abuse by a partner in clinical and community samples and found that those who reported multiple types of trauma had higher levels of a range of posttraumatic symptoms (Follette, Polusny, Bechtle, & Naugle, 1996).

There are several reasons why repeated or ongoing traumatic experiences would lead to more severe and long-lasting responses. Clearly, traumatic events such as sudden deaths of loved ones, rape, or combat exposure that occurred after an earlier trauma would be expected to further erode an individual's sense of controllability over negative events and to result in higher levels of psychiatric symptoms. According to Foa and Kozak's (1986) cognitive model for the emotional processing of fear, trauma victims develop memory or information networks in which a wide variety of cues are associated with threat or danger. This model implies that repeated traumatic events would result in greater psychological stress because more stimuli become associated with threat and danger.

Another reason why repeated traumatic experiences might lead to more severe responses is that repeated exposure to similar feared events would strengthen the connections between the cues for the events and anxiety and would result in more intense anxiety reactions to reminders of the events (Foa et al., 1989). In various studies of traumatized persons, the number of traumatic experiences has been positively related to posttraumatic symptoms (e.g., Beitchman, Zucker, Hood, & DaCosta, 1991; Carlson & Rosser-Hogan, 1991; Hartman et al., 1987; Kendall-Tackett et al., 1993). It is also worth noting that many, if not most, of those who experience chronic trauma are also experiencing severe and chronic stress and emotional deprivation. Consequently, symptoms seen in chronic trauma victims may be the result of the combined effects of trauma, chronic stress, and emotional deprivation.

Researchers' relative lack of attention to the cumulative effects of traumatic experiences over the lifetime seems to be the result of an arbitrary split between the fields of child abuse and PTSD. Researchers in the former field study traumatic child abuse experiences only while those in the latter field study adult trauma only. It seems increasingly apparent that it is important to study both childhood and adult trauma in order to understand the long-term effects of abuse.

All of the DSM-IV diagnoses that are observed following discrete traumas are also seen in those who have experienced chronic traumas. The diagnoses most commonly associated with chronic traumas in adults are PTSD and depression. High rates of PTSD have been reported in samples of combat veterans (Kulka et al., 1990a), refugees (Kinzie, 1993), concentration camp survivors (Yehuda et al., 1994), and prisoners of war (Crocq, Macher, Barros-Beck, Rosenberg, & Duval, 1993). High levels of depression have been found in combat veterans (Harvey, Stein, & Scott, 1995; Orsillo, Weathers, et al., 1996), refugees (Carlson & Rosser-Hogan, 1993; Kroll et al., 1989), and Holocaust victims (Yehuda et al., 1994). Depression may be a prominent response to chronic trauma because the chronic sense of learned helplessness that is manifested as depression remains even after the initial intrusive and arousal anxiety symptoms fade. The development of dissociative disorders in chronically traumatized children is addressed below.

Responses to Chronic Trauma in Children

For the most part, studies of the effects of chronic trauma in children have been limited to date to children who were physically and/or sexually abused. Since most abuse studies include children with both discrete and chronic abuse and children with both traumatic and nontraumatic abuse, most study samples inevitably include a large proportion of chronically and traumatically abused children.

In general, high levels of the high rates of reexperiencing and avoidance symptoms have been found in children who were physically and/or sexually abused (Fletcher, 1996a). Studies have found high levels of PTSD symptoms in physically abused children and in sexually abused children (Kiser, Heston, Millsap, & Pruitt, 1991; McLeer, Callaghan, Henry, & Wallen, 1994; McLeer, Deblinger, Henry, & Orvaschel, 1992). Evidence of reexperiencing and avoidance symptoms in several modes of experience has also been found. Affective reexperiencing in the form of aggression toward others and toward the self has been reported in studies of abused children (Burgess, Hartman, & McCormack, 1987; Herrenkohl & Herrenkohl, 1981; Herrenkohl, Herrenkohl, Egolf, & Wu, 1991; Monane, Leichter, & Lewis, 1984). Additional studies have found high rates of self-destructive behavior in abused children (Green, 1978; Shaunesey et al., 1993; Stone, 1993). High levels of cognitive avoidance in the form of dissociation have been found in children and adolescents who had been sexually abused (Aber & Zigler, 1981; Atlas,

Wolfson, & Lipschitz, 1995; Atlas & Hiott, 1994; Malinosky-Rummell & Hoier, 1991; Putnam, Helmers, & Trickett, 1993).

Studies of abused children have also found evidence of those effects we consider secondary or associated responses to abuse, including depression (Beitchman et al., 1991; Kiser et al., 1991; Koverola et al., 1993; Mennen & Meadow, 1994; Pelcovitz, Kaplan, Goldenberg, & Mandel, 1994; Stone, 1993; Toth, Manly, & Cicchetti, 1992), decreased self-esteem (Blake, 1994; Goodwin, Cheeves, & Connell, 1990; Grayston, De Luca, & Boyes, 1992; Mennen & Meadow, 1994; Toth et al., 1992), and disturbances in identity (Putnam, 1990; Putnam et al., 1993). Difficulties in interpersonal relationships have been found in the form of insecure attachment (Cicchetti & Barnett, 1991), confused patterns of relatedness (Lynch & Cicchetti, 1991), and social deficits (Pelcovitz et al., 1994).

Chronic traumatic abuse in childhood is thought to affect relationships because of the emotional deprivation that often accompanies such abuse. According to psychodynamic theories of attachment, in the course of normal development, infants and their primary caretakers form an emotional bond through reciprocal interactions. If the attachment is healthy, the caretaker will feel compelled to nurture the infant, and the infant will develop trust that the caretaker will provide for his physical and emotional needs. It is generally agreed that the nature of early attachments will shape the child's feelings of self-worthiness and trust in others throughout life (Aber & Allen, 1987; Alexander, 1992; Lynch & Cicchetti, 1991). A child who develops an unhealthy attachment with his caretaker is likely to have difficulties with relationships throughout life.

Alexander (1992) has noted that sexual abuse frequently occurs in the context of disturbed infant–caretaker attachments. If there is a poor attachment between the infant and the caretaker, the latter may not feel compelled to nurture and protect the child. Caretakers who are not nurturing or protective of their children are more likely to sexually abuse their children or to fail to protect them from abuse by persons outside the family. Poor attachment and the inability to trust caretakers are likely to lead to poor adult relationships. The nature of the difficulties in adult relationships varies according to the type of disturbed attachment formed in infancy (cf. Alexander, 1992).

Disturbances in attachment would also be expected in children who are physically abused (Aber & Allen, 1987; Cicchetti & Barnett, 1991; Cicchetti & Howes, 1991). Presumably, children who are physically abused are more likely than those who are not to be poorly attached to their caretakers and thus to experience difficulties in interpersonal relationships later on. In addition to this shaky beginning, core and secondary trauma responses of aggressive, avoidant, and depressed behavior are likely to further impede the development of stable relationships in a child who has been traumatized by abuse.

Some studies of children who experienced chronic trauma indicate that there are aspects to children's responses that are somewhat unique. According to Fletcher (1996a), chronically traumatized children generally experience lower levels of reexperiencing symptoms, higher levels of avoidance or numbing, and are more distressed by reminders of their experiences than are children who experience discrete trauma. Additional distinctive symptoms that have also been associated with the experience of chronic trauma in children include inappropriate sexual behavior, loss of beliefs, and loss of faith in authority or adults (Fletcher, 1996a; Nader, 1996).

The same DSM-IV diagnoses associated with chronic trauma in adults may also be seen in chronically abused children. In addition, prominence of particular posttraumatic symptoms may lead to diagnoses such as conduct disorder (when excessive aggression is present) or attention deficit disorders (when anxiety symptoms are manifested as problems with concentration) (Terr, 1991). Given children's distinctive trauma responses of regressive behavior, separation anxiety, and fears related to the trauma, traumatized children may meet DSM-IV diagnostic criteria for separation anxiety disorder, reactive attachment disorder, or specific phobia.

Some dissociative diagnoses associated with chronic trauma in adults may be less likely to occur in young children, while other dissociative diagnoses may be more likely. Dissociative amnesia may be extremely hard to detect in young children, given that they are not expected to have good autobiographical memory. Dissociative fugue seems unlikely on the basis of practicality: Young children are usually unable to travel on their own. But the more severe dissociative disorders of dissociative identity disorder (DID) and dissociative disorder not otherwise specified (DDNOS) have been observed in children (Hornstein & Putnam, 1992; Putnam, 1991a, 1994, 1997). Although specific diagnostic criteria for DID in children have been suggested (Peterson, 1991), no specific diagnostic criteria were included in DSM-IV. Consequently, the only available diagnoses are those for adult DID or DDNOS.

The DSM-IV criteria for DID specify the presence of two or more distinct personality states that recurrently take control of the person's behavior and an unusually extensive lack of recall of important personal information (American Psychiatric Association, 1994). DDNOS criteria specify the predominance of dissociative symptoms along with a failure to meet criteria for any other dissociative diagnosis. The diagnosis of DID (formerly called multiple personality disorder) has been quite controversial, with the main controversy focusing on the nature, veracity, and autonomy of the "personalities" manifested (Horevitz, 1994). These controversies are described in some detail in Chapter 9 (pp. 170–171). Setting aside the issue of whether those with severe dissociative disorders actually have distinct "personalities" that "take control" of their behavior, high levels of dissociative symptoms have been found in children and adolescents with dissociative diagnoses (Armstrong, Putnam, Carlson, Libero, & Smith, in press; Putnam et al., 1993). Those who study dissociative disorders in children have noted that their manifestation in children is particularly difficult to diagnose because of their extremely complex clinical presentations (Hornstein & Putnam, 1992; Putnam, 1991a).

The development of very severe dissociative disorders may be contingent on the developmental level of the person at the time of trauma. DID and some cases of DDNOS are generally thought to have begun in childhood (Putnam, 1989) and to result from the experience of severe and chronic trauma (Putnam, 1985; Putnam, Guroff, Silberman, Barban, & Post, 1986). One possible theoretical explanation for the development of severe dissociative disorders is that these extreme identity and memory disturbances result from repeated traumas occurring prior to the consolidation of identity in childhood. Continued traumas prevent normal consolidation of identity and autobiographical memory.

For example, a child who is severely and chronically sexually and physically abused over a period of years from the age of 4 might frequently experience depersonalization and amnesia. As described above, the abuse experiences would produce the initial response of cognitive avoidance in the form of amnesia and distortion in the sense of self (depersonalization). In other words, the child would try to avoid the emotional pain of abuse through forgetting abuse experiences or distorting self-perceptions to avoid being reminded of the abuse. Very frequent dissociation (involving cognitive, affective, behavioral, and physiological reexperiencing and avoidance) touching many aspects of a child's life might well lead to disturbances in identity (Cole & Putnam, 1992; Putnam, 1991a; Putnam & Trickett, 1993). Briere (1992) has made similar observations about the impact of childhood abuse on the self, suggesting that the process of development of a healthy sense of self is impaired in abused children because of the tendency to direct attention to others (as part of hypervigilance), impaired attachment, and the dissociation of fragments of identity.

For healthy identity development, one needs to have consistency in the sense of self and cohesiveness of biographical memory. Traumatized children might not have enough consistency or cohesion to allow consolidation of a clear identity. In extreme cases, severe identity disturbances might be manifested in the kind of global difficulties in establishing an integrated sense of self that are characteristic of severe dissociative disorders. Putnam and Trickett (1993) point out that a wide range of disorders associated with childhood sexual abuse all have disturbances in sense of self in common. Disturbances in identity and low self-esteem that occur in severe dissociative disorders and borderline personality disorder and distortions of body image that occur in eating and somatization disorders may all be the result of past abuse experiences.

In support of the connection between identity disturbance and early trauma, some research has reported an association between disorders involving extreme distortions in identity and early experiences of traumatic abuse. A sample of persons with DID (Putnam et al., 1986) and samples of persons with borderline personality disorder (Goodwin et al., 1990; Herman, Perry, & van der Kolk, 1989; van der Kolk et al., 1991) have been found to report high rates of childhood abuse.

If severe identity disturbances are largely associated with severe and chronic trauma that occurs before identity consolidation, then dissociative disorders such as DID would not develop in those older than 7 or 8 at the time of trauma. After that age, even severe and chronic trauma would result in PTSD rather than DID.

Some research has also linked chronic childhood abuse trauma to chronic and pervasive disorders such as borderline personality disorder (Herman et al., 1989). Along these lines, Terr (1991) has noted that disordered emotions, cognitions, and behaviors following chronic trauma in children may lead to profound characterological changes that are manifested in adulthood. A chronic psychiatric disorder called disorders of extreme stress not otherwise specified (DESNOS) has also been found to be associated with prolonged and repeated trauma (van der Kolk, 1996a). DESNOS has been delineated and was recommended for inclusion in DSM-IV, but it was not ultimately included in the diagnostic system (Brett, 1996; Herman, 1993). As described by Herman (1993), this disorder would include the posttraumatic stress symptoms described in Chapter 3. Among these symptoms, dissociation (cognitive avoidance), and self-harming behaviors (self-directed aggression) would be prominent. DESNOS would also be characterized by high levels of somatization and disturbances in relationships and identity. A detailed description of this proposed disorder can be found in van der Kolk (1996a).

Long-Term Course of Responses to Chronic Trauma

Studies of the long-term course of posttraumatic responses to chronic traumas indicate that posttraumatic symptoms can persist for years or even decades and that, in general, those who experience chronic traumas tend to be more symptomatic over time than those who experience discrete traumas. PTSD symptoms have been reported up to 50 years following chronic trauma in prisoners of war, Southeast Asian refugees, and veterans of World War II, Vietnam, and other wars (Crocq et al., 1993; Hunter, 1993; Kinzie, 1993; Op den Velde et al., 1993; Scurfield, 1993a; Tennant, Goulston, & Dent, 1993), and in adults with histories of childhood sexual abuse (Briere, 1988; Rowan & Foy, 1993; Wolfe et al., 1989; Yama et al., 1993). Specifically, elevated levels of affective reexperiencing in the form of aggression have also been observed in persons with histories of chronic trauma (Chemtob & Roitblat, 1994; Scerbo & Kolko, 1995). Avoidance in the form of dissociation has been found in combat veterans (Branscomb, 1991; Bremner et al., 1992; Hyer, Albrecht, et al., 1993; Orr et al., 1993) and appears to be particularly pronounced in those with chronic, early sexual abuse trauma (Chu & Dill, 1990; Irwin, 1994; Kirby et al., 1993; Sandberg & Lynn, 1992). Possible mechanisms for persistence of posttraumatic symptoms are discussed in Chapter 2 (pp. 40–43), and factors that will influence long-term responses to chronic trauma are discussed in Chapter 4.

Secondary and associated symptoms have also been found to be prominent long-term manifestations of chronic trauma responses. For example, elevated levels of depression have been found to be prevalent in refugees (August & Gianola, 1987; Carlson & Rosser-Hogan, 1991; Kroll et al., 1989), veterans (August & Gianola, 1987; Hovens et al., 1992; Kulka et al., 1990d), prisoners of war (Arthur, 1982; Harvey et al., 1995), and adults who experienced traumatic abuse as children (Bifulco, Brown, & Adler, 1991; Briere, 1992; Browne & Finkelhor, 1986; Bryer et al., 1987; Jehu, 1989; Yama, Tovey, et al., 1993). Decreased levels of self-esteem and self-efficacy have been found in adults who were sexually abused as children (Alexander & Lupfer, 1987; Finkelhor, 1990; Gold, 1986).

In terms of diagnosis, chronic trauma has frequently been associated with later diagnoses of PTSD (Rowan & Foy, 1993; Scurfield, 1993a) and depression (Bifulco et al., 1991; Carlson & Rosser-Hogan, 1993; Orsillo et al., 1996; Stone, 1993; Yama, Tovey, et al., 1993). As discussed above, chronic trauma in children has also been associated with diagnoses of DID, DDNOS, borderline personality disorder, and DESNOS.

SUMMARY

This chapter delineated prototypical patterns of short- and long-term responses to discrete and chronic traumatic experiences. Typical short-term responses to discrete traumas were reviewed for adults and for children, and diagnoses that correspond to these responses were identified. Common long-term responses to discrete traumas were reviewed along with associated long-term diagnoses. Common short-term responses to chronic traumas in adults and children and associated diagnoses were reviewed. Diagnoses that correspond to long-term responses to chronic trauma were also described.

Part II

PLANNING AND IMPLEMENTING ASSESSMENTS

Chapter 6

Challenges to Assessing Trauma and Trauma Responses

When you begin to assess a client who may be traumatized, you will have a number of concerns in mind. What can I do to encourage my client to give me a complete report of her trauma history and symptoms? What can I do to help my client report her history and symptoms accurately? How do I choose which measures of trauma and trauma responses to administer? What can I do to help minimize my client's distress during the assessment process? This chapter and the two that follow address these questions. This chapter discusses the challenges you will face in assessing trauma and trauma responses and offers suggestions for addressing these challenges. Chapter 7 then provides you with the information you need to plan an assessment strategy for a client. Chapter 8 describes the contents of the profiles of recommended measures and discusses practical aspects of administering measures and conducting therapeutic interviews.

Assessing traumatic experiences and responses to trauma can be particularly challenging for clinicians because they must try to minimize the likelihood that clients' reports will be inaccurate at the same time they maximize the likelihood that clients' reports will be complete. To meet these goals when assessing trauma, you must first understand what factors are likely to contribute to error in trauma reports and how accurate memories of trauma are generally thought to be. Although the accuracy of trauma memories has been the subject of intense debate, a convincing case can be made for routinely taking a trauma history and for using systematic methods to maximize the accuracy of clients' trauma reports. Accurate assessment of trauma responses can be a challenge as well, and systematic measurement can also help maximize the accuracy of symptom reports.

CHALLENGES TO ASSESSING
TRAUMATIC EXPERIENCES

Gathering information about clients' past traumatic experiences is an essential part of a trauma assessment, but it can create a clinical dilemma. While it is clearly necessary to ask specific questions about traumatic experiences in order to get information about trauma, it is also important that clients' reports about their experiences be fairly accurate so that you can plan effective treatments.

In most clinical circumstances, obtaining a highly precise report of past events is neither necessary nor particularly useful at the time of assessment. Usually, a therapist evaluating trauma histories of clients for purely clinical purposes is more interested in clients' memories about traumatic events than in a factual account of past events. For example, if your client reports being held up and seeing a gun in the hand of the mugger, there would be no therapeutic purpose to investigating whether the mugger was actually carrying a gun. Therapeutically, the important issue is your client's perception that there was a gun and that his life was threatened. You may be tempted to try to determine the veracity of clients' trauma memories so that you can make causal connections between those events and current symptoms. But you are not likely to be successful at precisely identifying cause and effect. As discussed in Chapter 4, there are a large number of variables that influence responses to trauma. Even if tracing the path of cause and effect for a particular client were possible, it would never be possible to confirm a particular understanding of how particular events and circumstances caused particular symptoms. Also, as discussed in Chapter 2, the client's perceptions of events are more influential in development of symptoms than the actual events themselves.

Nevertheless, there are several problems associated with assessing traumatic experiences that should be considered and anticipated. Sometimes, you may be concerned that a client's reports are extremely exaggerated or inaccurate, or you may be worried that a client has been led to make reports of events that did not occur. Also, some clients with memory loss for past events may be especially focused on determining the exact nature of their past experiences.

DISBELIEF OF TRAUMA REPORTS

Although it has only recently become a prominent issue, questioning the validity of trauma reports is not new. Herman (1992) reviews the past history of responses to trauma reports by American institutions and society. She describes a long and ongoing tendency to ignore and forget victims of traumatic events that were "man made" and discusses the societal forces that seem to encourage this. This is an issue for survivors of all types of trauma, but some trauma reports tend to be questioned more than others. Recently, attention has focused on the validity of reports of childhood sexual abuse, particularly reports of adults who say that they only recently remembered the abuse they experienced.

At one extreme pole of this debate, a group including cognitive psychologists, persons who say they are falsely accused of abuse, social psychologists, and some clinicians contend that it is relatively rare for victims of child abuse to have no memory for their experiences and that "recovered" memories of child sexual abuse are not likely to be valid ones. This group bases many of its arguments on results of laboratory studies demonstrating the fallibility of memory, and they are quite concerned about the possibility that clients can be influenced to report events that did not occur. The memory studies they cite do indicate potential sources of inaccuracy in memory, but most of them suffer from a lack of ecological validity. That is, the findings of most memory studies may not apply to "real life" trauma memories because the conditions of the study do not resemble "real life" trauma situations in a number of ways. For example, most studies focusing on the accuracy of memory involve recalling details of brief, one-time events of little personal significance to the individual. In contrast, many traumas that have been questioned (such as incest) involve events that were experienced repeatedly over long periods of time and that are of great personal significance. Further discussion of research on the fallibility of memory and its application to memory of trauma can be found in Read and Lindsay (1997), Pope and Brown (1996), Pope (1996), and Pezdek and Banks (1996).

At the opposite pole of the debate, trauma researchers and therapists contend that amnesia for child sexual abuse events is relatively common and that recovery of such memories is necessary for treatment. These researchers and clinicians base their opinions on clinical experience and on results of studies of memory for traumatic experiences (cf. Green & Wolfe, 1995). These studies have the advantage of directly addressing the memory for traumatic events, but they have the disadvantage of less control than some laboratory studies over extraneous variables that might influence findings. Further discussion of research on memory for trauma can be found in Green and Wolfe (1995), Read and Lindsay (1997), Pope and Brown (1996), and Pezdek and Banks (1996).

The term child sexual abuse usually is used to refer to repeated sexual assaults on a child, often by a family member or a person close to the child. One reason that child sexual abuse reports are sometimes questioned is because there is typically little evidence that sexual abuse occurred. Unlike traumas such as hurricanes or car accidents, sexual abuse typically occurs in secrecy and leaves no physical evidence that corroborates the victims' reports. What is more, family members may be motivated to deny the events in order to protect a family member who perpetrated the abuse or in order to spare the victim embarrassment. Given the high prevalence of child sexual abuse in the United States and the great recent concern about the accuracy of such reports, this discussion focuses on challenges associated with assessing this type of trauma. Most of the discussion also applies to reports of other types of trauma.

Error and Accuracy in Children's Trauma Reports

If a child experiences a traumatic event, how accurate will her reports of past trauma be? If a child reports a past traumatic event, how likely is it that the report is accurate? These questions are very difficult to answer, but research on the accuracy of children's memories sheds light on the general accuracy of their trauma reports.

Researchers have only recently begun to closely study children's memories of their personal experiences. It is almost impossible to study the accuracy of children's memories of actual abuse experiences because there is no unequivocal source of information on the exact details of the abuse. Instead, researchers study children's memories for controlled and well-documented events that closely mirror abuse experiences. An example of this is research on children's memory for medical examinations or invasive procedures. Like abuse, these experiences are both personal and distressing. In one such study, children between the ages of 3 and 7 were asked questions about details of an invasive examination of the urinary tract both immediately after and 6 weeks after the examination occurred (Ornstein, 1995). Overall, 6 weeks after the examination, these children correctly recalled 83% of the details of the exam and correctly denied 93% of the details that were asked about but did not occur.

It seems, then, that children may have very good recall of details of personal and distressing experiences. But to the extent that abuse experiences differ from the medical exam studied, so might the accuracy of memories for abuse. For example, abuse experiences might be much more distressing than the medical procedure, and perceptions of abuse are likely to be much more confusing. During a medical exam, explanations of what will happen are given to children that help them conceptualize and remember what happens. During most abuse experiences, a child may have no idea what will happen next or may have little understanding of what she is experiencing. Instead of facilitating understanding, abusers are likely to mislead a child with false statements. For instance, a father might tell his daughter that sexual activity with him is "okay" because he is "teaching" her about sex. Because of these confused perceptions, memories of events are likely to be more jumbled than memories for more structured, orderly events.

In addition, unlike children who have a stressful medical exam, children who are abused are usually not given any reassurance by a trusted adult. Consequently, some children are likely to be much more fearful during abuse events, and their extreme fear may interfere with memory consolidation (van der Kolk, 1996b). Furthermore, abuse that is so extreme that it is traumatic may lead to repression or dissociation of memories of the events (van der Kolk, van der Hart, et al., 1996). Although research has not yet given a definitive answer to the question of the accuracy of children's trauma memories, it seems reasonable to assume that when mild or moderate abuse does occur, memories of it will be fairly accurate in children who are old enough to have the cognitive abilities to process what happens to them. There is some evidence that children as young as three may give less accurate reports than older children (Ornstein, 1995).

But caution is still warranted in judging the accuracy of children's reports of abuse because, just like adults, children are capable of giving inaccurate or false reports. Children may misunderstand what is being asked of them, particularly if their cognitive abilities are not yet well developed. They can also intentionally lie, report misperceptions of events, report delusional beliefs, or report fantasies as though they actually occurred. Reports of bizarre events, however, should not be interpreted as evidence that abuse did not occur. Dalenberg (1996) has found that such reports are actually more common in cases of bona fide abuse than they are in cases in which abuse reports turn out to be unfounded. Research has also shown that leading or repeated questioning of children about events they have experienced can influence their memories for the events (Fivush & Schwarzmueller, 1995; Saywitz & Moan-Hardie, 1994). In a nutshell, while children appear to be generally able to accurately remember what happens to them, there is no guarantee that every reported abuse incident occurred, and we do not yet have any way to know what proportion of abuse reports by children might be false.

Unfortunately, most clinicians will have an obligation to form an opinion regarding children's reports of abuse, even when they do not feel they have enough information to do so. This is because clinicians in most states are legally compelled to report a case to child protection authorities if they have a reasonable suspicion of abuse. Given this obligation and the possibility that reports of abuse by some children will be inaccurate, it is critical that you conduct trauma assessments cautiously.

Error and Accuracy in Adults' Retrospective Abuse Reports

As described above, the accuracy of adults' retrospective reports of childhood sexual abuse has been questioned by some. Most of the concern about the veracity of child sexual abuse reports has focused on situations in which the idea that abuse occurred originated in the context of an assessment or during therapy. Doubts about reports of abuse seem to arise from three main sources. The first is that clinicians know that clients are capable of producing patently false reports of their experiences. The second is inconsistencies between a client's reports and some other source of information. The third is the suspicion that clients may be influenced to report past abuse by overzealous therapists.

Sources of Error in Retrospective Reports

As every experienced clinician knows, clients' reports of their experiences are not always wholly accurate and are sometimes patently false. A client might make an invalid report of childhood sexual abuse intentionally in order to obtain compensation, leniency when accused of a crime, attention, retribution, or some other gain. For example, it is possible that a man convicted of sexually assaulting a child might falsely claim to have been sexually abused as a child in order to obtain leniency in his sentencing. A very disturbed client may have delusions involving childhood abuse experiences. For example, a client might report that her parents were aliens from another planet who conducted experiments on her when she was a child. It is also possible that a client who has had childhood traumatic experiences could report some incidents of abuse that never occurred because of confusion over what was happening to her at the time of trauma. For example, a client might report that she was forced to drink blood in a cult ritual because she was made to believe at the time that she was drinking blood. Like reports of all other aspects of human experience, abuse reports can be the result of lying, delusions, or misperceptions of experience.

Sometimes, clients' reports of past abuse may not be supported by other sources of information. The reports may be inconsistent with reports of events by the client's family members. There may be no medical records or police records to document childhood violence experiences. Sometimes, a client's reports about past abuse may be inconsistent with his own prior statements. This can take the form of a gradual increase in amount of abuse reported because the client remembers more abuse as treatment progresses. Clients also can come to believe that they were mistaken in their reports and deny that abuse ever occurred. While, at first glance, these inconsistencies seem to be cause for concern about the accuracy of abuse reports, the presence of such inconsistencies is not at all unusual in bona fide cases of abuse. Family members of an abuse victim may be highly motivated to deny that abuse occurred or may be simply ignorant of the abuse and reluctant to believe it could have happened. Medical and police records may not document abuse because the abuse left no physical evidence on the child, because medical treatment was not obtained at the time of abuse, or because the abuse never came to the attention of authorities. Abused clients' own reports may be inconsistent because of gradual increases in access to memories of abuse, because of mixed feelings about facing the reality of what happened to them, or because of confused memories of abuse. It is certainly very painful to believe that one was abused, and some clients may retract reports of abuse because of a wish to deny that the abuse ever happened. Confusion over exactly what happened is also common in those who are sexually abused as children. In Williams's (1995) study of women with documented childhood sexual assault experiences, some aspects of their adult reports were inconsistent with accounts from the original documents. It is worth noting, however, that there were no more inconsistencies in reports of "recovered" memories of assaults than there were in reports of continuously recalled events. For all of these reasons, inconsistencies between abuse reports and other sources of information do not constitute convincing evidence that no abuse occurred.

Another source of concern about the accuracy of abuse reports that arise during assessment or treatment is the suspicion that some therapists may be inadvertently influencing their clients to overreport past sexual abuse. I use the term overreport instead of the terms "false memory" or "false report" because it seems likely that some clients who make inaccurate reports of extensive abuse did experience some abuse. It is easy to understand that a client with a history of early childhood trauma might be influenced to embellish or expand upon memories of abuse, but it is not possible to then conclude that no abuse occurred just because *all* of a client's reports do not prove accurate. Similarly, one cannot rule out the possibility that some abuse occurred when a client who initially reported abuse subsequently denies that the abuse took place. Because of the emotional upset and difficulties in family relationships that remembering abuse often causes, many clients are highly motivated to believe that they were not abused, even when they were.

Setting aside debate on whether abuse occurred in particular cases, it does seem evident that in the absence of spontaneous reports of sexual abuse, some therapists tell their clients, directly or indirectly, that past sexual abuse was possible or even likely. This state of affairs was probably influenced by a growing recognition of the long-term effects of sexual abuse combined with indignation over society's poor treatment of women and children. Having read books and attended workshops focusing on the effects of sexual abuse, some therapists may come to believe that a client who reports particular symptoms has been sexually abused, even when the client does not report any abuse.

This sort of error can occur because the subtleties of the connections between experiences and symptoms are not always emphasized in clinical presentations and writings. As described in Chapter 3, particular symptoms have been associated with traumatic experiences, including sexual abuse. But these same symptoms can also result from causes other than trauma. My own research on psychiatric inpatients and that of others indicates that no single symptom and no particular pattern of symptoms can be identified as definitive markers of trauma or abuse. For this reason, a clinician should never *assume* that abuse occurred because of the symptoms a client has. No set of symptoms make it possible to say for certain that abuse occurred. Furthermore, while it is true that a set of symptoms might lead a clinician to have a high index of suspicion that abuse occurred, one ought never to voice such a suspicion to a client. This is because voicing a suspicion of abuse might lead the client and therapist to a mistaken conviction that abuse did occur, and proceeding with treatment based on the assumption that abuse occurred when it did not would be detrimental to a client. A mistaken belief that abuse occurred is likely to cause great distress to a client, disrupt important relationships, and impede a more appropriate and effective treatment of psychological problems.

Telling a client that she "may" have been abused is likely to put some pressure on the client to concur, even when she has no memory of abuse experiences. Some clients are naturally very susceptible to suggestion, and some methods tend to increase the susceptibility to suggestion in most clients. Using hypnosis to "retrieve" memories of abuse as part of an assessment will leave open the possibility that the material obtained is a fantasy and not a memory (Lynn, Myers, & Malinoski, 1997). Under the influence of hypnosis, events that are suggested to a client can come to seem real. Other methods used in work with child abuse survivors that may have a similar influence on reported memories include dream analysis, sodium amytal interviews, and guided imagery (including age regression exercises). Another reason that a client may feel compelled to concur with a suggestion of abuse is that she may be actively seeking an explanation for her symptoms. While disturbing on many levels, the explanation that one's symptoms result from child sexual abuse is appealing in that it lays the blame for problems outside of oneself and allows one to feel justified in expressing extreme anger toward someone. Finally, clients may invest their therapist with great expertise and assume that the therapist must know better than the client herself. Clients may be extremely reluctant to contradict a therapist's belief that abuse occurred.

Even therapists who do not voice their suspicions that a client has suffered abuse must be cautious in their assessment methods so that clients do not misinterpret their questions about traumatic experiences. A client might misunderstand a therapist's sympathy and willingness to accept reports of traumatic experiences and infer that the therapist believes abuse or trauma did occur. If this should occur, a client's respect for the therapist's expertise and wish to be a cooperative client may lead him to concur that abuse did occur.

The danger of a client and therapist developing a mistaken conviction that abuse occurred is further exacerbated when the therapist is intellectually and emotionally invested in being an "expert" on identifying and treating abuse victims. A therapist may have read widely, attended professional workshops and conferences, and developed a reputation for success with clients who are abuse survivors. In this situation, there is always a danger that the financial incentive to find clients in need of the therapist's expertise may have an effect outside of the therapist's awareness.

On the other hand, it is important to allow clients ample opportunity to talk about experiences of abuse or trauma. Because of psychoanalytic formulations that females experience childhood fantasies of sexual activity, some therapists have disbelieved their clients' reports of childhood sexual abuse. Although it would be a mistake to ever assume that abuse did occur because of particular symptoms, it would also be a mistake to assume that it did not occur because a client does not spontaneously report such events or a particular set of symptoms. Clinicians can collect the most accurate information about past abuse or trauma by remaining objective and neutral and by not coming to conclusions prematurely when they have incomplete information.

Accuracy of Adults' Memories of Childhood Abuse

Clinicians and researchers question the accuracy of adults' memories of childhood abuse because they are concerned both that some adult clients may not remember or may underreport such experiences and that some may overreport or misreport childhood abuse experiences. Unfortunately, researchers interested in the accuracy of adults' memories of abuse experiences face the same kinds of challenges as those studying children's abuse memories. Since the difficulty of obtaining unequivocal sources of information on the exact details of abuse increases as the number of years since the abuse occurred go by, it is very hard to judge the accuracy of abuse memories after many years. Consequently, only a relatively small amount of research is available that sheds light on memory for traumatic childhood experiences.

Amnesia and Underreporting. The possibility that adults might not recall some or all of their early childhood experiences is suggested in part by the vulnerability of memory to forgetting. Some argue that adults might simply forget some or all of their early experiences of abuse. Studies of autobiographical memory in general shed some light on this question. In a review of research on autobiographical memory, Bradburn, Rips, and Shevell (1987) concluded that memory for emotional or important events is better than memory for everyday events. Similarly, Robins (1988) concluded from his review of retrospective longitudinal studies that recall of important events may be excellent.

In one example of a study of long-term autobiographical memory for important events, Damon, Damon, Reed, and Valadian (1969) compared women's recall of their age at the onset of menstruation to childhood medical records. After an average of almost 20 years later, just over three-quarters of the women reported an age that was within 1 year of the actual age, and about 90% reported an age that was within 18 months of the actual age. Studies like this one support the accuracy of memories of personally important childhood events.

As with children's memories for abuse, the traumatic nature of the events may influence the accuracy of adult retrospective recall. There seems to be evidence that the traumatic nature of an event may sometimes result in improved memory for the event. Christianson and Loftus (1987) have studied eyewitness memory for traumatic events and concluded that the traumatic nature of the events improved rather than reduced accuracy of recall. Similarly, from their review of the literature on the influence of affect on retrospective reports, Banaji and Hardin (1994) concluded that people are likely to have better memory for affectively intense events than for other events. The essential details of events were retained over a 6-month period, though peripheral details were not as well remembered. In a later review of the literature, Christianson (1992) concluded that real-life studies show that traumatic events are well preserved in memory. For example, memories for the central details of traumatic events such as witnessing a murder and living in a concentration camp were accurately recalled, the latter after periods as long as 40 years.

On the other hand, it is possible that people fail to remember some abuse events because they were psychologically distressing. So clients may remember fewer abuse incidents than they actually experienced. As mentioned above, clients may not remember details or the occurrence of some events because the information was not encoded normally due to extreme anxiety and arousal at the time of the event (van der Kolk, 1996b). A lack of memory may also be a result of forgetting because details of unpleasant events were not rehearsed for so many years, or it may result from repression or dissociation of memories for events that were overwhelming (van der Kolk, 1996b). There is evidence that adult abuse victims do fail to recall some childhood abuse events. Studies of adults who report childhood sexual abuse or who were documented to have been sexually abused as children show that people often fail to recall some or all of the abuse. In studies of general population subjects, persons in outpatient treatment, and persons in psychiatric hospitals, rates of partial or complete amnesia for abuse events have ranged from 31% to 64% (Briere & Conte, 1993; Carlson, Armstrong, Loewenstein, & Roth, in press; Elliott & Briere, 1995; Herman & Schatzow, 1987; Loftus, Polonsky, & Fullilove, 1994; Williams, 1995). As mentioned above, the traumatic nature of abuse events may interfere with memory for the events. My own research has shown that experiencing periods of partial or complete amnesia for childhood sexual abuse was associated with the severity of abuse experienced and severity of PTSD and dissociation symptoms in adulthood (Carlson, Armstrong, Loewenstein, & Roth, 1997).

Overreporting. It is possible that some adults might be influenced to have exaggerated memories of childhood sexual abuse experiences because of their level of emotional disturbance, because of a wish to find an explanation for their problems, or because of faulty thinking patterns. A study by Robins and colleagues (1985) bears directly on the question of whether people might have exaggerated memories of abuse because they are motivated to find explanations for their psychological problems or disorder. They studied agreement between retrospective reports of pairs of siblings for their childhood home environment. One set of siblings contained one sibling who was a psychiatric patient, and the control pairs were both nondisordered. Results showed that psychiatric patients agreed with their siblings at the same rate as nonpatient sibling pairs agreed. In other words, there was no evidence that the status as psychiatric patients or the presence of psychiatric illness affected the number of childhood environmental variables correctly recalled. In addition, Robins and colleagues (1985) found that the patients showed no bias toward either a more favorable or a less favorable assessment of childhood environment. The results of this study do not support the idea that people might overreport abuse because of their high levels of psychological disorder. Furthermore, Brewin, Andrews, and Gotlib (1993) reviewed the literature on retrospective reports with respect to the question of whether those with psychological problems are likely to exaggerate their early negative experiences. They concluded that there is little reason to think that findings of relationships between negative childhood experiences and later psychological symptoms are the result of patients' distorted memories.

A study by Mackenzie and Lippman (1989) bears on the question of whether clients might have distorted memories of abuse as a result of a wish to explain their psychological problems. They examined the influence of the knowledge of the outcome of a birth on retrospective reports of exposure to potential hazards (e.g., smoking). If knowledge of their current problems biases people to overreport prior negative events, then women with poor pregnancy outcomes would be expected to give negatively biased retrospective reports of exposure to hazards. But this did not occur: Error in memories was not associated with pregnancy outcome. These findings do not support the notion that knowledge of current problems influences people to give more negative reports of past events.

Another reason that people might exaggerate or overreport childhood abuse would be the common use of the inferential strategy called the availability heuristic (Bradburn, et al., 1987). With this strategy, the more easily an event can be brought to mind, the more frequent or recent the event will seem. Since vivid memories of abuse might be easily recalled, abused persons might overestimate the frequency of abuse experiences. Because of this possibility, we cannot expect retrospective reports of abuse to be very precise in terms of the details of early experiences. There is reason to believe, however, that the recollections of central features of early events will be reasonably accurate. In their review of the literature on retrospective reports, Brewin and colleagues (1993) conclude that recall of the central features of events is likely to be reasonably accurate so long as people are asked questions about specific events or facts, and they were old enough and well-placed enough to have knowledge of the events.

My review of research on retrospective reports leads me to conclude that, barring active attempts to persuade a client to recall past suspected, but not remembered, abuse, most adults' memories of past abuse are largely accurate. Not surprisingly, you cannot expect memories to be precisely accurate. There is plenty of empirical evidence, and you have evidence from your own experiences that memories are not factual accounts of past events. Furthermore, memory for traumatic events may be different from memory for other types of experiences. Recently, there has been a lot of interest in the cognitive processes involved in memory for traumatic experiences. Discussions of how traumatic memories are processed can be found in van der Kolk (van der Kolk, van der Hart, et al., 1996), Allen (1995b), Chemtob and colleagues (1988), Foa and Kozak (1986), Litz and Keane (1989), and McNally (1995). Also very useful is Harvey and Herman's (1994) discussion of the process of recall of childhood trauma in the context of treatment.

Even though memories of trauma may be largely accurate, you must always be mindful of the possibility that a client is intentionally making false reports or is reporting delusions about past experiences. Also, errors in reporting can result from a therapist's inadvertent influence on a client. While there is considerable debate about the prevalence of overreports of abuse resulting from the influence of therapists or other sources, even those who contend that amnesia for childhood sexual abuse is very common concede that it is possible for a therapist to mistakenly lead a client to report abuse events that did not occur (Berliner & Williams, 1994). Clearly, you want to do everything you can to avoid influencing a client's trauma reports.

Error in Trauma Reports from Using Nonsystematic Assessment Methods

In addition to the sources of error described earlier in this chapter, use of nonsystematic assessment methods could also contribute to inaccurate trauma reports. Underreporting and overreporting of trauma can both result from nonsystematic methods of assessment that lead to misunderstandings between the client and the clinician. Underreporting can occur when, because a general question about traumatic experiences is vague or unclear, a client does not report traumatic events that he did experience. For example, a clinician might use the DSM-III-R Criterion A to define a trauma and ask a client whether she had ever experienced an event outside the range of usual human experience. A client who experienced the sudden death of a spouse or chronic molestation as a child might answer "No" to the question because she did not conceptualize this as "Outside the range of usual human experience." Similarly, a client who is asked whether he ever had a traumatic experience might erroneously answer "no" because of his understanding of the word "traumatic." What constitutes a traumatic event is, after all, difficult to delineate, even for professionals.

Underreporting can also occur if a client is not specifically asked about the occurrence of traumatic experiences. You cannot assume that clients will volunteer information about these experiences if not asked. This is because clients may be unaware of the role of a past traumatic experience in their current troubles or reluctant to report events because of shame or because they wish to avoid the pain of discussing their trauma. A client may also report one or more traumatic experiences but neglect to report others. As discussed earlier, this might occur as a result of amnesia for some of the traumatic experiences or because of reluctance to report some events.

It is also possible for clients to overreport traumatic experiences because the questions they are asked are not absolutely clear. A client might easily misunderstand the word "traumatic" in that it is often used colloquially to mean any upsetting or disturbing event. People frequently refer to a negative life event such as a divorce or loss of a job as "traumatic," but these are not usually considered by clinicians to constitute truly traumatic events. Overgeneralizing the meaning of "traumatic" might lead a client to report events as traumas that were not truly traumatic. Overreporting can also occur because a client reports experiences that are within the realm of traumatic events but were not actually experienced that way. For example, there is evidence to suggest that people who were not conscious or aware during a traumatic event do not experience the event as traumatic. A study of traffic accidents found no cases of PTSD among those who had lost consciousness during a car accident (Mayou et al., 1993).

ADDRESSING CHALLENGES TO ASSESSING TRAUMATIC EXPERIENCES

The starting point for addressing the challenges to assessing traumatic experiences is to decide whether clinicians should routinely assess traumatic experiences. To decide this we must answer the question "Is knowledge of past trauma and memory for the trauma really necessary for treatment of traumatized persons?" Many authors of theories about traumatic responses, researchers who study the effects of trauma, and clinicians who treat traumatized people contend that access to and processing of traumatic memories is essential to an effective treatment of posttraumatic stress responses. There is empirical evidence to support this notion that is compelling. Controlled studies have shown that methods involving recall and processing of trauma memories are more effective in reducing symptoms of clients with PTSD than alternative methods that do not involve recall of trauma memories (Foa et al., 1991;

Gerrity & Solomon, 1996; Resick & Schnicke, 1992; Solomon, Gerrity, & Muff, 1992). Similarly, several studies have found a relationship between the extent of active oral or written processing of traumatic experiences and lower levels of psychological distress and physical symptoms (Foa, Molnar, & Cashman, 1995; Harber & Pennebaker, 1992; Pennebaker, 1988). On the other hand, gaining access to and processing *all* of the traumatic events experienced by a client may not be necessary or advisable (Briere, 1996c). For those with extensive trauma histories, it may be possible (and perhaps more practical) to effectively treat trauma responses by processing of a limited number of representative traumatic memories. Given these considerations, along with the absence of an empirically supported treatment for posttraumatic stress that does not include some accessing and processing of trauma memories, it seems reasonable to conclude that information about past traumatic experiences would be valuable to treatment planning.

Additional support for making trauma assessments a standard element of your routine clinical evaluations can be derived from areas of consensus among those debating the accuracy of adult memories of childhood sexual abuse. While there is much disagreement about the prevalence of childhood sexual abuse reports that are not accurate, even those who fear that a preponderance of the reports might be erroneous concede that research to date shows little reason to believe that illusory memories of abuse can be generated by careful, nonleading questions about past traumatic experiences (Lindsay & Read, 1993). If information about past trauma will be valuable to treatment and there is little danger that simply inquiring about past trauma in a neutral way will lead clients to overreport, then it seems wise to include a trauma assessment in your routine evaluations.

Using a Systematic Approach to Assessing Trauma

A systematic approach to assessing trauma will help minimize inaccuracies in reporting. Asking about traumatic experiences using methods that are standardized, neutral, and precise can help you eliminate reporting errors from a variety of sources.

Using standardized assessment methods means using measures that have been developed by experts in trauma and psychometrics and that have been established to be reliable and valid measures. Unfortunately, there are no measures of traumatic experiences that have unequivocally established validity. This is because, as discussed earlier, there are often no incontrovertible records or documents of trauma to which reports can be compared. Still, some trauma measures have been found to be reliable and to have some construct validity. Using one of these measures will ensure that you use a standard format when you inquire about traumatic experiences and that your questions are precise and neutral in wording.

Ideally, you should assess trauma before beginning treatment. If a client who has already been in treatment is referred to you, you should ask for any written records of a trauma assessment from the previous therapist. If such records are not available or appear to be an inadequate assessment of trauma, you should conduct a trauma assessment at the earliest possible opportunity. Assessing trauma before beginning treatment can assure you and the client that reports of traumatic experiences were not an inadvertent effect of treatment. It is important to follow any administration instructions closely when using a measure. Any departures from such instructions may diminish the validity of the results of the measure. For example, using hypnosis to "facilitate" recall during a trauma assessment may influence your client's memories and will invalidate the assessment. As mentioned earlier, although hypnosis may enhance recall, there is also strong evidence that hypnosis can cause people to have illusory recall so that memories are altered or memories are created of events that did not occur (Lynn et al., 1997).

Using standardized measures with questions that have neutral wording will minimize the chance of inadvertently influencing your clients. Questions about traumatic experiences in standardized measures are carefully designed to be nonleading. Although you may think that there is no danger of your asking leading questions of your clients, it is exceedingly difficult to monitor your words so scrupulously in a unstructured interview with a client. There may also be occasions when you do not realize that your wording of a question is leading a client. For example, you might ask a client who was physically punished as a child, "Was your father's harsh discipline ever abusive?" Your client may answer "Yes" to this question because she thinks you believe and want her to see that physical punishment constitutes abuse. It is much simpler and safer to use a standardized measure of trauma and avoid the possibility of leading questions altogether.

You may be concerned that using a standardized measure with neutral wording will be perceived as cold and unsympathetic by your clients. You certainly do not want to appear insensitive, indifferent, or skeptical of your clients' reports of trauma. This would be untherapeutic and is likely to make your clients reluctant to report traumatic events. But you also do not want to make the mistake of being so ready to believe and sympathize with your clients that you suspend your critical thinking skills. This may be a difficult dilemma for therapists who were trained to largely accept and "believe" what clients tell them. It is important to remember, however, that your clients are as much in need of your impartial and critical judgment as they are of your sympathy. For some clients, the greatest service you can give them is to help them be clear about reality and avoid misinterpreting or misremembering events. It could never be in the best interests of a client to believe or report that she had experienced a trauma if she actually had not done so. You can foster accurate reporting without appearing indifferent by conveying to the client that you take her trauma reports seriously. It may also help to educate the client about the vagaries of trauma memories. This issue is discussed in more detail below.

Using standardized trauma measures also allows you to gather very precise information about traumatic experiences. Gathering such specific information about traumatic experiences will help you avoid confusion about what a client has experienced. For example, knowing a client was mugged is not as useful as knowing that he was threatened with a knife and was afraid for his life. Obtaining specific information about traumatic events may also help you determine whether reports are delusional or the result of misperceptions. Although there is no assessment method that can prevent a client from reporting delusions or misperceptions or from knowingly giving false reports, detailed questions may reveal bizarreness that is indicative of delusions or reports of misperceptions.

Suggestions for Improving the Accuracy of Children's Trauma Reports

Obtaining accurate reports of trauma from children can be especially challenging because of the many factors described above that can influence their reports. Research shows that children are particularly susceptible to the influence of leading and repeated questioning (Fivush & Schwarzmueller, 1995; Saywitz & Moan-Hardie, 1994). Also, because of their lack of maturity, children may lie about their experiences without realizing the consequences.

Saywitz and Moan-Hardie (1994) studied children's resistance to leading questions and found that children acquiesce more to leading questions when they do not know that it is acceptable for them to say that they do not know or do not remember the answer to a question and when they expect negative consequences if they resist leading questions. Consequently, it is advisable to explain to young clients that they may not know the answer to some questions you will ask them or they may not remember some information from the past. Giving a child explicit permission to say "I don't know" and "I don't remember" will help avoid fabrication of answers by children who feel compelled to give some answer. Similarly, it is important for a child to understand that there are no "right" or "wrong" answers to the questions you will ask him about symptoms that he currently has. Sometimes, even when you do not intend to influence a child, he may feel compelled to answer a question in a particular way to please you. You can alleviate this problem by assuring the child that you are not expecting any particular answer to your questions and that you only want him to tell you the truth about what happended to him and how he feels now. Further suggestions for fostering accurate reports from children are offerred by Reed (1996). He suggests explaining to a child that you were not there, so you do not know what happened. Also, Reed suggests telling a child that you may ask a question more than once so that you can make sure that you got his answer right, not because his first answer was wrong.

Children also sometimes give inaccurate trauma reports when they have already made a false report of a trauma and are afraid to recant. For example, a child may have falsely accused someone of abuse in anger and is afraid of punishment for lying if he changes his story during the assessment. Similarly, a child may have reported abuse as a result of leading or repeated questions. This can happen in situations when parents are in custody battles and are motivated to find evidence of a spouse's wrongdoing. It can also happen as the result of inappropriate questioning by well-meaning, but poorly trained, teachers or counselors. You can help children to be honest with you by explaining that you can only help them and their family if they are completely honest with you about what has happened. You can explain to children that people sometimes make mistakes when they are trying to remember things and that they should be sure to tell you if they think that they made a mistake in an earlier report. Additional suggestions for maximizing the completeness and accuracy of children's reports of past events can be found in Saywitz, Geiselman, and Bornstein (1992), Saywitz and Snyder (in press), Saywitz and Goodman (1996), Saywitz, Snyder, and Lamphear (1996), and Reed (1996).

Educating Clients about the Validity of Trauma Memories

It is not uncommon for assessments of trauma to get sidetracked by a client's concerns about whether or not she experienced particular traumatic events or whether or not you believe her reports of traumatic events. This issue can be especially pressing if a client is seeking treating because of a desire to determine whether or not some trauma such as abuse or particular abuse incidents actually happened. Some clients may even request use of particular methods such as hypnosis or age regression to "retrieve" trauma memories. You can help relieve tension over these issues and lay a solid groundwork for later treatment by routinely educating your clients about the vagaries of human memory. Allen

(1995b) points out that many clients mistakenly believe that memory works like a tape recorder and that you can help them "play back" memories of traumatic events.

Meichenbaum (1994) offers several suggestions for educating clients about human memory. You should explain to clients that memories are not fixed, exact representations of past events, and, in fact, memories can be influenced by later events and feelings so that they become embellished or altered. When appropriate, you can also explain that methods to "retrieve" memories such as hypnosis or age regression can actively alter memories and create "memories" of events that were only imagined. Similarly, a person can "remember" having an experience that he did not have as a result of having been told about the experience. Clients need to understand that all of these illusory memories can seem very real. On the other hand, you should also explain to clients that there is no evidence that people can develop detailed memories of repeated traumatic events that did not occur. Although clients may *report* repeated abuse that did not occur, perhaps as a result of influence from a therapist or therapeutic methods, it is not clear that such clients have illusory memories of events. Those who make false reports may have come to believe that they were abused without having specific memories of the events. Finally, you can explain that some traumatic experiences may interfere with memory processing with the result that no coherent narrative memory of the event is ever formed.

After educating a client about the way memory works, you can make it clear that there may be no way to ever determine exactly what happened to her and that recovery of trauma memories ought not be the goal of therapy. Although this information may be discouraging to clients at first, you can reassure them that the success of treatment does not depend on determining the accuracy of trauma memories (Meichenbaum, 1994). Emotional issues related to traumatic events and memories can be worked through in treatment regardless of whether trauma memories precisely reflect past events. Furthermore, over the course of treatment, many clients do come to feel more certainty about past events in their lives. Many trauma therapists believe that helping a client to develop a coherent personal narrative that incorporates her trauma is a necessary part of recovery.

CHALLENGES TO ASSESSING RESPONSES TO TRAUMA

Most of the same challenges involved in assessing traumatic experiences apply to the task of assessing responses to trauma as well. The major sources of error in reports of trauma responses involve misunderstanding or intentional misrepresentation of symptoms. Since the reasons for error differ somewhat in adults and children, I will describe them separately for each group.

Challenges to Assessing Responses to Trauma in Adults

As with trauma measures, adults can sometimes misunderstand the questions being asked of them in measures of trauma responses. This can occur because the question is not worded clearly or precisely enough or because the client is not familiar with the type of symptom being described. If you ask a client if she has intrusive thoughts, she may not know what is meant by the term. This could lead to underreporting or overreporting of the symptoms. Overreporting can also occur when a client does not appreciate the distinction between a behavior or experience that is within the normal range and one that is truly disordered. For example, when asked about intrusive thoughts, a client might give a positive response. But upon further questioning, it might become evident that the client was reporting the normal experience of having thoughts come into her head about problems in her life rather than the posttraumatic symptom of repeated, unwanted thoughts about a traumatic experience.

As with reporting of trauma history, clients may intentionally misreport their responses to trauma. Reasons for this might include fear of the therapist's reaction, a desire for attention, or the pursuit of financial remuneration through legal action. A client might underreport symptoms that seem "crazy" such as intrusive images and depersonalization if he is worried that a therapist might think he is psychotic and hospitalize him. On the other hand, because of a wish to win the sympathy and attention of a therapist and show how distressed he is, a client may overreport his symptoms. Sometimes clients also report having symptoms in a misguided attempt to be cooperative and compliant. Since PTSD can be an issue in worker's compensation claims, criminal actions, and civil suits, some clients may be motivated to overreport their symptoms in order to obtain worker's compensation benefits or to win a legal battle.

Challenges to Assessing Responses to Trauma in Children

Children's reports of responses to trauma are even more subject to error than those of adults. Misunderstanding of the questions being asked can occur on several levels in children. On the most basic level, young children may simply not understand questions asked of them because of their undeveloped cognitive and language skills. This problem is exacerbated by questions that are unclear, overly complex, or involve vocabulary that is beyond the years of the child being assessed. Limited cognitive and language skills may also make it difficult or impossible for children to accurately report about their feelings, thoughts, and behaviors (Finch & Daugherty, 1993). Similarly, for some children, it may be beyond their cognitive skills to accurately report changes in feelings or behaviors since a particular event, as is required by several PTSD criteria. Furthermore, certain concepts that are pertinent to assessing trauma responses may not be well understood by young children. Assessing frequency or duration of symptoms over time may be problematic in children who do not yet fully understand concepts of time. For example, a 4-year-old may not be able to understand answer choices for frequency of a symptom such as "once every 2 weeks" or "twice a week."

Another reason for misunderstanding of questions can be the limited cognitive-emotional development of a child. For example, if asked about symptoms that require psychological insight into cause and effect, a child may not be able to make this judgment. This is particularly problematic in the assessing of PTSD symptoms because many of them involve a causal connection between the event and the symptom. A child may not realize, for instance, that he is avoiding reminders of an event and consequently would answer "no" if asked about that symptom.

Like adults, children can intentionally misreport their trauma responses. Such misrepresentation might be motivated by anger at someone or a desire to protect himself or others. A child may be afraid that he will get in trouble for reporting negative symptoms. For example, he may have the mistaken belief that he is being bad because he is avoiding thoughts or feelings associated with a traumatic event. Or he may be afraid that someone else will get in trouble if he endorses symptoms. For example, if a child is an incest victim, she might be motivated to minimize her symptoms in order to protect her father or out of fear of reprisal by the father. A child might also intentionally overreport symptoms in an effort to gain attention or to incriminate an accused person. In the case of the latter, the motivation for incrimination is probably more likely to originate in a parent than in the child, so that the child may exaggerate symptoms in response to prompting from a parent.

Because of the difficulties of obtaining accurate information from children about their trauma responses, clinicians often turn to parents, guardians, or others familiar with the child to obtain information about a child's symptoms. Section D in the Measure Profiles includes several such measures that are administered to parents or others. Information obtained from an observer can complement the information about symptoms obtained from the child. For example, while children are often poor reporters of "externalizing behaviors" such as aggression or misbehavior, parents are fairly good reporters of these behaviors (Putnam, 1996b). Conversely, children are fairly good reporters of "internalizing behaviors" such as anxiety and depression, while parents are poor reporters of these symptoms (Finch & Daugherty, 1993; Putnam, 1996b).

There are specific sources of error related to observer ratings, however, and you should be aware of these if you choose to use measures administered to parents or others. Finch and Daugherty (1993) describe three types of error that can affect observer ratings. The first, referred to as the halo effect, is the tendency for raters to be so influenced by a particular negative or positive characteristic that it colors the ratings of all of the child's behaviors. This type of overgeneralizng might result in underreporting or overreporting of symptoms by an observer. Another source of error is that observers are often reluctant to use the extreme points of rating scales. This tendency could also result in overreporting or underreporting of symptoms. The rater's frame of reference can also lead to error in reporting. For example, parents who live in a highly stressful environment where many children are exposed to violence may compare their child's behavior to that of more disturbed children and consequently underreport symptoms.

Evidence that the information obtained about symptoms from children and parents is of questionable accuracy includes several studies of the performance of structured interviews in assessing psychiatric disorders in children. Although these studies did not examine the performance of structured interviews for trauma responses in particular, it seems likely that the problems with other structured interviews for children will also occur in interviews relating to trauma responses. Two studies of structured interviews for children have shown high rates of overdiagnosis of psychiatric disorders (Breslau, 1987; Carlson, Kashani, & Thomas, 1987). Another study examined test–retest reliability of children's reports and found that children were not very reliable in reporting the onset and duration of their symptoms (Schwab-Stone, Fallon, Brigs, & Crowther, 1994). The poor performance of several structured interviews for children raises the very real possibility that children do not understand many of the questions asked in these interviews.

ADDRESSING CHALLENGES TO ASSESSING RESPONSES TO TRAUMA

As with assessing trauma, asking questions about trauma responses that are standardized, neutral, and precise will help minimize reporting errors from a variety of sources. Validated measures offer items with standardized and precise wording that reduce problems with misunderstanding of questions. It is still necessary, however, to be alert to signs of misunderstanding or lack of comprehension in both children or adults. Puzzled looks, long pauses, or examples of experiences that do not match the specified symptom are all indications that the client may not understand what you are asking. In children, it is important to take note of the child's level of cognitive and emotional development and to consider whether the questions you are asking are beyond a child's abilities to answer accurately.

Intentional misreporting motivated by a desire for attention or fears of negative consequences of reporting can be minimized by clarifying the purpose of the assessment, the importance of complete honesty in responding, and the fact that there are no right or wrong answers to questions. Essentially, you want to convey to your client that you really want to know what his experience has been, rather than what he thinks you may want to hear. With children, as described above, it is particularly important to clarify that it is acceptable for them to say that they do not know an answer to a question or for them to give any answer to a question.

Intentional misreporting motivated by secondary gain of the client (or perhaps the parent of a child client) is more difficult to prevent. It is important to inquire about any possible secondary gains that might result from a diagnosis of PTSD or any other motivations for exaggerating the effects of a traumatic experience. It is especially important for anyone assessing clients in a forensic context to be familiar with the literature on this topic (see Keane, 1995; Simon, 1995; Wilson, Keane, & Smagola, 1996).

SUMMARY

This chapter addressed the challenges involved in assessing traumatic experiences and trauma repsonses. Research was reviewed relating to error and accuracy in children's reports of trauma and adults' retrospective reports. Particular attention was given to the accuracy of reports of childhood abuse and to the interviewer's potential influences on such reports. Sources of error in abuse reports were discussed, and suggestions were made for addressing the challenge of accurately assessing past trauma. Accuracy of reports of trauma responses was also addressed, and suggestions were made for improving the accuracy of these reports.

Chapter 7

Developing an Assessment Strategy

As you develop your strategy for assessing the traumatic experiences and responses of your clients, there are a number of important issues that you should consider. Various potential sources of information are available about clients, and assessments conducted for different purposes may require use of different assessment methods. This chapter focuses on developing a strategy for conducting clinical assessments. First, you need to decide which domains of experience and symptoms to assess. Second, to choose which specific measures to administer to a client, you need to take into account factors such as your client's level of comprehension and the content, format, reliability, and validity of the measures you are considering. A general discussion of these measures characteristics is included in this chapter. Chapter 8 explains how to find information relevant to these characteristics in the Measure Profiles.

SOURCES OF INFORMATION

Your client is usually the primary source of information about past experiences and current symptoms. Although clients are seldom able to provide completely objective information about themselves and their experiences, they always provide important information about their own perceptions, recollections, and subjective experience of events. Obtaining such subjective information is essential to any assessment of trauma responses. There are several ways to obtain information from clients, and there are also other potential sources of information about clients.

Self-Reports and Interviews

Self-report measures and structured interviews have several advantages for the assessment of traumatic experiences and responses. First, they are readily available to clinicians, and they require no special equipment and relatively little training to administer. Compared to other sources of information from clients, more is known about the reliability and validity of self-report measures and interviews for assessing trauma responses, and more information is available about how to interpret results. Because of these advantages, this book focuses on these measures almost exclusively.

Psychological Tests

A variety of general psychological tests that measure cognitive functions and personality characteristics have proved useful in the assessment of responses to trauma. But since these tests were not designed to assess trauma responses, a full battery of psychological tests may not yield sufficient information to justify the time, effort, and cost of their administration. Often, though, psychological tests are routinely given as a means of assessing intellectual functioning and personality. When such tests results are available, they may provide some useful confirmation or elaboration of results of more specific trauma response measures. Sources are available that discuss use of particular types of psychological tests in evaluating trauma responses, including neuropsychological tests (Knight, 1996; Wolfe & Charney, 1991); intelligence tests (Allen, 1994); personality tests (Allen & Coyne, 1995; Allen, 1994; Armstrong, 1995; Briere, 1997); and the Rorschach inkblot test (Allen, 1994; Armstrong & Loewenstein, 1990; Briere, 1997; Carlson & Armstrong, 1994; Levin & Reis, 1996).

Physiological Measures

Physiological measures of trauma responses include relatively simple measures of physiological functions such as heart rate, blood pressure, and electrical responses of the brain, as well as more technically complex methods to measure cerebral blood flow, brain metabolism, stress hormones, and neurotransmitter function. Most of the research using physiological measures involves comparison of physiological functioning of those with PTSD to control subjects, and almost all of this research has been done on subjects who are veterans. Furthermore, this type of research is quite labor intensive, so studies involve fairly few subjects. To date, no markers of trauma responses have been found that definitively distinguish veterans with PTSD from others. Very little is known about use of physiological measures to assess traumatized civilians. Given the limited knowledge currently available about the use of physiological measures, and the fact that few clinicians have resources, equipment, or expertise to use physiological measures, they are not generally used for routine assessment of trauma responses. Those interested in further information about the use of physiological measures of trauma responses should see Litz and Weathers (1994), Orr and Kaloupek (1996), Allen (1994), and Kaloupek and Bremner (1996).

Alternative Methods for Obtaining Information from Children

Since children, especially very young children, may not have the cognitive or verbal skills necessary to describe and explain their experiences and feelings, you may need to use nonverbal methods of gathering information from children (Lipovsky, 1992). Some of the most common alternative methods used with children include interviews using anatomical dolls, observation of play, and analysis of drawings. These are frequently used to gather information from children who might have been sexually assaulted. Unfortunately, relatively little work has been done in this area, so that use of these methods has not been standardized. Consequently, the validity of indicators of trauma in play, drawings, or anatomical doll interviews is uncertain. Lipovsky (1992) cautions that interactions with anatomical dolls or behaviors observed during play cannot be taken at face value. Those evaluating children who are interested in these methods should realize that their use is still quite controversial. Some argue that having a child use anatomical dolls to "act out" what happened may introduce fantasy material into the evaluations. As an alternative, it may be better to use an anatomical doll, a body replica, or line drawings only as an aid to children in indentifying body parts. Before using any of these methods, it is advisable to read further about the methods and about alternative ways to assess trauma and trauma-related disorders in children (American Professional Society on the Abuse of Children, 1995c; Everson & Boat, 1994; Katz, Schonfeld, Carter, Leventhal, & Cicchetti, 1995; Koocher et al., 1995; McNally, 1991).

Official Records and Collateral Sources

Gathering information from official records and collateral sources may be useful and advisable under some circumstances. Official records might include records of prior treatment, testing results, medical records, police records, military records, school records, and news reports. An example of the use of official records might be the use of military records to obtain specific information about the combat experience of a veteran seeking treatment. This use of records to corroborate reports is recommended when assessing veterans or others seeking disability payments as some of these persons may intentionally misreport or exaggerate their trauma histories (Carroll & Foy, 1992; Sipprelle, 1992). Another example of using official records might be examining school records when evaluating a child to gather information about declines in functioning and disruptive behavior.

Information from collateral sources may provide useful information about a client's current functioning. Such sources may have information that is not available to the client because of cognitive avoidance or denial (Keane, Newman, & Orsillo, 1996; Newman, Kaloupek, & Keane, 1996). Collateral sources of information might include parents, family, friends, teachers, employers, and former therapists. It is easy to see how interviews with parents or teachers of a child might provide valuable information about the child's behavior. Some clinicians also suggest collateral sources be used to obtain information about adults. For example, Dutton (1992) mentions such interviews as potentially important sources of information about women who have experienced domestic violence. Most therapists will also want to obtain any records relating to prior treatment, although this may raise difficult ethical questions under some circumstances (see Dalenberg & Carlson, in press).

Use of official records and collateral sources can be a double-edged sword, however. Although they may be indispensable when evaluation serves a forensic purpose, they may be counterproductive and damaging to the therapeutic relationship when the evaluation is primarily made for clinical purposes. Obtaining information from other sources, even with your client's permission, may threaten the client's sense of control, reduce the client's trust in you, and make the client anxious about her privacy. With the possible exception of past treatment records, this cost may not be worth the benefit obtained. Furthermore, sometimes, it may not be in the client's best interest to question others. Sometimes the questioning has a negative effect on the client. For example, questioning a teacher about a child's behavior might violate the child's privacy and stigmatize the child as disordered.

Lastly, collateral sources may yield information that is difficult or impossible to interpret. While inconsistencies between client reports and reports from collateral sources may indicate that the client's reports are inaccurate, the inaccuracy may lie in the collateral sources. For example, Lipovsky (1992) notes that parents tend to underestimate emotional impact of sexual abuse on their children. Clearly some parents might be motivated to underreport or minimize abuse of their children because of guilt over failing to protect their children or because they want to protect the abuser from prosecution. Official records might also be inaccurate, incomplete, or misleading. For example, failure of medical records to show evidence of childhood sexual abuse might give the impression that abuse did not occur. Many times, however, sexual abuse leaves no physical evidence or abused children are not taken to doctors, so abuse goes undocumented. Furthermore, doctors with a low index of suspicion for sexual abuse may fail to look for or detect visible indicators of sexual activity in a child. For these reasons, if information from collateral sources in collected, its accuracy should not be taken for granted.

PURPOSE OF THE ASSESSMENT

Your strategy for assessment of trauma history and responses is likely to vary depending on the purpose of the evaluation. Because evaluations for research, forensic, and clinical purposes typically call for use of different measures and interview methods, it is important as you plan your assessment to consider what uses you will have for the information you gather. Although I briefly describe some of the issues that guide selection of measures for research and forensic use, this book focuses primarily on development of assessment strategies for clinical purposes.

Research Use

When measuring aspects of traumatic experiences and responses for empirical studies, it is desirable to use measures that have been standardized and validated. This means that norms have been developed for the measure so that scores of an individual can be compared to those of various specified populations and that the measure has been found to be reliable and valid. Reliability and validity of measures are discussed in more detail below. For most studies, it is also preferable to use measures that quantify the variables being studied. For example, a researcher can do more fruitful analyses of data representing the amount of intrusive thinking experienced than she can with data representing the presence or absence of intrusive thinking. A researcher is more likely to choose a more detailed quantitative measure, such as a scale that measures both frequency and intensity of symptoms, than a detailed qualitative measure, such as free responses from a structured interview. Researchers also often favor self-report measures over interviews because self-report measures take far less professional time and expertise to administer.

In the early 1990s, measurement of traumatic experiences has become an increasingly thorny issue for researchers as the validity of self-reports and retrospective reports of traumatic experiences have been challenged. Unfortunately, research on the accuracy of retrospective reports is extremely difficult to conduct. The available research tends to support the accuracy of the central details of self-reports and retrospective reports of traumatic events (Christianson & Loftus, 1987; Christianson, 1992). Recent studies of retrospective reports of childhood abuse seem to indicate that we should be more concerned about underreporting as a result of amnesia for traumatic events than we should be about misreporting or overreporting (Briere & Conte, 1993; Williams, 1995). For these reasons, researchers collecting retrospective reports of traumatic experiences will want to choose measures that are designed to maximize the accuracy of reports. Those interested in a detailed discussion of measurement of trauma and trauma responses for research should see Solomon and colleagues (1996), Norris and Riad (1996), and Newman et al. (1996).

Forensic Use

There are numerous examples of the need for assessment of traumatic experiences or responses in a forensic or legal context. The most common of these include assessment of responses to trauma when someone sues for damages or seeks disability compensation relating to a traumatic event, when a defendant wants to establish the presence of a trauma-related disorder as a mitigating factor in commission of a crime, and when the experiences of a child are assessed to determine if abuse occurred. In such forensic contexts, clinicians need to be especially scrupulous about their assessment strategies because secondary gain motivations make malingering more likely. Clinicians conducting forensic assessments should choose measures with the most scientific credibility and those that allow collection of the most detail. When forensic purposes are primary, clinicians should seek corroboration of symptom and experience reports from any official records and collateral sources available.

Perhaps the most challenging type of assessment that includes a forensic purpose is the evaluation of children who might have been abused. Lipovsky (1992) has noted that evaluation of children to assess abuse often means balancing the sometimes conflicting need to obtain information in order to comply with reporting laws and the need to provide a therapeutic environment for the child. Though an in-depth discussion of assessment for forensic purposes is beyond the scope of this book, clinicians would be well-advised to seek more information on forensic assessments before undertaking such evaluations. Good places to start include Wilson et al. (1996), Pitman and colleagues (Pitman, Sparr, Saunders, & McFarlane, 1996), Keane (1995), Quinn (1995), Simon (1995), Resnick (1995), and the practice guidelines of the American Professional Society on the Abuse of Children (1995a, 1995b, 1995c).

Clinical Use

Therapists conducting evaluations for clinical purposes will have a different set of needs than those conducting research or forensic assessments. The remainder of this chapter discusses in some detail those factors that clinicians should consider as they choose measures and conduct assessments. Here, I briefly contrast the assessment needs of clinicians with those of researchers and forensic assessors. Compared to the researcher and forensic assessor, clinicians are usually somewhat less concerned with obtaining detailed quantitative information about experiences and symptoms. For example, most clinicians will not feel the need to give a measure to every client they see that requires precise quantification of the frequency and intensity of PTSD symptoms. They might be more likely to use a very brief checklist to quickly single out those clients with trauma-related symptoms and to conduct detailed evaluations of PTSD for those clients only.

Clinicians are also usually more interested than researchers and forensic assessors in obtaining qualitative information about traumatic experiences and responses. Subjective, qualitative details about traumatic events such as what the client was thinking at the time of a traumatic event are needed to plan and provide appropriate treatment for a client. Clinicians should use detailed interviews to gather information about experiences and symptoms from clients who have had traumatic experiences.

Although clinicians are generally less concerned about gathering quantitative information and more interested in gathering qualitative information, you should always use scientifically validated measures and gather detailed, quantitative information. This is because it is important to be as sure as possible of the accuracy of the information you obtain about a client. Futhermore, forensic or legal aspects of the case can appear unexpectedly. It is advisable to be forearmed with data from well-researched and valid measures in the event of a forensic need.

In terms of evaluating trauma histories of clients for purely clinical purposes, therapists will generally find clients' memories about traumatic events more useful in treatment planning than a factual account of past events. This is because, as discussed in Chapter 2, the meaning of a traumatic event often shapes the psychological response more than the actual circumstances. An in-depth discussion of assessing for past trauma is included in Chapter 6.

DECIDING WHICH DOMAINS TO ASSESS

As discussed in Chapters 3 and 5, traumatic experiences can have a very wide range of effects in a person's life. In an ideal world, it would be helpful to assess all of the possible traumatic experiences, all of the potential symptoms, and all of the affected domains of your client's life. But realistically, you won't have the time or resources to do this for every client. So you must make sure you assess the most likely traumatic experiences and the primary posttraumatic symptoms. You can develop a basic set of measures of trauma and trauma responses, and, as time and resources allow, you can add measures of specific experiences and additional symptoms that are appropriate for each client.

Assessing Traumatic Experiences

Arguably, you should use some measure to assess traumatic experiences with every client you see. A brief, self-report measure will cost little time or money and may yield very important information. For those clients who are traumatized by past experiences, the time spent on a self-report measure is invaluable to planning their treatment (see Chapter 1, pp. 17–18). Clients who have not had traumatic experiences will not have to spend much time on the measure at all because they will simply answer "no" to most of the questions.

When you know a client has had a particular traumatic experience, such as a recent rape, it may be tempting to skip this step of the assessment. But this would be a mistake because you might miss valuable information about past traumatic experiences that have not been resolved. Very often, responses to recent traumatic events are exacerbated by unresolved earlier traumatic experiences. Even years after a posttraumatic response has been resolved, it can return in response to stressful or traumatic events that are reminders of the earlier experience (Sonnenberg, 1988). A detailed discussion of trauma assessment issues is included in Chapter 6.

Assessing Symptom Domains

Of the posttraumatic responses discussed in Chapter 3, PTSD and dissociation symptoms seem to be the cardinal responses to trauma. While other symptoms, such as depression, may frequently occur, PTSD and dissociative symptoms are most useful for distinguishing among posttraumatic reactions and other disorders. In other words, a symptom such as depression can develop from a wide variety of causes, but levels of depression cannot be used to distinguish between people who have a posttraumatic disorder and those who do not. PTSD and dissociation symptoms, on the other hand, seem to be uniquely related to the experience of trauma (Carlson, Armstrong, Loewenstein, & Roth, 1997; Carlson & Rosser-Hogan, 1991). For this reason, all of the symptom measures included in this book assess PTSD or dissociation symptoms.

PTSD Symptoms

Although there is some controversy over whether the symptoms listed in DSM-IV are the most apt for diagnosing PTSD, there is general agreement that, on the whole, they are the best available indicators of posttraumatic responses. Table 5.1 lists the DSM-IV criteria for PTSD. All of the PTSD scales and interviews described in this book include all of the symptoms in Table 5.1; however, the measures differ in some important ways. As described above, many of the measures specify that symptoms are related to a single traumatic event. This may limit their usefulness with persons who have had multiple traumatic experiences. Also, some measures that are keyed closely to the DSM criteria for PTSD begin with a screening question for Criterion A. If the client does not report such an experience, no further questions about symptoms are asked. Many clinicians find this method to be undesirable because a client may interpret the question too narrowly, erroneously denying having had a traumatic experience. Furthermore, some measures use the stressor criterion from DSM-III-R which defines a traumatic event as one "outside the range of usual human experience" that would be "markedly distressing to almost anyone" (American Psychiatric Association, 1987). Since this criterion is now thought to be inadequate as a definition of a traumatic stressor, measures that use it may be less useful. There is also a good deal of variation in the language measures use to describe symptoms, the length and complexity of the measure, and the requirement that the client connect her symptoms to the traumatic experience.

Because PTSD symptoms are fundamental to trauma responses, this is the most important domain to assess when evaluating clients. Although you may choose a brief self-report scale over a structured interview as a first step with clients, you cannot adequately assess trauma responses without finding out more about PTSD symptoms. This issue is discussed further in Chapter 8 where a step-by-step approach to assessment is outlined.

Dissociation Symptoms

Research on dissociation symptoms is not nearly so extensive as that on PTSD symptoms, but studies to date have shown that there is a clear relationship between traumatic experiences and later reports of dissociative symptoms (Putnam & Carlson, 1997). It is the more pathological forms of dissociation that seem to be strongly related to traumatic experiences (Putnam, 1995). The pathological forms of dissociation that have been studied to date include largely cognitive aspects of experience. The major dissociation measures used in research assess pathological dissociation in the form of gaps in awareness, depersonalization (defined as distortions in perceptions of oneself), and derealization (defined as distortions in perceptions of one's environment). Other manifestations of dissociation in affective, behavioral, and physiological realms of experience may also be related to traumatic experiences, but they have not yet been measured or studied.

Measuring pathological forms of dissociation can yield valuable clinical information about a person's response to trauma that will not be available from a PTSD scale or interview. Such information about dissociation symptoms may be useful in treatment. For example, results of a dissociation measure may help to identify a client's most commonly employed cognitive avoidance strategies and may detect disturbances in memory and identity. For this reason, it is advisable to measure dissociation for all clients who report past traumatic experiences or who show high levels of PTSD symptoms. It is important to be cautious, however, in interpreting high levels of dissociation in persons who report low levels of PTSD, because it is possible to have a high level of non-pathological dissociation with no history of trauma. This issue is discussed further in Chapter 9.

Other Domains

There are a few core trauma responses and many secondary and associated responses that are not adequately assessed by measures of

PTSD and dissociation. Of these, the two responses that are most prominent in traumatized persons are symptoms of aggression and depression.

Symptoms of aggression following trauma might be manifested as aggression toward others or toward oneself. Measuring aggression toward others is difficult because of limited development of measures in this domain. Some measures that might yield useful information about aggression include the Multidimensional Anger Inventory (Miller, Jenkins, Kaplan, & Salonen, 1995; Siegel, 1986), the Conflict Tactics Scale (Straus, 1979), and the hostility subscale of the SCL-90-R (Derogatis, 1983).

Aggression toward oneself can be expressed by a number of different forms of self-destructive behavior including suicidality, self-harming behaviors, substance abuse, sexual impulsiveness, and disordered eating. Many authors have noted the importance of assessing trauma victims for suicidality (Dutton, 1992; Resnick & Newton, 1992). Standard methods or measures of suicidality should serve for this purpose. It is a bit more challenging to measure the entire range of self-destructive behaviors. Gil (1988) offers suggestions for questions to evaluate self-harming behaviors, substance abuse, and disordered eating in traumatized people.

Depression is also not very well measured by PTSD scales and interviews. Although they do include items relating to decreases in interest in former activities, lack of hope about the future, sleep problems, and trouble concentrating, they do not include important aspects of depression such as depressed mood, feelings of worthlessness or excessive guilt, psychomotor agitation or retardation, weight gain or loss, fatigue, or suicidality. For this reason, you may want to assess your client's level of depression using some standard measure of depression such as the Beck Depression Inventory (Beck & Steer, 1993), the depression subscales of the MCMI (Millon, 1994), or the SCL-90-R (Derogatis, 1983).

Other secondary and associated symptoms that are worth investigating are guilt and shame and disturbances in self-esteem, identity, and interpersonal relationships. While it would be cumbersome to add detailed measures of all of these symptoms to your routine assessment battery, asking about these responses at some point in your assessment is likely to yield valuable information about the effects of core trauma responses and the trauma situation on your client's functioning.

Some measures are available that provide information about a number of the domains of interest when assessing traumatized people. These include the Trauma Symptom Inventory (TSI) and the Trauma Symptom Checklist for Children (TSCC). These measures allow you to obtain information in a number of diverse domains with only one measure and are described in more detail in the Measure Profiles section (see pp. 227 and 255).

It goes without saying that you should also assess your clients for other disorders and symptoms that are not trauma-related. Very often, those with trauma-related disorders also have other diagnosable disorders (Keane & Wolfe, 1990). Sometimes, the presence of comorbid disorders provides useful information about trauma responses. For example, substance use disorders may indicate efforts to avoid trauma-related symptoms such as intrusive thoughts and feelings (Newman et al., 1996). Further discussion of comorbidity in traumatized persons is discussed further in Chapter 9 (pp. 181–184).

CHOOSING MEASURES TO FIT THE CLIENT

There are numerous characteristics of measures that make them more or less suitable for use with a particular client at a particular point in time. Although this may seem like a large number of factors to consider at once, you will find that it is relatively easy to make your choices once you have become familiar with the issues and gained some experience with some scales and interviews. You may find that you can select a small number of scales and interviews that will serve for assessing the majority of your clients, or you may choose to have on hand a wide variety of measures that you can pick and choose among to fit each client. The advantage of using a small number of measures is that the more examples of responses you see to the same measure, the more expertise you will develop in interpretation of the measure's results. The advantage of using a wide variety of measures is that you may sometimes get more useful information about a client by using a measure that is particularly well-suited to her.

Comprehension

First and foremost, it is crucial that the client understands the questions that are asked in a scale or structured interview. Ideally, the questions should be asked in the client's first language. Unfortunately, most scales and interviews are only available in English, so assessing clients for whom English is not a first language becomes more challenging. If you find yourself in this situation, it is probably prudent to administer all measures and interviews verbally so that you will be better able to monitor the client's understanding of language and can clarify any uncertainties the client has about what words mean. The same method should be used with any clients who have limited reading skills or are illiterate.

It is also important that the level of language used in the scale or interview is appropriate for the cognitive capacities of the client. Certainly, most measures designed for adults would not be well understood by children. You may sometimes have to make a judgment call as to whether to use a measure designed for children or adults. For example, if you are assessing an adolescent for PTSD symptoms and you have a child interview and an adult interview, you should decide which to use based on the intellectual development of the adolescent. If you assess an adult who is retarded or developmentally disabled, an interview designed for children may work better than one designed for adults.

You may also find that measures in the same domain vary considerably in the level and complexity of language they use to describe symptoms. Many of the measures and interviews available were originally developed as research instruments and are written in fairly complex language that may be difficult for some clients to understand. In the profiles of scales and interviews in the Measure Profiles section, I have noted when a measure uses more simple language, and you may want to take this into consideration when choosing measures for clients who have less formal education.

Question Content

Experiences and Context

The questions asked in a scale or interview must be in the realm of experience of your client. Clearly, you would not give a child an interview that asks about symptoms in the context of adult activities. Similarly, you would not give a nonveteran a scale that asks about combat experiences. Many measures are available of trauma experiences that are designed for a particular population of traumatized people such as those who have been in combat or those who have been sexually assaulted. Some measures of trauma responses are also designed for particular populations and would not be suitable for all clients. In this book, I focus on measures and interviews that can be used with most clients, regardless of the type of trauma they experienced, but you may find more specific measures to be useful. Sources of information about more specialized measures include Stamm (1996) and Meichenbaum (Meichenbaum, 1994).

The context in which questions are asked may also be of concern when choosing measures. Since most measures of PTSD are based on the criteria for the disorder listed in the DSM-IV (American Psychiatric

Association, 1994), they follow the convention of assuming that the client has experienced a single traumatic event. Every symptom is then inquired about in the context of that event. For example, a scale might ask if the client has "amnesia for the event." Some clinicians believe that such a context for questions limits the usefulness of such scales with clients who have experienced multiple traumatic events. One group of clients for whom this is particularly problematic is adults who have histories of chronic childhood abuse. For these clients, it may be difficult to answer questions focused on a single trauma. Commonly, clinicians and researchers who use single-event trauma response measures ask clients to identify the single worst traumatic event and to respond to scale or interview questions in reference to that event. But since many assessments occur at a point when the therapist does not know if a client has experienced multiple traumatic events, this may not be a viable solution. Furthermore, many believe it is unwise to place such limitations on symptom reports. If a client has nightmares about one event and intrusive thoughts about another, you certainly want to know about all of these symptoms. There is, in fact, some controversy over the basic assumptions of the PTSD diagnosis and criteria. These are explored in detail in Chapter 9.

Level of Insight Required

The level of insight required for answering questions about symptoms should also be appropriate for the client. This is another controversy that is related to the structure of DSM criteria for PTSD. Some of the DSM criteria require the client to recognize a link between the symptom in question and the traumatic event she experienced. For instance, one criterion is that the client experiences intense psychological distress at exposure to cues that symbolize or resemble an aspect of the traumatic event. But clients may not see a connection between the distress and reminders of a traumatic event. As Solomon and colleagues (1996) point out, it may be preferable to use measures that do not require clients to have this high level of insight.

Cultural Background

Cultural background may be an important issue in the choice of measures. Although scales and interviews were not intentionally designed for clients of any particular cultural background, it seems reasonable to assume that they were developed using middle- and upper-middle-class American subjects as the norm. Consequently, to the extent that your client's cultural background differs from that of middle-class America, a scale might be inappropriate for him. This is particularly true of scales and interviews measuring past traumatic experiences. An example of how culture might affect responses to a measure would be if you gave a measure of traumatic experiences to a refugee from Vietnam. The traumas asked about in that measure are unlikely to be those most relevant to the experience of this client. For example, standard U.S. trauma interviews would not inquire about many traumatic experiences common to refugees such as losing all of one's possessions, witnessing torture, or having one's family members disappear. Discussion of ethnocultural issues in the assessment of mental disorders can be found elsewhere (Keane, Kaloupek, & Weathers, 1996; Lu, Lim, & Mezzich, 1995; Manson, 1996).

One could also argue that some of the symptoms of PTSD listed in DSM-IV are also culturally bound. The core responses of reexperiencing and avoidance are likely to be manifested in different behaviors in different cultures. For example, in a society where sanctions for violent behavior are extreme, an aggressive response to trauma might be manifested verbally, by angry yelling, rather than physically, or it might not be expressed at all. Further discussion of this issue is included in Chapter 9 (p. 175).

Format of Measure

Self-Report versus Interview

Because self-report measures and structured interviews vary greatly in their characteristics, they differ in their usefulness at various points in the assessment process and for different purposes. I briefly describe some important characteristics of self-report and structured interviews here. A more detailed discussion of when in the assessment process you might want to use each type of measure follows in Chapter 8. Self-report measures have several clear advantages. As mentioned earlier, they take very little of the patient's or clinician's time to administer, and they often cost little or nothing to use. In addition, some clinicians believe that self-report measures may yield better disclosure from clients than face-to-face interview questions because clients may be less inhibited in written self-reports (Newman et al., 1996). These qualities make self-report measures a good choice for a first step in the assessment of traumatic experiences and responses. If a client scores high on a self-report measure, you will certainly want to continue your assessment with a structured interview.

Structured interviews have several advantages as well: They enable the clinician to obtain more detailed information about experiences or symptoms; they typically include collection of qualitative information as well as quantitative information; and they allow the clinician to observe the client's interpersonal behavior and affective responses. These qualities make structured interviews particularly useful for obtaining detailed trauma histories and detailed information about symptoms after you have established that a client has had some sort of traumatic experience or has some posttraumatic symptoms. It is also highly advisable to conduct structured interviews with any clients who are being evaluated under special circumstances such as for disability compensation, as part of a law suit claiming damages from traumatization, as part of a criminal defense, or as part of a custody evaluation. In such circumstances, the more detailed information obtained from a structured interview is of much more help in determining the veracity of responses than the results from self-report measures would be.

Length and Complexity

As may be seen in the Measure Profiles, the self-report measures and structured interviews described in this book vary considerably in their length and complexity. For example, some self-reports of traumatic experiences include more detail and more questions than others. The differences between these measures may matter little, since, even if you initially use a briefer measure, you will need to gather this type of detailed information about any reported traumatic experience before you can plan treatment.

Self-report measures of symptoms also vary in length and complexity. For example, some of the self-report measures of PTSD have the client rate both the frequency of PTSD symptoms and the intensity of the symptoms, whereas others measure only one of these or a combination of the two. The self-report measures that tap both frequency and intensity naturally take longer to complete than those that ask for a single rating. Clinicians who know they will be unable to conduct a structured interview with a client might prefer to use one of the more complex self-report measures for PTSD so that they can get as much information about symptoms as possible. Descriptions of self-report measures in the Measure Profiles include information about the length and complexity of the scales.

Structured interviews for trauma assessment also vary considerably in their length and complexity. Longer interviews usually yield a good deal more detailed information about a client's traumatic experiences and his subjective appraisal of the experiences. Structured interviews to measure symptoms vary in the length of time they take to administer primarily because of the range of symptoms they assess. For example, in addition to collecting information about PTSD symptoms, one PTSD interview, the Clinician-Administered PTSD Scale (CAPS) also collects information about a number of symptoms associated with PTSD and about the impact of symptoms on the social and occupational functioning of the client. Given the limits on time and resources faced by most clinicians, the length and complexity of interviews are likely to be important factors in deciding which interview to administer. In the Measure Profiles, descriptions of structured interviews include information about the domains assessed and the length of time to administer and score.

Why You Should Care about Reliability and Validity

Many people who use psychological measures and interviews to gather information about their clients' histories and symptoms have little or no formal training in psychometrics or the validation of measures. Others may have had training but remember few specifics about the validation of clinical instruments. The lack of interest in psychometrics seems to be exacerbated by the fact that many practicing clinicians find these issues to be rather dry and tedious. For those of you in any of these categories, I briefly review some aspects of validation of measures. I hope to convince you that the reliability and validity of the measures you use really do matter and can have practical consequences for your ability to accurately assess and effectively treat your clients. In addition, attention to the reliability and validity of measures you use will be invaluable should you unexpectedly be called upon to defend the accuracy of your assessment in a legal setting.

Reliability

The reliability of a measure refers to the consistency of responses to the measure. There are different kinds of reliability indices that address consistency of scores of the same person across time (test–retest reliability), across different items in the same measure (internal reliability), and across different scorers (interrater reliability).

If a measure shows good test–retest reliability, that means that studies have found that a person tends to earn the same score if she completes the measure on two different occasions. This kind of reliability is established by giving the measure to a person on two occasions that are far enough apart so that the person cannot remember what answers she gave before but not so far apart that the symptom being measured would be expected to change. Usually a test–retest period is 1–2 weeks long. In the case of measuring trauma history or trauma symptoms, you would expect a client's score to be about the same one week as it would be the next. If the scores are very different, that inconsistency may indicate some problem with the measure. Perhaps the questions are ambiguous so that a person does not interpret them the same way each time she answers them. Although scores on the same measure at different times may not be perfectly correlated (with a correlation of 1.0), there should be a strong relationship (i.e., a correlation between .7 and .9) between the scores on the first and second administrations of a measure. This would be evidence of good test–retest reliability.

If a measure shows good internal reliability, that indicates that there is consistency in peoples' answers to questions across different items in the measure. This kind of reliability is typically established by calculating the average correlation for all possible pairs of items in a measure or a measure subscale. This average correlation is reported as a Cronbach's α value. In general, these will vary from 0 to 1.0 with values of .7–.9, indicating good to excellent internal consistency. The idea here is that if all of the items in a measure or subscale are measuring the same construct, then the scores on items should tend to vary together. For example, if a client is experiencing a lot of physiological reactivity to reminders of trauma, then you would expect his responses to different physiological reactivity items to be similar to each other. If he gave very different answers to different questions about physiological reactivity, then you would wonder whether the items were really measuring the construct you thought they were measuring. Perhaps some of the items are unclear in their meaning. This type of reliability is also considered to be evidence for the construct validity of a measure. In other words, internal reliability also gives you information about whether a measure accurately measures the construct that it was designed to measure.

Because internal reliability is an indicator of the consistency of measurement of a construct, it is arguably only relevant to measures of constructs or specific psychological phenomena. This means that it is not relevant to a measure of experience such as frequency of traumatic experiences because those types of measures do not measure any under-lying construct. Instead, they gather information about past experiences that are not necessarily expected to vary together. For example, you wouldn't expect someone's experience of combat to be related to his experiences with hurricanes.

If a measure shows good interrater reliability, that means that the scores determined by two different interviewers or scorers of the same measure would be consistent with one another. This type of reliability applies largely to measures that are administered by an interviewer or that require some judgment in scoring. Interrater reliability might be applied to a measure that is scored objectively (such as adding up ratings to items), but this is not usually thought to be an issue unless a measure is extremely complicated and difficult to score. An example of a measure that would be tested for interrater reliability would be a structured interview that gets scored to determine a diagnosis. If two clinicians administered the same structured interview to a client and each came up with a different diagnostic status or score, then you should be very concerned about whether the administration and scoring criteria for the interview are clear and precise.

Validity

The validity of a measure refers to whether the measure accurately assesses the construct or set of experiences it is designed to measure. There are many different kinds of validity, and what kind of validity is most relevant will depend on the purpose you have for using the measure. Some types of validity that are important in your choice of measures of trauma and trauma responses include convergent validity and concurrent validity. The validity of trauma measures is particularly difficult to determine. A detailed discussion of the validity of trauma reports is included in Chapter 6.

Convergent validity is used to determine if two scores on two different measures of the same construct are strongly related. This type of validity is very relevant if you are using a measure that you want to be sure works as well as another measure. A common example would be that you want to use a very brief measure of PTSD to save time, but you want to be sure that it gives you scores that would be comparable to those on a more detailed and longer measure of PTSD. Usually, longer measures are more accurate because there are more measurement points involved. For example, if you wanted to measure a person's knowledge on a topic, the more questions you asked, the more precisely you would be able to gauge their knowledge. Another use of convergent validity is to establish whether scores on a new measure of a construct relate strongly to scores on an established, psychometrically strong measure. Although scores on two measures will never be perfectly related (with a correlation of 1.0), good convergent validity would be indicated by strong relationships (e.g., correlations between .6 and .9) between scores on the two measures.

Convergent validity would only be expected if the two measures in question were designed to measure exactly the same construct. For this reason, it would be misleading to judge a measure that inquires about symptoms related to multiple traumas by its convergent validity with a measure that inquires about symptoms from only a single trauma. Inconsistency in scores across the two measures might be a result of the difference in the construct being measured and not the result of a measure's lack of validity.

Concurrent or criterion-related validity is used to determine whether scores from a measure are consistent with some other criterion related to the construct you are measuring. An example of the use of concurrent validity would be determining whether the diagnosis of PTSD made from a brief self-report scale was the same as that made by a very lengthy and thorough diagnostic process. In this case, you would want to be sure that those getting a PTSD diagnosis from the scale also got the diagnosis from the longer process and that those who did not get a PTSD diagnosis from the scale did not get the diagnosis from the longer process. In other words, you want the measure to be accurate in identifying those who do have PTSD (called the sensitivity of the measure) and to be accurate in identifying those who do not have PTSD (called the specificity of the measure). Generally, you would want to see sensitivity and specificity rates of .7 or higher for a measure, meaning that at least 70% of the time, the measure accurately identified subjects who did have PTSD and accurately identified subjects who did not have PTSD.

The caveat regarding the appropriateness of assessing the convergent validity of a measure by comparing it to one that assesses a somewhat different construct applies to concurrent validity as well. For example, if the measure you are validating inquires about symptoms related to multiple traumatic events, it might not make sense to use DSM-IV PTSD diagnosis as the criterion because that diagnosis is based on symptoms related to only one traumatic event.

Threats to Reliability and Validity

Many, many factors can interfere with a measure's capacity to reliably and validly assess a construct or set of experiences. As mentioned above, the test–retest or internal reliability of a measure might be compromised by ambiguous wording of items. The interrater reliability of a measure might be impaired because administration or scoring instructions are unclear or inconsistently applied.

Validity of a measure can be threatened by a wide variety of factors. A few sources of error are most relevant to measures used to assess trauma and trauma responses. A measure might not be valid because clients and the measure's designer do not understand questions in the same way. For example, one should not ask a client, "Have you ever been raped?" because your definition of rape and the client's may differ. A measure might not be valid because items do not accurately represent the construct intended. For example, suppose you want to ask about intrusive thoughts, and you ask, "How often do you have thoughts about the past that are unpleasant?" You are likely to get overreporting on this item because it is overly general and does not specify that the thoughts are unbidden and about a traumatic event. A measure might also lack validity because its items are not properly distributed across the construct to be measured. For example, suppose you had a 50-item measure of PTSD, and 20 of the items related to problems with sleep, concentration, or physiological reactivity. Persons with depression or anxiety disorders might score high on such a measure and reduce the specificity of the measure in identifying those who do not have a PTSD diagnosis. Some additional threats to the validity of trauma measures are discussed in Chapter 6.

You can never assume that a measure is reliable or valid unless it has been systematically studied to establish its reliability or validity. Even if it appears that the items would accurately measure the construct, this cannot be assumed. Furthermore, you cannot assume that a measure is reliable and valid because it is widely distributed, published in a journal or a book, or published by a test publisher. None of these guarantee the reliability and validity of a measure. Unfortunately, there are countless measures of constructs and experiences that have been widely distributed and published, but have not been validated. So it is up to the individual clinician to investigate measures she intends to use and to judge their reliability and validity. An excellent source of further information on reliability, validity, and related measurement issues can be found in Weathers, Keane, King, and King (1996).

SUMMARY

This chapter reviewed a number of sources of information about clients and various purposes for conducting assessments. The remainder of the chapter focused on using self-report measures and structured interviews to gather information from clients for clinical purposes. First, various domains were described that are key in making assessments of trauma and trauma responses. Next, issues important to choosing measures were discussed, such as the client's level of comprehension and the measure's content, format, reliability, and validity. Explanations were given as to why clinicians need to be mindful of these measure characteristics when choosing measures.

Chapter 8

Selecting and Administering Measures

This chapter provides information and suggestions relevant to selecting and administering the measures described in the Measure Profiles of this book. The general parameters used to select measures for this book included the availability, overall quality, and unique features of the measures. Additional parameters for selection were specific to the different types of measures included. When choosing which measures to administer in a particular assessment, information about characteristics of specific measures should be helpful to you. This chapter includes an explanation of the categories of information about measures that are provided in the profiles. When choosing the sequence of administration of measures in a particular assessment, flowcharts can be used to follow a stepwise screening and interview process. Once the measures to be used in an assessment have been chosen, it is time to consider the process of conducting assessments. In planning procedures for administering your assessments, you should consider the timing and the setting of various elements of the assessment. Finally, though it is easy to get caught up in the measurement process as an investigatory endeavor, it is critical that you be mindful of clients' emotional needs during an assessment so that you can make your assessments as therapeutic as possible.

PARAMETERS FOR SELECTING MEASURES INCLUDED IN THIS BOOK

There are literally hundreds of measures of traumatic experiences and trauma responses in existence. These range from questionnaires that have never been systematically studied to published measures that have extensive norms and have been carefully validated. To select the measures included in this book, I used several criteria. First, I have only included measures that are readily available to you. Along with each measure's description is the name and address of a contact person or publisher to whom you can write to obtain the measure. When available, a citation for a published source that includes the measure itself is also included. In choosing the measures for the book, I have also favored measures that are particularly well developed or show promise, that have special qualities, or are unique. In addition, I have tried to select those measures that were most carefully constructed, those with the most evidence of their reliability and validity, and those that are most widely used.

For some types of measures, some of the instruments included are very similar to one another. The discussion in Chapter 6 of factors to consider when choosing a measure should be helpful as you select which measures to administer to a client. In the end, however, you may find one of the measures to be more appealing to you simply because you prefer the wording of items or format. Many measures that are not included in the book are also clinically useful and accurate. Information about other measures of trauma and trauma responses can be found in Briere (1997), Stamm (1996), Wilson and Keane (1996), Nader (1996), Resnick and colleagues (Resnick, Falsetti, Kilpatrick, & Freedy, 1996), Solomon and colleagues (1996), Newman et al. (1996), and Meichenbaum (1994).

I first briefly introduce the types of measures I have included in the book and then describe some general parameters that I used to select the specific measures. The Measure Profiles are divided into four sections covering different types of measures: trauma measures; self-report measures of trauma responses; structured interviews of trauma responses; and measures for children and adolescents.

In the section on trauma measures, self-report measures are listed first, followed by structured interviews for trauma. In its coverage of trauma measures, this book focuses on global trauma measures that query about a wide range of traumatic experiences that a person may have had. Some measures also contain fairly in-depth assessments of specific types of traumatic experiences (such as sexual assault). Development in the area of global measures of traumatic experiences has only recently begun to expand in terms of the validation and publication of measures. In part, the limited development of trauma measures to date is due to the great difficulties in establishing validity of trauma measures (McFarlane & de Girolamo, 1996). While researchers have only just begun to solve the problem of how to establish validity of measures of experiences when no incontrovertible records are available, clinicians and researchers have become more aware of the necessity of inquiring about a person's trauma history before interpreting their symptoms or planning treatment. Because of increased research efforts in the area of trauma measurement, some of the measures described here that are in the early stages of development are likely to prove valid and useful in the future. In addition, although this book is focused on more global trauma measures, many measures are also available to measure details of specific types of traumatic experiences. For example, there are measures that assess combat experiences, abuse experiences, and refugee experiences. Some sources of information on more specific measures of trauma are Briere (1996a), Stamm (1996), and Meichenbaum (1994).

Because adult self-report measures of trauma responses are fairly well-developed and validated, you have many options for measuring these symptoms. This book includes profiles of measures of PTSD symptoms, dissociation symptoms, and of multiple domains. For the domain of PTSD, there are many measures available that are very similar in content and format. Because of these similarities, I have chosen only a few to include in the book. The PTSD self-report measures are all ones that measure the full range of DSM PTSD symptoms and can be used to assess responses to any type of trauma. All of them can serve you well as screens for trauma responses. Specific measures are also available for those who have been through particular traumas. Such measures ask about PTSD symptoms in the context of the particular event or type of trauma. For example, there are measures of trauma responses following combat that ask about intrusive thoughts about combat. Many such trauma-specific measures are described in Stamm (1996) and Meichenbaum (1994).

Structured interview measures for PTSD are fairly well developed and have been in use for the past decade. There are several structured interviews for PTSD available, and these vary considerably in the amount of detail that is collected about symptoms. Only two structured interviews are available for dissociative disorders, but they have both been validated and in use for several years. All of the measures profiled in this chapter are readily available for use by clinicians. The PTSD structured interviews all measure the full range of DSM PTSD symptoms, and one of the dissociation interviews inquires about DSM symptoms for all dissociative disorders in detail.

Two structured interviews for PTSD worth noting that are not included in this book are modules of more extensive diagnostic interviews. Both the Diagnostic Interview Schedule (DIS) and the Structured Clinical Interview for DSM-IV (SCID) contain PTSD modules, but neither is as strong a measure of PTSD symptoms as the interviews described in the profiles. Several reviewers of trauma response measures have raised questions about the performance of these interviews in diagnosing PTSD (Meichenbaum, 1994; Newman et al., 1996; Weiss, 1996). Because of these concerns, profiles of the DIS and the SCID were not included in this book.

Section D of the Measure Profiles includes self-report and structured interview measures of both trauma and responses to trauma for children. All of the other measures described in the book are designed for use with adults with the exception of the Evaluation of Lifetime Stressors, which can be used with adolescents. If your client is a child or a developmentally disabled adult, you should use measures in Section D. It may be tempting if you already have an adult trauma measure in hand to "translate" it to a lower level for use with children. This method is likely to be a very poor substitute for using a measure designed for children. A measure that is valid for one population is not necessarily valid for another. Furthermore, measuring characteristics and experiences of children is particularly challenging because of their limited verbal abilities and because of great individual differences in behavior across children and differences in children of different ages. Accordingly, making a valid measure of children's experiences is a task best left to those with experience and expertise in design and validation of psychological measures.

Development of measures of children's experiences of trauma and trauma responses has expanded very rapidly over the past few years. Consequently, there are many self-report and structured interview measures available for assessing trauma and trauma responses in children, but there is less psychometric information available about most of these measures than is available for comparable adult measures. I have included those measures that are available and that appear promising with the hope that evidence of reliability and validity will be forthcoming for most of the instruments. Additional information on measures of traumatic experiences in children can be found in Nader (1996). In addition, when assessing children, it is often useful to gather information from a parent or another person who is in a good position to observe the child. Within the sections on trauma response measures, those measures that are administered directly to children are listed first, followed by measures administered to parents or other observers.

As discussed in Chapter 7, the reliability and validity of a measure are critical to its capacity to accurately assess trauma or trauma responses. Accordingly, I favored measures for which there is good evidence of their reliability and validity. In an ideal world, when an measure is developed, all of the different types of reliability and validity that are relevant to the measure would be established. But research on instruments is difficult to conduct, and funding for such research is hard to come by. Consequently, most of the instruments available have some evidence of their reliability and validity, but all of the types of reliability and validity that one would want to know about might not have been studied. Also, some measures have stronger evidence of their reliability and validity than others. Older measures that have very well-established reliability and validity and are widely used often also have the advantage of having well-established norms. This means that large numbers of subjects from different populations of people have been given the measure, and the average scores earned have been established. For example, an older measure of PTSD might have been given to large samples of combat veterans, rape victims, hurricane survivors, and car accident victims, so that the average scores for subjects in these groups would be known.

The sheer number of studies of reliability and validity should not be the only consideration in choosing measures, though, because newer measures have generally been the subject of the fewest studies. Despite this lack of research, some newer measures may be superior to older ones because advances in our understanding of trauma and trauma responses have been incorporated into them. For example, measures that assess symptoms from multiple traumatic experiences instead of keying to one event are very new, so they have less-established reliability and validity than older measures. If you value that innovation, however, you may decide to use a newer measure that assesses multiple traumas despite the limited information about its reliability and validity. This is usually a safe bet as long as the measure has been developed by a researcher who has experience developing reliable and valid measures. It is not wise, however, to use a measure with no evidence of its reliability and validity, no matter how innovative it is, if it has been developed by a person with little expertise in measurement development. In keeping with these ideas, I have included some measures in the book that have relatively little established reliability and validity because they are innovative and were developed by trauma measurement experts.

You should also keep in mind that the trauma field is relatively new and is rapidly evolving. This means that information about the reliability and validity of measures of trauma will continue accumulating as they are studied further. You can check on the development of new measures, new norms for an existing measure, and new evidence for the reliability and validity of measures in a number of ways. The resources mentioned below can help you stay abreast of these developments in trauma measurement. Information about all of these resources is included in the Appendix. Two very valuable resources are the *PTSD Research Quarterly* and the *PTSD Clinical Quarterly*, both published by the National Center for PTSD. These publications are also available electronically via the Internet as is an international trauma literature database called PILOTS. Using the PILOTS database, you can specifically search the trauma literature for studies that used particular measures, read the abstracts of those studies, and find out where you can obtain the articles. Another good source of information is through membership in a professional organization such as the International Society for Traumatic Stress Studies (ISTSS). The ISTSS publishes a newsletter and the *Journal of Traumatic Stress* and holds annual meetings that include educational workshops and research and clinical symposia relating to measurement. It is also a good idea to keep an eye out for review articles or book chapters on the subject of measurement of trauma or trauma responses.

CATEGORIES OF INFORMATION IN THE PROFILES

The profiles of measures in this book are designed to make it easy for you to find specific information about the measures. The categories of information are uniform across the profiles, and they contain the kinds of information you will need to make a decision about which instruments will be most appropriate for each of your clients.

Each measure profile begins with the name and acronym of the measure. Sometimes, when measures are being developed, they are referred to with a number of different names. You may have the experience of reading about two different measures by the same group of authors, only to find later that they are referring to the same measure at different points in its development. Conversely, you may assume that two measures with very similar names are the same, when they are, in fact, different and unrelated measures. The names of the authors of the measure may help you clear up mysteries about the identities of measures. You should also be aware that acronyms for measures are frequently used and that very small differences in an acronym may be very important. For example, the TAA-SR and the TAA-I are different versions of the same measure, but the TAA-I is a structured interview, whereas the TAA-SR is a self-report version.

The "Recommended Uses" category contains suggestions for the settings and clients that each measure is particularly well suited for. Some recommendations are my own, and some have been offered by other authors. These suggestions are in all cases in keeping with the uses suggested by the measure's authors. You will find similar recommendations for use of many of the measures. In that case, your decision about which measure to use can be guided by the special features of the measures (see below) or by the format, length, or wording of the questionnaire. Of course, the suggested uses given here are not the only possible uses, and you may find additional and alternative suggestions for use elsewhere.

Some of the recommendations for use of measures are influenced by changes in our understanding of trauma and trauma responses that have come about in recent years. For example, a brief scale developed some years ago to assess responses to trauma might have been based on the assumption that the client had only one traumatic experience. Since the first PTSD measures were developed, it has become increasingly clear that many individuals experience multiple traumatic events over a lifetime. In fact, exposure to one traumatic event has been found to increase the risk of exposure to future traumatic events and the likelihood of developing PTSD after the second event (Newman et al., 1996). Research has also indicated that clients seeking treatment often do not spontaneously report previous traumatic events (Jacobson et al., 1987). Given these conditions, measures that focus on only one traumatic event may not adequately assess trauma responses. Newman and colleagues (1996) have suggested routine assessment for multiple significant stressors in clients who present for a clinical assessment following a traumatic experience. For these reasons, I have suggested more limited uses for PTSD measures that were developed to assess responses to a single traumatic event.

The "Special Features" category alerts you to aspects of each measure that are relatively unique. For trauma measures, you should check this category for information about specific traumas that are assessed by the measure and the type of detail elicited about each event. You may want to choose a measure that has particularly strong probes for details in an area that you know is relevant to a particular client. For example, if your client reports a sexual assault as her presenting problem, you might choose a measure that includes specific inquiries about various sexual assault experiences.

The "General Descriptive Information" categories are designed to give you a good idea of what each measure "looks like." For trauma measures, the "Events Assessed" category gives you information about the types of traumatic experiences that the measure inquires about. As mentioned above, the trauma measures included in this book are global measures of traumatic experiences. Measures that inquire about more types of events have the advantage that they may elicit more information than a questionnaire inquiring about fewer traumatic events. However, they have the disadvantage of taking longer to administer or complete. For trauma response measures, the "Symptoms Assessed" category gives you information about the range of symptoms a measure covers.

The "Number of Items Assessed" is listed along with the "Time Required to Administer or Complete" the measure because these two factors should be considered in conjunction with one another. A measure with fewer items does not necessarily take less time to administer or complete because it may have more detailed probes of experiences. It is also worth noting that the complexity of the client's trauma history and responses will largely determine the administration time for all interview measures. Consequently, the category for "Time to Administer or Complete" provides a range of amounts of time: The shortest time listed refers to a client who has had no traumatic experiences and few symptoms, while the longest time listed refers to a client who has had multiple traumatic experiences and extensive symptoms. These are, of course, only estimates. It may take even longer to administer a structured interview to a client with an extremely complex trauma history or to a client who takes a long time to answer questions.

The "Response Format" category tells you what the client's options are for answering questions. Response formats vary from dichotomous "Yes/No" formats for screening tools to free-response formats for structured interviews.

The recommendation in the "Training Required to Administer" category represents the suggestions of measure authors when they have given specific recommendations in this regard. Often, however, measure authors do not specifically address the issue of how much training is required to administer the measure. Self-report measures may require no special training or expertise to administer. Some structured interviews are designed to be administered by clinicians or paraprofessionals, and some are designed to be administered only by trained mental health professionals. Needless to say, those with the least clinical experience and expertise will need the most supervision in their interviews with clients. Also, the training level necessary to administer a measure is often not the same as that necessary to interpret the results of a measure. All of the measures discussed in this book should be interpreted only by experienced mental health professionals who are knowledgeable about assessment methods and interpretation. Ideally, those interpreting measure results should have completed graduate level courses in psychological assessment and measurement.

A sample item is provided for each measure to give you an idea of the format of questions and the complexity of the language used. For many of the measures, the sample item is representative of all of the questions. The "Type of Outcome Measure Provided" category tells you what kinds of scores can be obtained from the measure results. For example, results from measures that are in the form of "Yes/No" questions can provide a count of traumatic stressors experienced. A measure that inquires about details of traumatic experiences may provide a rating of the severity of trauma. Some measures yield subscale scores as well as total scores.

For trauma measures, the "Aspects of Trauma Assessed" category lists the kinds of details that a particular questionnaire probes for. This category is also helpful in estimating the time required for administering or completing the measure. In general, the more probes used to explore each type of trauma, the more time the interview is likely to take.

The "Time Frame Assessed" category tells you what portion of the client's life will be assessed by the measure. Most of the general trauma measures assess events over a client's entire lifetime. The structured interviews for specific types of traumatic experiences may assess only a circumscribed part of the client's life, such as abusive experiences during childhood or spousal abuse experienced in the past 6 months. Trauma response measures vary widely in terms of the time frame assessed.

The "Development Notes" category provides information about the development of the measure. In most cases, this information describes the origin of the measure or specifies when a previous version of the measure by another author was adapted to create the new measure. This category may be omitted when no previous versions existed.

The last category of general descriptive information provides information about how closely the measure corresponds to DSM criteria for PSTD. For trauma measures, it is often useful if the measure probes match the language of Criterion A so that you can determine if the client's traumatic experience will meet the criterion. For example, measures that inquire about threat of or actual injury or death and the experience of fear, horror, or helplessness would allow you to determine whether an event meets DSM-IV Criterion A. For measures of trauma responses, this category specifies which of the relevant DSM symptom criteria are assessed.

The "Psychometric Information" categories provide a brief overview of research findings relevant to the psychometric properties of each measure. This includes information about which populations the measure has been normed and validated on and a summary of the measure's reliability and validity. While this review of psychometric research will not be detailed or exhaustive, it will give you a good idea of the current stage of development of each measure. When you consider the information about populations that the measure has been normed on, it is important to remember that further research may be in progress or recently completed on additional populations. Furthermore, as mentioned above, a measure that is valid for one population is not necessarily valid for another. That means that a measure normed for use with a community population sample may perform differently if you use it with clients in another setting.

Two types of reliability that are relevant to measures of traumatic experiences and responses are test–retest reliability and interrater reliability. As described in Chapter 6, establishing the test–retest reliability of a measure is done by administering it on two separate occasions and comparing the results of the two administrations. Good test–retest reliability indicates that clients' reports of traumatic experiences or responses on a particular measure are consistent over time. Some authors caution, however, that the finding of a low test–retest reliability for a trauma measure might be misleading because there is a tendency for an initial trauma assessment to cue memories of forgotten events and because people may be more willing to disclose events to an interviewer with whom they have previously spoken (Newman et al., 1996; Resnick et al., 1996). On the other hand, a compelling need for avoidance may prompt some clients consciously or unconsciously to avoid remembering and reporting a traumatic event during the retest measurement (Resnick et al., 1996). All of these factors would reduce the consistency of the reports over two administrations and would tend to lower test–retest reliability, even when properties of the measure are not causing a lack of consistency over time.

Interrater reliability is relevant to structured interviews for traumatic experiences and responses. As described in Chapter 6, establishing the interrater reliability of an interview is done by having two clinicians administer and score the interview and comparing the results of the two administrations. Good interrater reliability indicates that there is consistency in responding and scoring of interview questions across interviewers. For trauma measures, this type of reliability may also be adversely affected by the memory, disclosure, and avoidance factors described above, even when properties of the measure are not causing a lack of reporting consistency across interviewers.

Studies of the internal consistency or internal reliability of measures are relevant to measures of trauma responses but not to measures of traumatic experiences (Norris & Riad, 1996). This is because internal consistency studies examine the consistency of responses across the different items of a measure. While one would expect responses to similar symptom items to be fairly consistent, one wouldn't expect one's experiences across a variety of traumas to be consistent. In other words, while traumatic stress symptoms should "hang together" and reports should show good internal consistency, traumatic events can occur randomly.

Methods used to assess the validity of measures include concurrent or criterion-related validity, convergent validity, and other forms of construct validity. For all of these types of validity, measure results are compared to some other source of information to establish their accuracy. These types of validity are described in detail in Chapter 7 (pp. 138–139). In general, all of these validation methods are well suited to studying the validity of trauma response measures. Evidence of a measure's validity can also be established by comparing prevalence of traumatic experiences or responses found when using a measure in one study to results of similar studies (Resnick et al., 1996). As discussed in Chapter 6, establishing the validity of trauma reports and trauma measures is extremely problematic (Norris & Riad, 1996). For example, it is very difficult to establish the criterion-related validity of a trauma measure because often no certain criteria such as documents or records of the event are available for comparison.

Key references for obtaining more detailed descriptive or psychometric information about each measure are also provided in each profile. It is noted here when a publication contains a measure in its entirety. Lastly, information is provided about how to obtain each measure. At the time of publication, all of the trauma measures and most of the trauma response measures in the book were available at no cost or at a very reasonable cost, and no costs were associated with using most of the measures with clients.

For some measures, the appropriate contact is a test publisher. When this is the case, there are costs associated with the use of the measure. Some measures that are now obtained through individual authors are likely to be published (and available for sale) in the next few years. In such cases, the contact person listed will be able to direct you to the appropriate test publisher.

USING THE ASSESSMENT FLOWCHARTS

Given the high prevalence of potentially traumatic events, the case could easily be made that every client ought to fill out either a PTSD or a traumatic events brief measure as a screen at the outset of assessment. The small cost in time and effort would likely be well worth the benefit to those with unreported trauma or trauma-related symptoms who were "flagged" by the screening measure. Remember, though, that neither a report of a traumatic event nor a high score on a PTSD screen is sufficient evidence to diagnose PTSD. No single measure alone can definitively assess responses to trauma (Newman et al., 1996). Also, it is possible for people to score low on a brief scale for PTSD, even when they do meet criteria for PTSD.

The flowchart in Figure 8.1 provides a suggested order for administering measures of trauma and trauma responses in adults. A separate flowchart is provided in Figure 8.2 for assessments of children. I recommend that you begin the assessment with either a measure of traumatic experiences or a measure of PTSD symptoms. Your choice of which to start with may be dictated by the presenting problem your client brings to you. If she is aware of and concerned about a traumatic experience that has affected her emotionally, it would make sense to begin with a brief trauma questionnaire. If you are aware of a history of multiple traumatic events, you might want to skip the brief questionnaire and begin with a more detailed structured interview for traumatic events. If the client does not mention any traumatic events, but is troubled by some PTSD symptoms, it would make sense to begin with a brief screen for PTSD. Here, too, if you are already aware of considerable PTSD symptomatology, you might want to skip the brief scale and begin with a structured interview for PTSD.

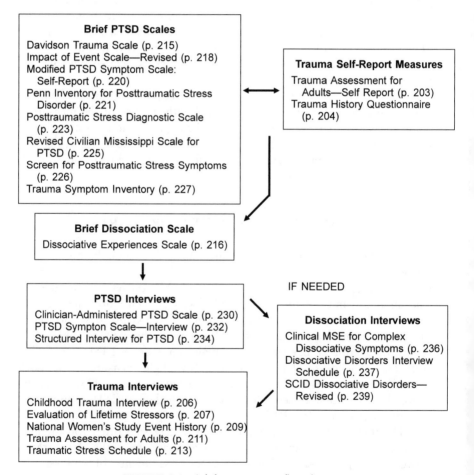

FIGURE 8.1. Adult assessment flowchart.

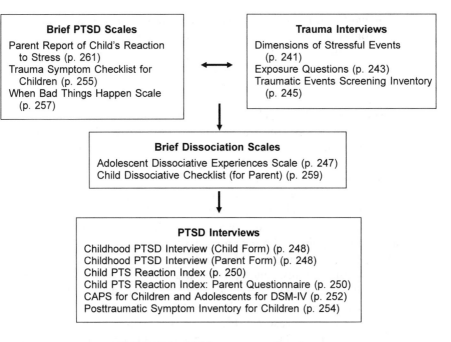

FIGURE 8.2. Child assessment flowchart.

If you give a trauma experiences screen as the first measure, you should give a brief PTSD scale as the second measure and vice versa. After administering the brief measures, you can proceed to structured interviews as necessary. The flowcharts provide one possible sequence of measures, but minor deviations from this plan are unlikely to change the results significantly and may, in some circumstances, be desirable. If you do choose to use both a brief scale and a structured interview to assess experiences or responses, the brief measure should always be administered *before* the structured interview.

The amount of time that the assessment for a particular client will take to complete will, of course, depend on the complexity of the client's trauma history and the degree and extent of symptoms experienced. Low scores on self-administered PTSD and dissociation scales and reports of no traumatic experiences on trauma questionnaires might mean that the assessment would take little or no clinician time. On the other hand, a person with a complex trauma history and many symptoms might need scales and structured interviews for trauma, PTSD, dissociation, and other related symptoms or experiences. That kind of evaluation could take several sessions to complete. In general, the results of self-report measures will help you gauge the number of sessions that will be needed to make a complete assessment.

It is worth noting that there are some times when you may need to deviate from the instructions of a structured interview in order to make a complete and therapeutic assessment. One of these times is when you are using a structured interview that requires the client to meet Criterion A before assessing any PTSD symptoms. It is advisable to conduct the interview if the client does not seem to meet Criterion A because there may be a Criterion A event that the client does not remember or does not interpret as meeting Criterion A. Unfortunately, for most structured interviews for PTSD, an identified traumatic event is an integral part of many items. If you use brief measures for PTSD and trauma before conducting the structured interview, you may be able to avoid this dilemma altogether. If you do continue a structured interview that requires a Criterion A event with a client who reports no such event, remember that this method may invalidate the results of the interview and may make it inappropriate to compare your client's results to published norms for the interview.

As the flowcharts indicate, if your client reports any past trauma on an initial self-report instrument, you should follow up the self-report measure with a structured interview for trauma experiences in order to gather more detailed information. If your client reports only one traumatic event on a self-report measure of traumatic experiences, it is probably safe to use a self-report PTSD measure or interview that is keyed to one trauma. If clients report multiple traumatic events, however, a structured interview that is not keyed to a single event may yield more useful information about the range and severity of your client's current symptoms.

If your client reports significant posttraumatic symptoms on an initial self-report instrument, you should follow-up the self-report measure with a structured interview for PTSD in order to gather more detailed information. It is also important to measure dissociation in those clients who report any past traumas or who show high levels of PTSD. As described in Chapter 7 (p. 129), information about dissociation symptoms may be very useful in treatment. High dissociation scale scores do not always reflect traumatization, however. As is discussed in Chapter 9 (p. 177), a client might have a high dissociation score on some measures even when she is not traumatized because of high endorsement of nonpathological dissociation items. Guidelines for comparing your clients' scores on self-report measures to norms and making decision rules for what constitutes a "high" score are discussed in Chapter 9 (pp. 176–178).

ADMINISTERING MEASURES

The remainder of this chapter addresses issues relating to administering assessments. Suggested procedures are reviewed for administering self-report and interview measures. Therapeutic issues relating to interviews of traumatized people are also discussed.

Procedures for Conducting Assessments

Ideally, self-report measures are administered as part of a two-session evaluation process. In the first session, you might gather the usual information about the client's presenting problem and psychosocial history. After this session, you should have a better idea about which measures would be most appropriate for this particular client. Administering self-report measures of trauma experiences and trauma responses as a second step in the assessment process also allows you to have a more conversational first interview with your client because it frees you of the necessity of asking a series of questions about possible experiences and symptoms. It is not a good idea to ask clients to complete the measures before the first interview because they may be more hesitant to disclose information before they have met you and established some rapport with you.

Between the first and second assessment sessions, the client can come to your office to complete the self-report measures that you have selected for her. You may be tempted to give or mail self-report measures to your client for her to fill out at home in order to save her the trouble of coming in to your office. This is not advisable because a small minority of clients may become extremely distressed when filling out self-report measures of trauma experiences or symptoms.

The ideal setting for a client to complete self-report measures is in a quiet, private room in an office where a therapist is available (or can be called) if the client becomes extremely distressed. If a private room is not available, your office waiting room may be suitable as long as there are not other clients waiting there. If it is not possible for your client to come to your office on a separate occasion to complete self-report measures, the next best arrangement is for the client to complete the measures at the end of the first appointment. A separate occasion for completing the self-report measures is optimal, though, because clients are often fatigued or emotionally "spent" after an initial assessment session. Coming back at another time to complete questionnaires also allows the client some time to process his meeting with you and to give you a more thoughtful response to self-report measures than would be possible immediately following the first session.

Before the second meeting with your client, you can review and score the self-report measures and determine which additional measures you want to administer. The preceding sections that describe the assessment flowcharts should be helpful in deciding which additional measures to use. The second session can be used to review the results of the self-report measures with your client and to complete any additional assessment interviews. It may be possible at the end of the second session to make a treatment plan or you may need to do this during a third session, depending on the complexity of the client's presenting problems and trauma history.

Structured interviews for trauma responses should be administered in a quiet, private room. If administered by a lay interviewer, a therapist should be readily available if the client becomes extremely distressed. In general, it is important to follow the administration instructions of a structured interview closely. Some clinicians, as they become more familiar with the questions that constitute the interview, are tempted to move to a more open-ended interview format. They may want to begin with a less-structured approach and finish by consulting a checklist of symptoms to make sure none of the relevant symptoms have been missed. These clinicians desire a less-structured approach because it allows for a more naturally flowing conversation with the client. But it is important to give serious thought to the possible consequences if you are tempted to depart in any way from a structured interview.

Any departure from the order and wording of an established structured interview may seriously compromise the usefulness of the assessment. Changes you make may render the interview less accurate than its original form in quantifying symptoms or assigning a diagnosis. Furthermore, a systematically administered structured interview will be more useful to another clinician if the client is referred for treatment or seen at some time in the future. When conducting assessments for forensic or research purposes, you should never depart from the exact methodology of the chosen structured interview as the results of an interview that was not systematically administered would certainly be challenged. The fact that forensic or legal issues can unexpectedly arise in any clinical case also serves as a caution against departing from the instructions for administration of a structured interview. Also, it is not feasible to conduct an open-ended interview at first and another systematic interview later on if needed. This is because the experience of the first interview is likely to influence responses to the second, rendering it less valid.

Conducting Therapeutic Assessments
of Traumatized People

When you assess a person's traumatic experiences and responses to trauma, you need to be sure that your interviews are therapeutic as well as informative. Disclosing information about past traumatic events and about psychiatric symptoms can be particularly stressful for people who have been exposed to traumatic events. In addition to employing all of your clinical interview skills and using standard methods for making assessments, there are several considerations that particularly apply to assessing traumatized people.

Fostering Clients' Feelings of Control

As discussed in Chapters 2 through 5, the controllability of events plays a key role in the development and maintenance of posttraumatic stress responses. Several authors have noted that the need to feel in control is an important issue for people who have endured traumatic experiences (Courtois, 1988; Gil, 1988; Herman, 1992). There are a number of ways that you can help foster your client's feelings of control during an assessment interview. Before beginning the interview, you can explain the assessment process in detail including descriptions of the self-report measures you will ask the client to fill out. This will help your client know what to expect during the assessment process and will allow her to make a decision about whether she wishes to participate in the assessment process. It is important to remember that some clients may not wish to discuss or may not be emotionally prepared to explore trauma-related issues (Pearlman & McCann, 1994). Making it clear that she has a choice about whether to participate will ensure an ethically defensible approach to assessment and will also help maximize a client's cooperation as a partner in the assessment.

During the assessment of traumatic experiences, control of the pace of inquiry is particularly important (Newman et al., 1996). Before asking any questions, you should make it clear to your client that she should let you know if she is becoming upset. You will need to be sensitive to any signs of discomfort in case a client is reluctant to speak up. Some traumatized clients may be very compliant even when they are in distress. Sometimes, you might even need to stop a client who expresses a willingness to go on with an interview, since she may be having trouble knowing how much distress is too much. This may be a difficult distinction for you to make too, and you should enlist your client's help in deciding if she is too upset to go on. As in other clinical decisions, you will have to rely on your intuition to some extent. Certainly, you would not interrupt a client's report just because she is crying, is becoming agitated, or appears angry, but if nonverbal behaviors lead you to wonder whether the client is feeling out of control, you can simply ask the client whether she feels in control and is comfortable going on.

If you do stop a line of questioning because you see that your client is becoming overwhelmed, you will help her learn how she can protect herself emotionally by interrupting escalating anxiety. Be sure, however, that stopping the questioning process in a trauma interview is in the client's best interests and not for your own comfort. Since listening to clients recount traumatic experiences can be very distressing, you may feel tempted to protect yourself emotionally and inadvertantly give the client the message that you have heard enough. It is as important to avoid prematurely cutting off a client's account as it is to avoid allowing her to continue too long.

If a client asks to stop talking about a particular event, you should reinforce this self-protective coping behavior. Explicitly noting to your client that she has some good emotional coping skills will encourage her to use them more and will remind her that she is not completely helpless. It is a good idea to ask the client for permission to come back to the question or topic at some later time when she feels up to it. In this way, you convey that avoidance of the traumatic content is not a good long-term strategy, even if it is a wise choice in the short term. Clients whose avoidance of traumatic material is predominant should be informed of the role of avoidance in posttraumatic stress responses and the impediment such avoidance may be to progress in treatment.

Finally, toward the end of the assessment process, it is beneficial to clients to point out some of their strengths and successes in coping with their traumatic experiences (Dutton, 1992; Herman, 1992). Many traumatized clients are to be congratulated on their fortitude for surviving a traumatic experience and remaining as emotionally intact as they have. Highlighting this strength can help reduce the feelings of helplessness and hopelessness that typically accompany a posttraumatic stress reaction.

Promoting Trust and Openness

It is not surprising that the issue of trust should be a major concern for those with trauma histories, particularly those who have experienced an intentionally inflicted trauma such as assault or rape (Newman et al., 1996). For this reason, you need to be especially careful about establishing rapport and building a trusting relationship with these clients before asking them for details of a traumatic experience. This is probably of less concern when the traumatic experience is relatively impersonal in nature such as a fire or a car accident, but it is of much more concern for experiences that are deeply personal such as rape or incest. For a client whose trauma involved violation of his privacy, protecting his privacy is likely to be a major issue, and threats to privacy may be quite distressing. Some clients may feel that they have "survived" psychologically by not disclosing or by not thinking about events, so they will be understandably reluctant to tell you about them.

It is best for your client, of course, if he can be very open with you about his experiences and current symptoms. The more information you can get from him about his experiences and symptoms, the more likely you will be able to plan an effective treatment. There are a number of things you can do to encourage trust and promote openness with traumatized clients. Clearly, your therapeutic manner will be important. It goes without saying that your manner should convey a serious interest in what your client tells you. Resick and Schnicke (1993) advise that you should avoid erring in the direction of underreaction because you don't want to give the client the impression that you don't think the event was important. They also advise against overreaction when you are told about traumatic experiences. Becoming visibly upset yourself or appearing alarmed when a client becomes upset may give your client the impression that you think the trauma is insurmountable. Rushing to give a client a tissue may give her the message that you want her to pull herself together and stop crying. She may think that you do not want to hear any more about her experience or that you cannot handle even hearing about what happened to her. Both underreaction and overreaction are likely to stifle a client's openness and reduce the amount of clinical information you are able to collect. Worse yet, such negative reactions can also greatly discourage a client from pursuing treatment.

As with any client, it will be important for you to provide social support. This is particularly important after a client has been willing to trust you with the details of a very personal trauma. As described in Chapter 4, social support can be a powerful ameliorating influence for trauma victims. Maintaining a calm and reassuring manner will make your client feel supported while telling you about traumatic experiences. It is also supportive to assure a client that he is not overreacting to the traumatic event nor "going crazy." You can provide education about posttraumatic responses and help your client see that his symptoms are typical of those who experience trauma.

Maintaining an Accepting Attitude

There may be some aspects of interviewing traumatized people that make it hard for a clinician to maintain an accepting and therapeutic attitude. One of these circumstances is when the client expresses intense anger and agitation when recounting traumatic events. Sipprelle (1992) has observed that this is common when working with clients who are war veterans, and it applies to clients with many other types of trauma as well. He cautions that the clinician must be prepared to be exposed to intense anger and agitation without responding in a challenging or provocative way. In this situation, Sipprelle (1992) notes that a therapeutic stance of detachment and objectiveness will not be effective. This is easy to understand if you look at it from the client's point of view. You can imagine how upsetting it would be if you described a terrifying, disturbing, and infuriating experience to someone and she remained neutral and detached.

It may also be difficult to maintain an accepting attitude in situations when a client tells you something you find hard to believe. This may be because something in the client's manner gives you the impression that he is not being truthful or because you find the event itself implausible. There is little to be gained, however, by expressing doubt or disbelief of a client's reports during an assessment. If it is the client's manner that troubles you, be sure to make note of whatever verbal or nonverbal cues you observe. If you continue to doubt what you hear, you can always challenge the client later when you have a more firmly established relationship and more information about the client's motivations and general credibility. It is important to remember, though, that clients' demeanors when relating a traumatic event may vary greatly. For example, a client who relates a horrifying experience with little or no affect might well be experiencing the PTSD symptom of emotional numbing.

Sometimes during assessments, clients report events that are hard to believe because they are so horrible or extraordinary. In part, these events are hard to believe because we do not want to believe that such a thing could or would happen. Such reports might include experiences of inhumanity such as torture or the abuse of a child by a parent. You might have become even more skeptical of extreme reports given the widespread publicity and challenge in the 1990s to reports of adults who say they were abused by cults as children. These kinds of reports certainly require careful consideration and sometimes raise difficult ethical issues. Discussions of ethical issues relating to assessment and treatment of child abuse victims and to handling reports of delayed memories of trauma are available in Dalenberg (in press-b) and Dalenberg and Carlson (in press).

Helping Clients Overcome Avoidance

As discussed in Chapter 3, avoidance of traumatic reminders is a core response to trauma. Accordingly, traumatized people often have a powerful urge to avoid thinking about their trauma, even when they have come to you to for help (Newman et al., 1996; Resick & Schnicke, 1993). Your client may be very afraid even to talk about what has happened to her. She may avoid traumatic material directly by changing the subject or refusing to talk about it, or indirectly by dissociating and not hearing what you ask. You can help your client to overcome such avoidance by openly discussing fears and reluctance to discuss traumatic material at the beginning of the assessment process. Normalizing such fears and discussing them may help dispel them enough to allow assessment to proceed. You might introduce the notion to your client that a lot of people are hesitant to talk about terrible things that have happened to them and ask if that is true for her as well. It may also help to discuss what it is that makes it hard for her to talk about the trauma. Gil (1988) offers additional suggestions for beginning interviews with cleints who seem uncomfortable getting started.

If a client continues directly or indirectly to avoid traumatic material despite your efforts to dispel her anxiety, that may mean that she is not willing or not yet ready or able to discuss these details. It is important that you not push a client to go faster than is comfortable for her. Some clients become very disturbed when uncovering traumatic memories so that it is not possible to probe for details during the initial assessment (Litz & Weathers, 1994). Other clients are unable to verbalize their experience because they are so emotionally numb or withdrawn. Litz and Weathers (1994) suggest focusing first on developmental history with those who have difficulty discussing their trauma. In this way, you can establish rapport with your client and ease into the more difficult material later on. You should be especially cautious with clients whom you suspect are psychologically fragile or deteriorating as such clients may decompensate if stressed too much. As long as the purpose of the evaluation is clinical and not forensic, you can usually put off gathering details of traumatic experiences until later in treatment. Although it may be undesirable, you may sometimes have to proceed with treatment recommendations when you have incomplete information about a client's traumatic experiences.

Special Therapeutic Considerations for Particular Populations

If you assess clients you know have been through particular types of traumatic experiences, you should read further about special considerations and cautions when interviewing such clients. This is especially important to do if you are treating the client as well as assessing him. For example, establishing trust may be a major challenge with those clients who have experienced intentionally inflicted interpersonal traumas, such as rape, while maintaining an accepting attitude may be the greatest challenge with clients who are angry and aggressive, such as some combat veterans. There are readings available about interviewing and treating sexual assault victims (Harvey, Orbuch, Chwalisz, & Garwood, 1991; Resick & Schnicke, 1993; Resnick et al., 1996);

childhood sexual abuse survivors (Courtois, 1988; Gil, 1988; Herman, 1992; McCann & Pearlman, 1990); veterans (Carroll & Foy, 1992; Keane et al., 1996; Sipprelle, 1992); battered women (Dutton, 1992); bereaved persons (Raphael & Martinek, 1996); Asian American survivors of violence (Lee & Lu, 1989); children (McNally, 1991); and the elderly (Falk, Hersen, & Van Hasselt, 1994).

SUMMARY

This chapter began with information relevant to selecting measures for assessments. The parameters used to select the measures described in this book and the categories of information used in the measure profiles were explained. A step-by-step approach was then described that offers possible paths to pursue as you progress in the assessment of a client. This system includes flowcharts that you can use as guides in the assessment process. In regard to administering measures, suggestions were made for procedures to follow and for conducting therapeutic interviews with traumatized people.

Part III

MAKING USE OF
ASSESSMENT RESULTS

Chapter 9

Interpreting the Results and Making a Diagnosis

Once you have administered and scored the trauma and trauma response measures you have chosen for a client, you will be faced with the task of interpreting the results of your assessment. To most effectively interpret results and diagnose clients, it is important to be aware of a number of controversial issues regarding diagnosis of trauma-related disorders. When you examine the results of an assessment, they will sometimes paint a clear picture, and you will feel fairly certain that your client either does or does not have a diagnosable posttraumatic response. But for many clients, there will be ambiguities in the results of the assessment that make interpretation difficult. The first issue you must consider is the overall accuracy of the reports you have obtained in your assessment. Once you have made a determination about the accuracy of reports, you will be able to make quantitative and qualitative interpretations of the overall results of the measures used. These interpretations may need to be supplemented with additional information in order to make an accurate diagnosis. Finally, you need to consider how to discuss the results of the assessment with your client.

CONTROVERSIES RELEVANT TO DIAGNOSIS OF TRAUMA-RELATED DISORDERS

There are a number of controversies relating to assessment and diagnosis of trauma-related disorders that are important to keep in mind as you assess clients' traumatic experiences and responses. Many of these questions relate to whether the DSM-IV PTSD criteria are valid and adequate, and others relate to the difficulties in objectively assessing the criteria for dissociative disorders. Each of these controversies is discussed below along with its implications for assessment and diagnosis of trauma-related disorders.

Controversies Relevant to Diagnosis of PTSD

Should Criterion A Be Required?

Criterion A of the DSM-IV PTSD diagnosis essentially defines what is considered a traumatic stressor for the purpose of diagnosis of PTSD (see Chapter 2, p. 27). In response to concerns about the adequacy of Criterion A in DSM-III-R (Davidson & Foa, 1991; March, 1993), the criterion elements were altered considerably for DSM-IV. In DSM-III-R, a traumatic stressor was defined as an "event that is outside the range of usual human experience and that would be markedly distressing to almost anyone" (American Psychiatric Association, 1987, p. 250). This definition was thought to be inadequate, in part, because it did not permit inclusion of many stressors that do seem to produce traumatic stress. For example, some events that are within the range of usual human experience, such as being the victim of a crime, do often produce PTSD (Davidson & Foa, 1991). Furthermore, some events that are not "markedly distressing to almost anyone" also result in PTSD (Davidson & Foa, 1991; Scott & Stradling, 1994). The definition was also considered inadequate because it did not take into account a person's subjective perception of the event (March, 1993). The essential changes made to Criterion A for DSM-IV were to define the stressor event in terms of specific features or characteristics of events that are known to relate to PTSD development and to add a criterion element that reflects subjective perceptions by requiring that the response to the event involve fear, helplessness, or horror (American Psychiatric Association, 1994).

While these changes to Criterion A are considered an improvement over previous criteria by most trauma researchers and clinicians, there is still some question as to whether the stressor definition is sufficiently broad to accommodate all of the kinds of events that can produce PTSD. There are events that most clinicians would consider potentially traumatic that still do not seem to meet Criterion A-1. For example, it is unclear whether an incident of acquaintance rape actually meets Criterion A-1 if the victim did not fear physical injury or death, but, arguably, most women would experience this as a traumatic event. A case has been made that Criterion A should either be eliminated altogether or defined solely in terms of a subjective response to the event of shock (Solomon & Canino, 1990). On the other hand, some argue that broadening the criterion of a traumatic event to this extent would make the diagnosis potentially applicable to anyone experiencing intrusive recollections of even a mildly distressing event (March, 1993). Such a broad criterion might result in an unacceptably high number of false positive diagnoses.

This controversy becomes important to the assessment of traumatic events when a client's symptoms meet DSM-IV PTSD Criteria B, C, and D, but he has either experienced an event that does not seem to meet Criterion A-1 or reports no potentially traumatic events. In the first case, Criterion A-1 may simply be inadequate to accommodate a genuinely traumatic event. In the second case, because of disruptions of memory associated with trauma, a client may not recall a traumatic event that did occur (van der Kolk, 1996b). In both cases, clinicians must choose between following the DSM-IV criteria to the letter and making an exception to the criteria based on their diagnosis or clinical judgment. This choice is particularly problematic in forensic settings where strict adherence to DSM-IV criteria may be the norm.

Should the Diagnosis Focus on One Event?

Another controversy relating to the assessment and diagnosis of PTSD involves the measurement of symptoms in relation to a single traumatic event. Solomon and colleagues (1996) point out that the DSM-IV PTSD diagnostic criteria and most measures of PTSD symptomatology assume that the individual has had only one traumatic experience. If clients report symptoms related to a single traumatic event when they have experienced multiple traumatic events, they may underreport their symptoms and not appear to meet criteria for a diagnosis of PTSD when they are experiencing a full-blown PTSD response.

The other side of the controversy would be the position that symptoms should be measured in relation to only a single event. While I have not come across any arguments in the literature in favor of this position, the position clearly has advocates since the DSM-IV diagnostic criteria reflect this position.

The dilemma here for clinicians is that using a measure that allows reporting of symptoms that relate to multiple traumatic events (such as the Modified Posttraumatic Stress Symptom Scale or the Screen for Posttraumatic Stress Symptoms) means a departure from a strict application of the DSM criteria. This kind of departure seems to be one that trauma researchers and clinicians are increasingly willing to make. For example, the most recent edition of the CAPS allows reporting of symptoms related to up to three traumatic stressors (Blake et al., 1996).

Should the Patient Be Required to Connect C and D Symptoms to an Event?

Another controversy pertaining to the relationship between a DSM-IV PTSD Criterion A event and Criteria B, C, and D symptoms involves the necessity of linking the event to the symptoms. Most measures of PTSD symptoms have interpreted the PTSD diagnostic criteria in such a way that the client must identify a causal connection between the traumatic event and several of the current symptoms in order to meet the symptom criteria. For example, a client might be asked if he experiences physiological arousal in response to stimuli connected to the traumatic event. But some argue that this method of measurement will result in a failure to identify some symptoms that actually are present because the client may not see the connection between the symptom and the event (Solomon et al., 1996).

In this case, it seems that the clinician is not faced with too much of a dilemma. Since the DSM criteria specify only that the symptom and event are related and not that the client recognize this relationship, it seems in keeping with the criteria to measure symptoms more broadly and have the clinician determine whether there is a connection between the symptom and the event. For example, the client might be asked whether he is experiencing sudden unexpected increases in physiological arousal. The difficulty here lies in the fact that it may not be easy or possible for the clinician to make such a determination. Also, if symptoms are measured more broadly, measure scores might be erroneously high for some symptoms. Furthermore, some symptoms may be impossible to measure without a connection to trauma. For example, it may be impossible to measure behavioral avoidance of reminders of trauma if a client is not aware of the behavioral avoidance.

Do DSM-IV Criteria Accurately and Adequately Describe PTSD?

The publication of the DSM-IV diagnostic criteria for PTSD constitutes endorsement of the symptom criteria as accurate and adequate in describing posttraumatic stress reactions of duration of a month or more. There are several ways in which the particular symptom criteria for PTSD are controversial. First, Solomon and colleagues (Solomon et al., 1996) maintain that the categorization of PTSD symptoms in the DSM and the number of symptoms required for each category of symptoms are arbitrary. van der Kolk and McFarlane (1996a) make the point that avoidance and numbing symptoms, although in the same category in the DSM criteria, probably have very different physiological bases. In regard to the number of symptoms required to meet category criteria, it has been suggested that the required number of Criterion C (avoidance) symptoms should be only two rather than three (Davidson & Foa, 1991).

Another controversy involves whether there are particular symptoms of PTSD that are not adequately represented in the diagnostic criteria. For example, dissociation symptoms, while a prominent feature of the diagnostic criteria for ASD, are not well represented in the PTSD criteria. Arguably, dissociative symptoms should be included in criteria for PTSD, since they have been found to be prominent in persons experiencing a range of traumatic events (Classen et al., 1993; Putnam, 1995; Putnam & Carlson, 1997). Other symptoms observed in trauma survivors, but not included in the DSM criteria, include personality changes and self-harming behaviors. These symptoms are part of the DESNOS diagnosis described in Chapter 5 (p. 93). Field trial studies have supported the validity of this diagnostic category, but it has not yet been added to the DSM diagnostic system.

This raises the issue of whether posttraumatic symptoms vary in relation to the type of trauma experienced. As described in Chapter 5, Terr (1991) has proposed that PTSD may be manifested differently in those who experience a single traumatic event and those who experience a series of traumatic events or a prolonged traumatic stressor. Differences in the specific traumatic stressor experienced may also have an impact on the symptoms that follow. For example, PTSD symptoms in combat veterans and disaster victims may be different from those that follow rape. Whereas the DSM PTSD criteria seem to accurately describe the symptoms of combat veterans and disaster victims, it is less clear whether they adequately assess the sequelae of traumas such as rape. Rape experiences generally have profound impacts on self-esteem, identity, and relationships that are not well-represented in the DSM criteria. Similarly, it seems possible that PTSD symptoms may vary as a function of sex. For example, whereas aggressive behaviors might be a common symptom in male trauma survivors, female survivors may be more likely to direct aggression toward themselves in the form of self-harming behaviors. My own research shows a fairly strong and significant relationship between severity of childhood sexual abuse experiences and adult self-destructive behaviors in female psychiatric patients.

Clinicians have little choice, however, about which particular symptoms can be considered to constitute PTSD. It certainly is not practical to use a unique categorization system for symptoms or to choose your own cutoff criteria for the number of symptoms needed in each category. Similarly, you cannot add symptoms to the diagnostic criteria or use a diagnostic label that has not been officially recognized. Still, these issues are important for clinicians to keep in mind because, regardless of whether you determine that your client meets DSM criteria for PTSD, their actual posttraumatic symptoms will be of importance to your understanding of their trauma response and to treatment planning. Consequently, you should consider assessing symptoms such as dissociation symptoms, personality changes, and self-harming behaviors in addition to the PTSD symptom criteria.

Controversies Relevant to the Diagnosis of Dissociative Disorders

While the controversies relating to PTSD diagnosis revolve around the specific diagnostic criteria for PTSD, the major controversies that are relevant to the diagnosis of dissociative disorders focus on the very existence of dissociative disorders and their etiology. In particular, the validity of the diagnosis of dissociative identity disorder (DID, formerly multiple personality disorder) has been questioned, and the etiology of the disorder and its phenomenology have been the subject of much debate. Horevitz (1994) has provided a detailed discussion of these issues that highlights the fact that the debate over DID has tended to be polemical with those on all "sides" sometimes making errors in reasoning and logic as a result of strong identification with a particular conceptual paradigm. I briefly review the major controversies about the validity, etiology, and phenomenology of DID here, but clinicians who diagnose and treat dissociative disorders are encouraged to read Horevitz's discussion in detail.

Questions about the validity of the DID diagnosis have been accompanied by hypotheses about the phenomenology and etiology of conditions that clinicians label DID. The initial question raised is whether DID is, in fact, a bona fide clinical syndrome or whether the symptoms and behaviors associated with DID are the result of the influence of overzealous therapists. Some propose that therapists who are fascinated with the concept of "multiple personalities" or who believe that DID is highly prevalent among those with particular trauma histories may inadvertently cue their patients to report dissociative symptoms such as identity disturbances and memory deficits (Orne & Bauer-Manley, 1991). According to this model, what clinicians identify as DID is actually a pattern of reports and behaviors that have resulted from the combined effects of the client's suggestibility, social and interpersonal influence, expectancy effects, and demand characteristics (Horevitz, 1994). In this view, those diagnosed with DID are best understood as playing the role of a person with "multiple personalities."

Horevitz (1994) notes that this etiological explanation has not been applied to any other psychological disorder, despite the fact that the processes thought to produce DID operate similarly in interactions between clients with other diagnoses and their therapists. Furthermore, to date, no studies of identified DID patients have supported this etiological hypothesis. Results of laboratory studies of normal subjects that relate to the effects of suggestibility and social influence on behavior (from the fields of hypnosis, social psychology, and cognitive psychology) have arguably been overgeneralized in their application to DID (Horevitz, 1994).

On the other hand, many clinicians and researchers consider DID to be a bona fide psychological disorder (Michelson & Ray, 1996). This position is supported by the inclusion of DID in the DSM system and by empirical studies of those diagnosed with DID (Putnam, 1991b; Ross, 1997). Most of those who study and treat dissociative disorders believe the etiology of DID to be traumatic in nature, but understanding of the relationship between traumatic experiences and the kind of severe disturbances in identity and memory observed in DID has been limited to date. The development of detailed and testable theories about the precise mechanisms involved in the development of DID has been hampered by a lack of clarity in the definitions of traumatic experiences and of the phenomenon of dissociation.

Until recently, there has been little discussion of what makes events traumatic and exactly how the experience of such events interacts with an individual's perceptions, developmental level, and subsequent experiences to create a dissociative identity disorder. In addition, as discussed in Chapter 3, there is much confusion over the definition of dissociation. Very different definitions of dissociation are used by those studying the phenomenon in the context of hypnosis, in relation to cognitive processes, and in clinical settings. It may well be that these researchers are actually studying distinct, if related phenomena that have all been given the label of dissociation but that vary in terms of their psychological function and etiology.

Until issues surrounding the validity, etiology, and phenomenology of DID are clarified, it seems wise for clinicians to approach the diagnosis and treatment of DID with some caution. The power of therapist and client beliefs and expectations should not be underestimated. Although it is debatable how frequently it occurs, it certainly does seem possible that a therapist and client could unwittingly "collude" to convince themselves that the client has DID. This possibility is all the more worrisome in light of the likelihood that those with childhood histories of severely traumatic abuse may be particularly prone to suggestibility as a result of profound disturbances in identity and memory. Caution is warranted, then, in both the process and methods of assessment for DID and the interpretation of assessment results and diagnosis of DID. Sources of advice regarding diagnosis of dissociative disorders are offered below.

INTERPRETING THE RESULTS

Evaluating the Accuracy of Trauma and Symptom Reports

It is important to consider the overall accuracy of your client's reports of trauma and symptoms before interpreting results of particular measures. Your appraisal of the accuracy of these reports should inform your interpretation of the assessment results.

As discussed in detail in Chapter 6, it is possible for people to give inaccurate reports regarding both traumatic events and posttraumatic symptoms. Factors that might contribute to inaccuracy in reports include misunderstanding of the questions asked during the assessment; reporting of misperceptions, delusional beliefs, or fantasies; errors in reporting due to distortions in memory; and intentional misreporting. All of these factors should be kept in mind during the assessment process.

During the assessment, you should be alert to indications of your client's possible misunderstanding of the questions being asked. An example of such a misunderstanding might be if a disaster victim answered "Yes" to having feelings of estrangement or detachment from others but was really only feeling estranged from a few people who he felt "wouldn't understand" (Weiss, 1993). There would, of course, be no way to detect this type of misunderstanding from the results of a self-report measure. That is one reason why it is so important to follow up a high brief scale score with a structured interview. One way to detect such misinterpretation of questions in a structured interview is to ask for clarification or elaboration. You can prompt a client to clarify by saying, "I'm not sure I understand exactly what you mean." To prompt for elaboration, you might ask a client to tell you more about a particular experience of a symptom or you might ask for a different example of a symptom. Use of such prompts for clarification should not affect the results of a structured interview as long as you have already asked the initial question in its original form.

A client's report of an event that is outside the realm of the possible is an indication that she may be reporting a misperception, delusion, or fantasy. For example, a client might report having been traumatized by an alien abduction as a child. As mentioned in Chapter 6, it is important to keep in mind, however, that reports of fantastic events are not necessarily an indication of a lack of credibility of all of the client's reports. In fact, a recent study of children's abuse experience reports found that reports containing fantastic elements were more frequent in reports of those known to have been abused than in reports from a control group of children whose reports had not been corroborated (Dalenberg, 1996).

Errors in reporting due to inaccuracies in memory might include either underreporting or overreporting of past events. One possible indicator of such errors might be an extreme discrepancy between the trauma experiences reported and the symptoms associated with them. For example, a client who reports no past traumatic experiences, but reports severe PTSD symptoms, may be amnestic for past trauma experiences or may be overreporting PTSD symptoms. Similarly, a client who reports severe and distressing traumatic events, but denies any related PTSD symptoms, may be overreporting traumatic events or underreporting symptoms. It is important to remember, however, that because there is great individual variation in responses to trauma, an unusually mild or severe response to trauma may occur in some of your clients. Therefore, a discrepancy in trauma and response reports alone is not necessarily an indicator of misreporting. If you observe such discrepancies, it is advisable to gather additional information to clarify the reason for the discrepancy. For example, perhaps a client who reports no PTSD symptoms following a traumatic event received a great deal of social support that ameliorated symptoms within a few weeks. Or perhaps a client who reports extremely severe PTSD symptoms following a relatively mild trauma has experienced an earlier trauma that went unresolved, or perhaps he was under stress from other sources at the time of a mild trauma.

Another way that memory distortions might lead to misreporting is that a client may come to believe that traumatic events happened to him because of the influence of previous experiences in therapy. If a client reports that traumatic memories surfaced during therapy with another therapist, it is a good idea to find out more about what methods were used to explore traumatic memory. You can ask the client about this, but you should also try to obtain permission to talk directly with the previous therapist to get more information about the context in which the traumatic memories emerged. Causes for concern about the credibility of memories might include memories that arose only during hypnosis, during sodium amytal interviews, or as a result of pressure from a therapist. Another cause of concern might be a client's expression of doubt over whether the traumatic experiences really happened or not. Although one study has found no relationship between a person's level of certainty about past early abuse experiences and the actual occurrence of abuse (Williams, 1995), in another study, clients' doubts were found to significantly predict the likelihood of finding no supportive evidence for abuse (Dalenberg, in press-a). It is still unclear, then, whether doubt about traumatic experiences is an indicator of the accuracy of trauma reports.

You should also be alert to any indications of intentional misreporting that might be the result of the desire for personal gain, attention, retribution, or leniency when the client is accused of a crime. You typically have no information about the veracity of reports from clients on any subject, and traumatic experience or responses are no exception. Usually, this is not of great concern, and you tend to take reports either at face value or with a grain of salt given your knowledge of the client's general credibility. But you may feel especially pressed to determine the credibility of a trauma report under some circumstances. For example, if you are assessing a child, you will need to make a judgment about the credibility of a report of child abuse because you may be legally required to report suspicion of abuse to authorities.

One aid in making a judgment about the credibility of a client's reports is your assessment of that client's credibility on other issues. You may want to interview a client about other aspects of his life in order to assess his overall credibility. Information about a client's response style may also be useful. Validity scales of inventories such as the MMPI, the MCMI, and the TSI (see p. 255 in the Measure Profiles) may shed light on an unusual reporting style (Newman et al., 1996). Caution is warranted in such interpretations, however, since results of validity scales can sometimes be misleading. For example, a high F scale score on the MMPI might be an indication of overreporting, but research has shown that F scale scores are elevated in trauma survivors because the F scale contains trauma-related symptom items (Carlson & Armstrong, 1994).

The possibility of secondary gain can also be explored directly by asking clients about possible financial gain, retribution motives, or desire to reduce culpability for some offense. If you suspect that secondary gain issues may be influencing a client's reports, you should seek guidance specific to assessments in a forensic context, since those assessment methods focus more on the issue of credibility. A number of good sources on conducting forensic assessments are cited in Chapter 6 (p. 126).

Challenging or questioning a client's reports at the time of assessment is unlikely to clarify accuracy of reports and is likely to damage the therapeutic relationship. While you should certainly ask whatever questions you need to to help you establish the credibility of client reports, it is almost always advisable to wait until you know a client well to address issues of credibility directly. Also, you should keep in mind that some things clients tell you are hard to believe because you have a strong desire not to believe them. Some reports of intentional harm might be especially difficult to believe because, if they are true, it means that the world is a more dangerous place and people are more evil than you would like to believe. An example of this is the initial widespread disbelief in the United States about reports of Holocaust death camps. This example illustrates how even extremely horrible and extremely unlikely events do sometimes occur.

The Influence of Cultural Background and Situational Factors on Symptom Reports

A person's cultural background and current situation can have a strong influence on her symptom reports. Clients who are from another country or from an American subculture such as an urban Hispanic culture might underreport symptoms for a number of reasons. One reason might be differences in cultural norms for a particular symptom. For example, it would be difficult to apply the PTSD criterion for restricted range of affect to a Japanese American client because norms for expressing emotions are very different in Japanese culture than in "mainstream" American culture. Another reason for underreporting of symptoms might be the client's lack of familiarity with some of the symptoms you are asking about. For example, if you were using the CAPS to inquire about a client's sense of a foreshortened future, you would ask, "Have there been times when you felt there is no need to plan for the future, that somehow your future will be cut short?" (Blake et al., 1996). If your client were a Southeast Asian immigrant who believes in reincarnation, it might be very difficult for him to answer the question. The answer to the first part would be "Yes" and the answer to the second part would be "No," but neither answer might actually be related to a traumatic experience. Similarly, situational factors might make a question difficult to answer or might make the question moot. If a disaster victim has lost his home and had his life disrupted, it might not make sense to ask whether he has lost interest in former activities since the event.

There is also cultural variation in willingness to report psychological symptoms. In fact, mainstream U.S. culture probably has fewer prohibitions against such reports than almost any other culture or any American subculture. For example, according to researchers studying trauma responses in Southeast Asian refugees, clients from Southeast Asian and Chinese cultures will more readily report somatic symptoms than psychological symptoms (Lee & Lu, 1989). Awareness of cultural variation in responses to trauma will be especially important if you are assessing or treating clients who are from a culture that is very different from mainstream U.S. culture. Good resources for cultural considerations in the assessment of trauma are Keane and colleagues (Keane, Kaloupek, et al., 1996), Manson (1996), Lu and colleagues (1995), and Marsella and Kameoka (1989). Some good general resources for information about cultural variation in responses to trauma include Marsella and colleagues (Marsella, Friedman, Gerrity et al., 1996), deVries (1996), Dinicola (1996), Wilson and Raphael (1993), and Krippner (1994).

Interpreting the Results of Self-Report Symptom Measures

In addition to serving as screening devices to determine who you need to assess further, most self-report symptom measures of trauma responses can provide useful information about the level of severity of symptoms. In order to decide whether the results of a self-report measure indicate a need for further assessment or to judge the level of severity of symptoms, you need normative information about the measures you use. Norms allow you to compare your client's score on a measure to those of a large sample of subjects from a given population. You can use norms to determine how many standard deviations your client scored above or below the average for a given population. For some measures, such norms are well-developed and extensive. For example, the TSI and TSCC have norms for both sexes and different ages for large general population samples (Briere, 1996a; Briere, 1996b). Usually, norms are established that allow comparison to general population samples rather than to a treatment or clinical sample.

For most trauma response self-report measures, formal norms are not available. For these measures, you can use the means and standard deviations for various clinical groups and normal control groups for comparison. For example, if you gave the Posttraumatic Stress Diagnostic Scale to a woman who had been raped, you might compare her score to the mean score of a sample of rape victims and to the mean for a sample of nonclinical control subjects. Standard deviations of scores in these comparison groups would be useful for determining how far from the mean of a particular group your client scored. You can adopt a decision rule for further assessment based on such comparisons. For example, a reasonable criterion for further assessment might be a score that is either one or more standard deviations above the mean for a control group or is within one standard deviation of the mean for a traumatized group. Suggestions for decision rules for further assessment may be given in a measure's manual or in an article about the scale.

There are a number of cautions for the interpretation of self-report measure scores. First, the best comparison group for norms or group means is one that is appropriate for your particular client. For example, if your client is a rape victim, a sample of combat veterans will not be the appropriate comparison group. Also, you should be aware that there is a great deal of individual variation in scoring on self-report measures.

Means reported for groups of subjects sometimes obscure this fact. It is usually the case that some individuals who are traumatized will score relatively low on a self-report measure, and some individuals who are not traumatized will score relatively high. Also, as Weiss (1993) notes, the relationship between mean scale scores on a self-report measure and membership in a particular diagnostic category can vary as well. For example, the mean score of different samples of disaster victims diagnosed with PTSD might be very different on the same scale, depending on aspects of the trauma and how long after the traumatic event the measure was administered.

You should keep in mind that a self-report measure is never a definitive indicator of diagnosis and can sometimes be misleading. A client may not appear to meet criteria based on the results of a brief scale but may still have PTSD. For example, a client may not report high levels of anxiety or intrusive thoughts or images because she is using drugs or alcohol to dampen her emotions and cognitive processes (Dutton, 1992; Newman et al., 1996). Such a client might not currently meet criteria for PTSD, but she would if she stopped using alcohol and drugs. Other PTSD symptoms might be masked in a similar manner, such as lack of anxiety in someone who takes antianxiety medication.

Similarly, a very high score on a self-report measure does not necessarily indicate that the client fits into a particular diagnostic category. This is particularly true of measures that include symptoms that occur in people with various disorders. For example, if a client reports on a PTSD screen that she has difficulty concentrating, poor sleep, physiological arousal, and loss of interest in former activities, but she does not endorse any reexperiencing or avoidance symptoms, you might reasonably conclude that the results probably reflect problems with anxiety or depression rather than a posttraumatic response. Similarly, a high score on a dissociation scale does not necessarily mean that the client has a dissociative disorder. Persons with other diagnoses, such as PTSD, can also score fairly high on a dissociation scale. Also, because of the different forms dissociation takes, a high score can result from high levels of normative or nonpathological dissociative experiences rather than from pathological dissociation symptoms. Technically, a person who scores high on a measure, but does not have the target diagnosis, is referred to as a "false positive." That is because the scale score indicates that the person is "positive" for the diagnosis when she actually does not have the diagnosis.

Consideration of the relationship between false positive diagnoses and the positive predictive value of a measure makes a convincing case that one can never rely on self-report measure results to make a diagnosis. The positive predictive value of a measure is the proportion of the number of people who score high on the measure and who really do have the target diagnosis (the "true positives") to the number of people who score high ("true positives" plus "false positives"). It turns out that even if a measure has a very favorable true positive rate (sensitivity) and a very good true negative rate (specificity), it can still have a low positive predictive value. That is because the positive predictive value is affected by the base rate of the target disorder in the population being studied. The base rate of a disorder is simply the prevalence of the disorder in the population of interest. A low disorder base rate will drive down the positive predictive value of a measure regardless of the measure's capacity to accurately identify persons with the target diagnosis or persons who do not have the target diagnosis.

An example of this phenomenon is the relatively low positive predictive value of dissociation scales to predict a dissociative disorder diagnosis despite acceptable levels of sensitivity and specificity. Because dissociative disorders are fairly rare, even in psychiatric populations, most of those with high dissociation scale scores will actually be "false positives." These persons may have PTSD or some other trauma-related disorder, but they do not have a dissociative disorder. Although this problem is greatest for measures that do not specifically assess diagnostic criteria for a disorder or that target diagnoses that are rare (such as dissociative disorders), it also affects measures that closely parallel diagnostic criteria and target diagnoses that are less rare (such as PTSD). A false positive in the form of a high score on a PTSD measure can easily occur because many of the symptoms for PTSD are not specific to PTSD. This issue is discussed further below on p. 181. The bottom line is that one must always gather detailed information and use clinical judgment to make a diagnosis.

Interpreting the Results of Structured Interviews

Structured interviews provide the kind of detailed information about the experience of potentially traumatic events and posttraumatic symptoms that a clinician needs to make a DSM diagnosis of a trauma-related disorder. DSM criteria for both PTSD and ASD specify that exposure to a traumatic event is required for the diagnosis. Although the DSM does not specify a trauma criterion for any of the dissociative disorders, these are generally thought to be trauma-related disorders (Putnam, 1985; Putnam, 1995; Ross, 1997; Steinberg, 1994). Furthermore, although the criterion of exposure to a trauma is controversial (as discussed above), many clinicians still find it very useful to assess traumatic experiences carefully.

Traumatic events checklists or self-report scales for traumatic events can be used to determine whether the client has been exposed to a traumatic event, but you will need more information to determine whether the client fully meets Criterion A. To fully meet Criterion A, the client must have experienced both an event that involved actual or threatened death (Criterion A-1), and he must have had a response involving intense fear, helplessness, or horror (Criterion A-2) (see DSM-IV PTSD Criteria in Chapter 5, p. 78) (American Psychiatric Association, 1994). Clinicians need to be careful of error in either direction when making Criterion A determinations. Error in the form of believing that someone has experienced a traumatic event when he has not might occur if a client understands the word "traumatic" to mean "very bad or upsetting." Frequently, traumatic events reported in the "other" category on self-report measures or trauma interviews are actually upsetting experiences that do not meet Criterion A (Norris & Riad, 1996).

On the other hand, you also want to avoid believing that someone has not experienced a traumatic event when he has. It is possible for a seemingly nontraumatic event to cause considerable PTSD symptomatology (Litz & Weathers, 1994). This can happen because a client's subjective appraisal of an event is a key factor in the development of PTSD. For example, the sudden death of a pet might be traumatic to someone who was very emotionally attached to her pet or who felt responsible for the death. It is also possible that a client does not report a traumatic event that actually occurred because of a reluctance to report (for instance, reluctance to report a rape) or because of amnesia for the event (see Chapter 7). In addition, as noted earlier, recent stressful events can trigger PTSD responses in those with unresolved prior traumas.

In determining whether clients have a particular trauma-related disorder, you must also decide if they meet the symptom criteria for a particular disorder. As discussed in detail above, one difficulty with the DSM symptom criteria for PTSD and ASD is that they link symptoms to a single traumatic event. Arguably, one should assess symptoms related to any Criterion A event, not just one (Resnick et al., 1996). For all trauma-related disorders, it may be relatively easy to decide whether a client meets a particular criterion, or it may be difficult. There are many trauma-related symptoms that are very similar to symptoms of other disorders. For example, it may be hard to distinguish between intrusive thoughts of a traumatic experience and obsessive intrusive thoughts. Similarly, in the diagnosis of DID, the presence of two or more distinct identities or personality states may be difficult to distinguish from the kind of extreme variations in personality and behavior seen in disorders such as Borderline Personality Disorder (BPD). Sources of detailed advice about making distinctions about symptoms include Weiss (1993) (for assessing criteria for PTSD) and Steinberg (1994, 1995) (for dissociative disorders).

MAKING A DIAGNOSIS

There are several diagnoses specific to trauma listed in DSM-IV. Prominent among these are PTSD, ASD, and the dissociative disorders, which are all described in Chapter 5 (pp. 77–82, 91–92). Many other DSM diagnostic categories may also apply to traumatized clients. And while you may or may not have confidence in the validity of DSM diagnoses, most clinicians find it useful and often necessary to be knowledgeable about them.

Ideally, a diagnosis of a trauma-related disorder should be made based on information from a variety of sources and should never be made based on the results of only one measure (Finch & Daugherty, 1993). Collecting additional information about a client's psychosocial history and other symptoms will be necessary to put a client's traumatic experience into the context of his entire life. It is also important to note that some structured interviews allow you to obtain much more diagnostically relevant information than others. You might well have enough information from a very extensive interview such as the CAPS or the SCID-D to make a diagnosis, but other interviews are not likely to provide all the information you would need.

Newman and colleagues (Newman et al., 1996) suggest that clinicians look for convergence in the results from several measures and sources of information when making a diagnosis. When results of different measures or from different sources of information conflict, more evidence can be sought to reconcile differences. For example, one should be sure to assess functional impairment by finding out about the degree of disruption in a client's work or social functioning. Although this is one of the diagnostic criteria for PTSD, it is not measured explicitly in many self-report and structured interview measures of PTSD. Physiological measures can also be used to obtain diagnostic information that is independent of the client's self-report. Litz and Weathers (1994) offer suggestions for measures of physiological reactivity that do not require use of standardized stimuli or expensive equipment. Independent information about a client's symptoms might also be obtained from family members of a client who are in a position to observe the client's behavior.

Another source of information that might help reconcile conflicting results from scales and interviews might be information about response style from general inventory validity scales (Newman et al., 1996). As noted above in regard to assessing the credibility of a client's reports, the MMPI, the MCMI, and the TSI all have validity scales that may shed light on a client's response to symptom measures. In addition to providing information about possible overreporting of symptoms, validity scales can sometimes detect a reporting style characterized by guardedness and underreporting of symptoms. Caution is warranted, however, regarding use of the F scale of the MMPI (see discussion on p. 7).

Conflicting results of measures can also occur because many trauma-related symptoms are not specific to trauma-related disorders. Endorsement of these items can lead to erroneously high scores on measures. The most problematic nonspecific symptoms are those PTSD symptoms that overlap with anxiety disorders and affective disorders. In some ambiguous cases, information about the presence of comorbid disorders may be very helpful in making a differential diagnosis of a trauma-related disorder (Newman et al., 1996). For example, careful assessment of premorbid anxiety symptoms may be helpful in making a differential diagnosis between PTSD and other anxiety disorders. Suggestions regarding the differential diagnosis of PTSD and other disorders can be found in Blank (1994) and McNally and Saigh (1993).

Assessment of other factors may also help clarify conflicting results of trauma and symptom measures. For example, assessment of a client's social support following a traumatic event may help explain inconsistencies between reported events and symptoms. A person who experienced a mildly traumatic event may have great symptomatology as a result of receiving no social support following the event. On the other hand, a person who experienced a severe traumatic event may show relatively little symptomatology as a result of receiving extensive social support following the event.

As discussed in Chapter 7 (p. 131), diagnosis of trauma-related disorders should also involve the consideration of other psychological disorders. Research has shown that people who meet criteria for PTSD also often meet criteria for a number of other psychological disorders (Keane & Wolfe, 1990). Personality disorders that are diagnosed on Axis II of DSM are also important because they may affect the presentation of a trauma-related disorder. Whether Axis II personality disorders might also be traumatic in etiology or whether they simply co-occur with trauma-related disorders, they are likely to have a considerable impact on interpretation of assessment results and treatment planning. Comorbid conditions may occur because traumatized persons are at greater risk for developing psychological disorders or because those with psychological disorders are at greater risk for being traumatized after a highly stressful event. Consideration of the possible etiology of comorbid disorders is important because symptoms with different causes may require different treatment approaches.

Diagnosis of dissociative disorders is somewhat more difficult than for PTSD or ASD, in part because self-report measures of dissociation and structured interviews for dissociative disorders do not closely parallel the DSM diagnostic criteria for these disorders. In addition, the diagnostic criteria are far less detailed for dissociative disorders and do not include a great number of symptoms and behaviors that are thought to be characteristic of the disorders. Detailed advice for translating results of assessments into a diagnosis can be found in Cardeña and Spiegel (1996), Steinberg (1994, 1995), Allen and Smith (1993), and Carlson and Armstrong (1994). Finally, the controversies about the diagnosis of DID discussed above (pp. 170–172) should be kept in mind when you are making diagnoses of dissociative disorders.

Diagnosis of trauma-related disorders in children is particularly difficult, largely because the manifestation of these disorders in children is not yet well understood. The fact that measurement development for trauma-related symptoms in children has lagged behind development of measures for adults has further hampered progress in this area. There are considerable difficulties in the diagnosis of both PTSD and dissociative disorders in children.

In the case of child clients, even information obtained from an extensive interview such as the CAPS-CA is unlikely to be adequate for diagnosis of PTSD because of children's more limited insight and verbal abilities and because of the ambiguity of many trauma symptoms in children. Finch and Daugherty (1993) note that trauma-related avoidance may be especially hard to assess in children. Children may not be aware of the connection between a traumatic event and their avoidance behaviors, or they may attempt to minimize the importance of the traumatic event by denying avoidance symptoms. Another symptom that may be especially difficult to assess in children is a sense of foreshortened future (McNally, 1991). The symptom is difficult to assess partly because of varying definitions of researchers and of children of what constitutes a "foreshortened" future and partly because it is still unclear how many nontraumatized children experience a sense of foreshortened future because of realistic appraisals of dangerous living environments.

Most of the work on diagnosis of dissociative disorders has focused on the diagnosis of DID and DDNOS. As discussed in Chapter 6 (pp. 116–118), there are great difficulties inherent in assessing children's internal states and external behaviors. Added to this problem is the fact that the kind of fluctuations in internal states, identity, and behavior that are central to a dissociative disorder are also part and parcel of normal children's behavior. The extremely complex clinical presentations of children diagnosed with dissociative disorders make differential diagnosis particularly difficult (Hornstein & Putnam, 1992). More detailed discussions of the diagnosis of dissociative disorders in children are available in Putnam and colleagues (Putnam, 1997; Putnam, Hornstein, & Peterson, 1996), Hornstein (1996), Steinberg (1996), Lewis (1996), and Peterson (1990, 1991).

DISCUSSING ASSESSMENT RESULTS AND DIAGNOSIS WITH YOUR CLIENT

Discussing the results of assessments and diagnosis with clients can be difficult and challenging. Some clients may be very concerned about determining exactly what happened to them early in life. While you want to take your client's concerns seriously, you do not want to give the impression that you know or can find out exactly what a client has experienced. Some clients may be certain that abuse or some other events occurred and may put pressure on you to confirm their beliefs. Others may come into treatment with the hope or expectation that you will be able to tell them or help them determine what really happened to them in the past. Still others may hope that examination of their memories or hypnosis will lead to certainty about past events. With all of these clients, it is important to explain that you do not know what happened to them and there is no way to determine this for certain through therapy. Regardless of whether you believe that the events did occur or you have doubts about their veracity, you should try to maintain neutrality on this question. At the same time, it is important to be sensitive to clients' strong desire to be believed and to have their memories validated. It may be helpful to explain to your client the intricacies of memory and the reasons why people sometimes believe they "remember" events that did not actually happen. Suggestions about educating clients about these issues in Chapter 6 (pp. 114–115) should be helpful to you in this regard.

In discussing assessment results with your clients, it is helpful to demystify the assessment process and dispel the notion that a scale or test somehow "knows" what is "wrong" with a client. You can explain to clients that scales, inventories, and interviews are simply tools to gather the answers to a large number of questions and to analyze those answers for particular patterns. If the pattern of answers about current symptoms that your client reports matches that of a group of people with a particular diagnosis or condition, then the two of you should consider whether that diagnosis may be an accurate description of the client's current psychological condition. It is also helpful to explain that results on a particular measure are not necessarily definitive as they can be affected by a wide range of individual and situational factors.

Discussion of diagnosis with your clients should also be undertaken with care. You may find a diagnosis to be helpful to you in conceptualizing your client's response and planning treatment, but information about diagnosis can lead to problems if clients misunderstand the purport of a diagnostic label. Many clients may ascribe characteristics to having a diagnosis that are not valid. For example, a client may believe that if she "has" a particular diagnosis, then she is not fully responsible for her symptoms. A client may feel less empowered to change if she has a diagnosed "condition." For this reason, it is important to explain that the diagnosis may simply be a descriptive label for a pattern of symptoms rather than an explanation of the cause or reasons for your client's difficulties. Along with information about a diagnostic label, be sure you convey your understanding of your client's psychological problems and your ideas about addressing them.

SUMMARY

In this chapter, controversies relevant to diagnosis of trauma-related disorders were described so that they can inform the interpretation of assessment results and diagnosis. Advice was offered on interpretation of the results of trauma and trauma response measures. This includes information about evaluating the accuracy of trauma and symptom reports, being sensitive to the potential influence of cultural background, interpreting the results of self-report measures and structured interviews, and making a diagnosis. Suggestions were also offered about discussing the assessment results and diagnosis with your client.

Chapter 10

Where to Go from Here: Treatment Options

Once you have administered and interpreted the results of an assessment, you can begin treatment planning. A wide variety of treatments have been developed for trauma-related disorders, and many of these are described in detail in books and articles that are readily available. Although it is beyond the scope of this book to describe treatment options in detail, this chapter briefly reviews some of the most well-developed treatments. Sources of more comprehensive information about treatment of trauma-related disorder include Williams and Sommer (1994a), Meichenbaum (1994), Wilson and Raphael (1993), van der Kolk and colleagues (van der Kolk, McFarlane, & Weisaeth, 1996), Foy (1992), Saigh (1992), Kluft and Fine (1993), and Lynn and Rhue (1994).

The material in this chapter is organized to correspond to the path you are likely to follow when making choices about treatments. Since the first consideration is whether you are treating an adult or a child, these treatments are covered separately. The next treatment decision is likely to involve a choice between individual treatment and group treatment. Within the section on adult treatments, I have first described some more generic or global approaches to treatment and then reviewed treatments that are specific in terms of their theoretical orientation. The next sections cover individual treatments designed for specific trauma populations and group treatments for adults. Much less professional literature is available describing treatments for traumatized children. The section on child treatment includes coverage of general individual treatment models, individual treatments for specific populations, and group treatments.

Before you choose a treatment method, you certainly want to know something about its effectiveness in treating trauma symptoms. The efficacy of treatments for PTSD have been studied, and many approaches appear to be promising or clearly effective in the populations studied. Solomon and colleagues (Gerrity & Solomon, 1996; Solomon et al., 1992) reviewed the results of randomized, clinical trials of various treatment methods. They report that behavioral methods involving systematic desensitization and flooding have been effective in reducing intrusion symptoms in several controlled studies. Cognitive methods have been demonstrated to be effective in reducing a range of PTSD symptoms. Results of the one study that has investigated psychodynamic methods of trauma treatment indicate that these methods may also be effective in reducing PTSD symptoms. But definitive conclusions about the *relative* efficacy of treatments for particular traumas or populations are not yet possible because of methodological limitations of studies (Gerrity & Solomon, 1996; Solomon et al., 1992). Because studies examined treatment effects in subjects with different trauma types, gender, and trauma recency, and because they assessed the efficacy of treatments with different measures and different follow-up periods, it is not possible to compare the effectiveness of treatment methods across studies. Until more controlled studies are completed, clinicians should understand that results of a treatment study may not generalize to populations other than that studied. In other words, a treatment that was studied and found to work well for combat veterans or rape victims may not work as well for victims of other traumas.

In addition to choosing a treatment method, a number of other decisions must be made before beginning treatment. Litz and Weathers (1994) offer valuable advice on ways to incorporate the results of assessments into your client's treatment. Litz and Weathers (1994) also discuss several essential questions that you need to address. These questions involve: the safety of your client's environment, your client's current capacity for tolerating the stress of uncovering trauma memories, the need to address concurrent problems such as substance abuse before beginning treatment, and the need for pharmacotherapy. While you may or may not have the training to administer pharmacotherapy as part of treatment, you should be knowledgeable about biological and pharmacological aspects of treatment. If pharmacotherapy seems indicated for a client, you may want to collaborate with a psychiatrist in order to provide this as an adjunctive treatment. Good sources of information on biological and pharmacological aspects of trauma treatment include Davidson and van der Kolk (1996), Friedman (1993, 1994), Marmar and colleagues (Marmar, Foy, Kagan, & Pynoos, 1993), and Lin and colleagues (Lin, Poland, Anderson, & Lesser, 1996).

Another issue that you need to consider regardless of the treatment method you choose is the possible role of ethnic and cultural factors in your client's symptoms and treatment. Introductions to ethnocultural aspects of posttraumatic responses can be found in Marsella and colleagues (Marsella, Friedman, & Spain, 1996) and Kirmayer (1996). Chapters in Marsella and colleague's book on ethnocultural aspects of PTSD (Marsella, Friedman, Gerrity, et al., 1996) examine the phenomenology of PTSD in various ethnic minority groups including African Americans (Allen, 1996), Hispanic Americans (Hough, Canino, Abueg, & Gusman, 1996), American Indians (Manson et al., 1996; Robin, Chester, & Goldman, 1996), Asian Americans (Abueg & Chun, 1996), and children (Dinicola, 1996). Good sources of information about ethnocultural aspects of trauma treatment include Draguns (1996), Gusman and colleagues (1996), and Krippner (1994).

Finally, there are a number of issues related to the process of psychotherapy that are important to all trauma treatments. Turner and colleagues (Turner, McFarlane, & van der Kolk, 1996) discuss many of these issues including intimacy and interpersonal safety, intuitive aspects of treatment interventions, the "victim" and "patient" roles that clients play, barriers to successful treatment, and countertransference issues. Other useful sources that focus on the client–therapist relationship in trauma treatment are Pearlman and Saakvitne (1995) and Stamm (1995). One other psychotherapy process issue discussed by van der Kolk and colleagues (van der Kolk, McFarlane, & van der Hart, 1996) that applies to all therapies is planning for and dealing with client noncompliance.

TREATMENTS FOR ADULTS

Despite the lack of definitive evidence for the efficacy of most adult treatments for trauma-related disorders, a wide variety of treatments and methods have been developed and described in the professional literature. These include: individual treatment models that are general or eclectic and interventions grounded in particular theoretical orientations; individual treatments designed for specific trauma populations (including those with dissociative disorders); and group treatments.

Individual Treatment Models

Several authors have described general approaches to treatment of traumas. These generic models can provide a framework for treatment regardless of the particular treatment techniques used. Williams and Sommer (1994b) have proposed a four-stage model for treatment based on the techniques, methods, and strategies described by various authors in the chapters of the *Handbook of Posttraumatic Therapy*. In stage one of the model, the goals are to establish a safe environment, a therapeutic relationship, and an initial diagnosis; to educate the client about trauma responses; and to begin to establish control over self-destructive behaviors and the symptoms of PTSD. Stage two includes working with traumatic memories and using adjunctive therapies including medications. The tasks of stage three involve restructuring of maladaptive belief systems and working on social skills and emotional intimacy. The fourth and final stage of the model focuses on finding intellectual and spiritual meaning in the trauma, initiating social action relating to the trauma, efforts toward preventing future distress, and termination.

van der Kolk and colleagues (van der Kolk, McFarlane, & van der Hart, 1996) describe a general approach to treatment of PTSD that is similar in many ways to the model proposed by Williams and Sommer (1994b). In their model, van der Kolk et al. set forth the basic principle that the aim of therapy with traumatized clients is to help them move from being haunted by the past and reactive to traumatic stimuli to being fully engaged in life and capable of reacting adaptively. To accomplish this aim, the authors propose that psychotherapy must both decondition anxiety responses and reestablish feelings of personal efficacy. According to their model, treatment should proceed through five phases of stabilization: education and identification of feelings, deconditioning of traumatic memories and responses, restructuring of personal schemas, reestablishment of secure social connections and interpersonal efficacy, and accumulation of restitutional emotional experiences (van der Kolk, McFarlane, & van der Hart, 1996).

Ochberg (1993) has described a general model for treatment that is holistic and eclectic in nature. The treatment he calls posttraumatic therapy rests on three fundamental principles. These principles emphasize the importance of normalizing traumatic responses, the role of a collaborative therapeutic relationship in helping clients overcome reexperiencing symptoms and negative emotions, and the notion that each client will follow a unique path to recovery from traumatic stress. The guidelines for treatment detailed by Ochberg are likely to be particularly useful to clinicians with little previous experience or training in the treatment of trauma survivors.

Behavioral and cognitive-behavioral approaches to the treatment of traumatic stress are based on a behavioral theoretical foundation. According to behavioral theory (explained in Chapter 3, pp. 41–42), through classical and operant conditioning, previously neutral stimuli become associated with traumatic events, and avoidance of trauma-related stimuli increases because it is reinforced by a decrease in anxiety. Cognitive and emotional aspects of traumatic experiences also seem to play important roles in the development and maintenance of traumatic responses (see Chapter 3, pp. 42–43). A number of interventions based on behavioral and cognitive-behavioral models have been developed for the treatment of PTSD. Although some may conceptualize behavioral treatments of PTSD to operate primarily by reducing fearful associations to trauma-related stimuli, it seems that cognitive and emotional aspects of trauma responses are also elicited and treated during behavioral interventions (Foa & Kozak, 1986). Consequently, some interventions that are very similar in nature may be considered behavioral by some and cognitive-behavioral by others. Other interventions that focus directly on modifying cognitive elements of trauma responses (usually in addition to addressing traumatic associations) are referred to as cognitive-behavioral or cognitive interventions. With these vagaries of nomenclature in mind, I refer to interventions that focus directly on modifying cognitions as cognitive-behavioral and those that do not as behavioral.

Rothbaum and Foa (1996) provide a detailed review of behavioral and cognitive-behavioral interventions, along with suggestions for successful use of these techniques. I briefly describe several prominent and related behavioral techniques and two popular treatments that have major cognitive components. It is worth noting that, in general, the behavioral and cognitive-behavioral treatments are time-limited treatments with the number of sessions ranging from just a few to as many as 20.

One behavioral treatment method called "systematic desensitization" involves gradual imaginal exposure to feared stimuli combined with training in relaxation. Even though systematic desensitization methods have appeared to reduce PTSD symptoms in a number of studies, Rothbaum and Foa (1996) favor the use of exposure to traumatic stimuli without relaxation because they found that the relaxation component is not necessary to obtain symptom reduction and may actually reduce the effectiveness of the exposure for some people. Exposure techniques can be either imaginal or *in vivo;* those involving extended exposure or exposure to high-intensity stimuli are often referred to as "flooding." Some caution is recommended in use of exposure-based techniques (Falsetti & Resnick, 1994; Kilpatrick & Best, 1984; Solomon et al., 1992) because of concern that the techniques may exacerbate some symptoms in some clients (Pitman et al., 1991) and because some flooding techniques do not address faulty cognitions or coping skills (Kilpatrick et al., 1985). Descriptions of exposure and flooding techniques are provided in Keane and Kaloupek (1982), Rothbaum and Foa (1992, 1996), and Meichenbaum (1994).

A widely used cognitive-behavioral approach called stress inoculation training (SIT) incorporates a variety of cognitive and behavioral techniques. Originally developed in the 1970s as a treatment for anxiety disorders, SIT has more recently been used to treat PTSD (Meichenbaum, 1994). SIT involves three phases of treatment including an education phase, a skills acquisition phase, and an application phase. During the first phase, the client is educated about the effects of trauma, and coping strategies are developed. The second phase focuses on training in coping skills such as relaxation, guided self-dialogue, problem solving, and attention diversion. The third and final phase involves imaginal and behavioral rehearsal of the newly acquired coping skills. A detailed description of the methods of SIT are provided in Meichenbaum (1994). Results of studies that incorporated both a prolonged exposure technique with SIT indicate that this combination of methods may be optimal for treating PTSD (Rothbaum & Foa, 1996).

A very popular cognitive-behavioral treatment method that is also extremely controversial is eye movement desensitization and reprocessing (EMDR; Shapiro, 1995). During EMDR, the client is asked to imagine an anxiety-provoking scene that represents the trauma while following the therapist's moving finger with her eyes. Although the method seems to be a form of exposure therapy, the theoretical basis for why this treatment would be effective is as yet unclear (Shapiro, 1995). Because there is no clear theoretical foundation for EMDR and because proponents claim that it can greatly reduce or eliminate severe PTSD symptoms in only a few sessions, EMDR has been very controversial. Empirical support for EMDR is inconsistent, with some studies reporting positive treatment effects (Vaughan et al., 1994; Wilson, Becker, & Tinker, 1995) and others reporting no superior effect over a control condition treatment (Jensen, 1994; Renfrey & Spates, 1994). Conclusions from reviews of empirical studies of EMDR have also been inconsistent. Some authors have concluded that research has supported the efficacy of the treatment (Greenwald, 1994; Shapiro, 1994). Others, however, conclude that eye movement is not actually an essential component of the treatment and that studies finding treatment effects are methodologically flawed (Herbert & Mueser, 1992; Lohr, Kleinknecht, Tolin, & Barrett, 1995). The greatest concern about EMDR is that subjective reports of its effectiveness are the result of clients' and therapists' expectations, rather than the treatment itself. This concern has not yet been adequately addressed empirically because most studies of EMDR have not included adequate control groups and have relied on clients' and therapists' subjective reports of improvement instead of using independent raters of effectiveness who are blind to the treatment condition.

Psychodynamically oriented treatments of PTSD have been less widely used than behavioral and cognitive-behavioral treatments. Psychodynamic treatments generally emphasize the need for traumatized persons to integrate traumatic events into their lives and their views of themselves and the world (Solomon et al., 1992). PTSD intrusion and avoidance symptoms are seen as defenses against psychological conflicts that are created or exacerbated by traumatic events. In one controlled study of a psychodynamic treatment approach, the therapy was found to be more effective than a wait-list control and more effective in reducing avoidance symptoms than intrusion symptoms (Brom, Kleber, & Defares, 1989). More detailed descriptions of psychodynamic approaches to the treatment of PTSD can be found in Lindy (1993, 1996), Marmar, Weiss, and Pynoos (1995), Marmar and Freeman (1991), and Weiss and Marmar (Weiss & Marmar, 1993).

Marmar and colleagues (Marmar et al., 1993) offer a unique multimethod approach to treatment. They review the common and contrasting change mechanisms of psychodynamic, cognitive-behavioral, and pharmacological trauma response treatment methods. They then offer suggestions for combining treatment methods from these three orientations with different strategies for those with normal stress responses, acute responses to catastrophic events, PTSD without comorbidity, PTSD with Axis I comorbidity, and chronic PTSD with secondary Axis II comorbidity. This tailored and eclectic approach to treatment seems to combine the most effective aspects of a variety of treatments.

Individual Treatments for Specific Populations

There is a considerable literature available describing individual psychotherapy treatments for specific populations of clients. Many of these are designed for persons who have experienced a particular traumatic stressor, such as combat or sexual assault. Others are designed for persons who fit into a particular diagnostic category, such as those in the acute stage of a trauma response or those with dissociative disorders. In some cases, a specialized treatment may be more effective than a general treatment approach because the specialized treatments address key aspects of responses to particular traumas that more generic treatments may not. For example, combat veterans may benefit from a special focus on survivor guilt and rape victims may benefit from a special focus on self-esteem issues. Similarly, most clinicians who treat persons with dissociative disorders suggest specialized treatment methods that focus on issues of identity disruption and memory deficits. For these reasons, I strongly recommend that you educate yourself about treatment issues and caveats for any specific trauma or diagnostic groups that you frequently treat. While detailed coverage of specialized trauma treatments is not possible here, I briefly review some examples as starting points for exploring the trauma literature. As described on p. 263, the PILOTS database offers an inexpensive and easy means of locating additional sources of information on particular trauma-related topics.

Treatments for Acute Responses

Special approaches have been suggested for interventions during the acute phase of the trauma response that immediately follows the traumatic experience. These interventions are designed to minimize trauma responses and, if possible, to prevent development of a full-blown PTSD. Turnbull and McFarlane (1996) and Foreman (1994) offer strategies and principles for treating clients who have recently been exposed to traumatic events and are experiencing extreme distress. Caution in use of early or "preventive" interventions is recommended, however, by Raphael and colleagues (Raphael, Wilson, Meldrum, & McFarlane, 1996) who describe and critically review a number of these approaches. They note that there is little controlled research of acute preventive interventions, and available studies showed mixed results with some indicating a possibility that such interventions may actually have negative effects under some circumstances.

Treatments for Adult Survivors of Child Abuse

An extensive literature is available on the subject of treatment for adult survivors of child abuse. The focus of most of this literature is on treatments for those who experienced sexual abuse or incest. The treatments, for the most part, are not specific to particular diagnostic groups but are appropriate for clients with a variety of diagnoses including PTSD, depression, or dissociative disorders. Some of the issues that are especially critical for survivors of childhood abuse include self-esteem, self-image, self-efficacy, and trust in interpersonal relationships. Good places to start your exploration of this literature include Briere (1996a, 1996b), Davies and Frawley (1994), Herman (1992), Gil (1988), Courtois (1988), and McCann and Pearlman (1990). In addition, Smucker and Niederee (1995) describe a brief treatment for incest survivors that combines imaginal exposure with mastery imagery.

Treatments for Adult Assault Victims

The literature on treatment of adult assault victims focuses almost exclusively on women who have been sexually assaulted. These women struggle with many of the same issues as adult survivors of child sexual abuse. In addition to problems relating to sense of self and relationships, they are also often acutely anxious about their personal safety. In treating women who have been assaulted, it is important to remember that those who experience multiple assaults or who live in constant danger of assault are likely to have unique treatment needs. Consequently, treatment for a woman who experienced a single incident of rape might differ considerably from treatment for a woman who was battered and raped by a spouse for a period of years. Similarly, those who experienced physical assaults are likely to have different therapeutic issues than those who experienced sexual assaults. Good sources of information on treatment for sexual assault includes Resnick and Newton (1992), Foa and Riggs (1993), and Hartman and Burgess (1993). Sources of information on treatment of battered women include Dutton (1992, 1994).

Treatments for Other Traumas and Diagnostic Subcategories

Fewer treatments have been developed that are designed especially for clients in diagnostic subcategories or clients with other types of traumatic experiences. Specialized treatments have been described for clients with PTSD and substance abuse problems (Abueg & Fairbank, 1992), for those with chronic PTSD (Hyer, McCranie, & Peralme, 1993), for refugees (Kinzie, 1993), and for combat veterans (Carroll & Foy, 1992; Scurfield, 1993b; Sipprelle, 1992).

Treatments for Dissociative Disorder

Treatments for dissociative disorders are fairly well-developed and described in the literature, particularly those designed for clients with DID (previously MPD). Unfortunately, empirical studies of these treatment methods are lacking, and the controversies surrounding the diagnosis of DID (discussed in Chapter 9, pp. 170–172) have called into question some treatment techniques. For example, given the possibility that some clients' beliefs that they have multiple identities can be inadvertently socially facilitated or encouraged, some have suggested that treatments for DID clients should not include naming or addressing individual "personalities." Similarly, given the possibility that highly dissociative persons are also highly suggestible, some have questioned the use of hypnosis in the treatment of DID clients.

Good sources of information about treatment methods for DID are Allen and Smith (1995), Barach and Comstock (1996), Horevitz and Loewenstein (1994), Putnam (1989), Ross (1997), Kluft and Fine (1993),

Kluft (1993, 1996a), and Fine (1993, 1996). Treatment of clients with DID is considered particularly challenging because of the chaotic psychological life of dissociatively disordered persons and because of the characterological disorders that often are seen in these clients. Accordingly, Loewenstein (1993) has written about the need for special attention to transference and countertransference issues in the treatment of DID clients.

Group Treatments

Group treatments have been widely used for those with trauma-related disorders, particularly PTSD. Traumatized patients can benefit greatly from some of the unique characteristics of group psychotherapy. As discussed in earlier chapters, social support appears to promote healing after traumatic experiences. Group members who have been through similar traumatic experiences can offer each other social support that is all the more powerful because it comes from someone who has "been there." Group members can also serve as role models for one another as they successfully cope with trauma symptoms. van der Kolk (1987d) points out that group psychotherapy can also help trauma victims to feel more empowered as they have the opportunity to be helpful to others in the group. The relative benefits of individual and group psychotherapy for trauma victims are discussed in detail in van der Kolk (1987d) and Meichenbaum (1994).

Group treatments can be open-ended with turnover in group membership or time-limited with closed group membership. Herman (1992) has proposed that different types of group are appropriate at different stages of recovery from traumatic experiences. In her book, she describes both purposes and structures of both types of groups. Open-ended groups have also been described for adult incest survivors (Herman & Lawrence, 1993) and adult sexual abuse survivors (Mennen & Meadow, 1992; Webb & Leehan, 1996).

Time-limited group treatments have been developed for clients with abuse histories (Gil, 1988) as well as clients with all types of trauma (Flannery, 1987). Resnick and Schnicke (1993) have developed a 12-session, cognitive-behavioral treatment for rape victims that has been empirically validated. The treatment is described in great detail in their book, including detailed homework assignments and worksheets that can be copied. The treatment program could be easily adapted for use with persons with other types of traumatic experiences. A number of other group treatment options are described by Meichenbaum (1994).

TREATMENTS FOR CHILDREN

Development of treatments for traumatized children has lagged behind that of treatments for adults. This is due, in part, to the added complications of treating children. Just as with treatment for other disorders, clinicians treating children for traumatic responses must contend with many practical issues that can hinder treatment efforts. For example, clinicians treating children are dependent on family members to bring the child to treatment. This can prove a significant barrier to treatment, especially if the parent is directly or indirectly responsible for the traumatic event(s). Desires to avoid thinking about or to deny such responsibility can make parents uncooperative in the treatment process. Other challenges unique to treating children include children's limited abilities to understand the purpose of treatment, children's limited insight into their feelings and responses to traumatic events, and children's limited abilities to verbalize their feelings and describe their experiences.

For the most part, treatments of traumatized children have focused on the individual treatment modality. Pynoos and Nader (1993) discuss therapeutic issues in the treatment of traumatized children as they apply to short- and long-term therapy and various treatment modalities. Guidelines for determining the treatment needs of particular traumatized children are provided in James (1994). Sources of information are provided below for generic treatment models for traumatized children and for specific treatment methods for children who were sexually abused or who have a dissociative disorder.

Williams and Sommer (1994b) have described a generic trauma treatment model that can be applied to children as well as adults (see p. 188 for a description). However, most treatments for traumatized children are designed for particular trauma groups or diagnostic groups. The most work has been done in the area of treatment of children who have been sexually assaulted or abused. Finkelhor and Berliner (1995) have reviewed the research on these treatments and made recommendations to clinicians. Specific suggestions for methods and techniques for treating children traumatized by sexual abuse are provided by Lipovsky (1992) and James (1989). A time-limited, cognitive-behavioral treatment program that involves offending parents in treatment is described in detail by Deblinger and Heflin (1996).

Treatments for children with dissociative disorders have also been developed. Comprehensive discussions of treating highly dissociative children can be found in Putnam (1997) and Kluft (1986, 1996b). Use of play therapy in the treatment of children with dissociative disorders is described by McMahon and Fagan (1993). Suggestions for inpatient treatment methods for this population of children are provided in Hornstein and Tyson (1992).

MONITORING TREATMENT PROGRESS AND OUTCOME

No matter which treatment methods you use with a particular client, it is important to monitor the progress of your client during treatment. Your subjective impression that treatment is going well is not sufficient evidence that it is. Unfortunately, there is ample evidence that positive impressions of both client and therapist about the effectiveness of treatment can be mistaken (van der Kolk, McFarlane, & van der Hart, 1996). If you have done a careful assessment of your client at the outset of treatment, you will be in an excellent position to determine treatment progress. Readministration of brief symptom measures every 4 to 8 weeks can give you a good idea of progress in reduction of trauma-related symptoms. You can also reassess your client's occupational and social functioning to determine whether treatment has led to positive changes in these areas.

Along with monitoring progress of individual clients, you should stay alert to developments in treatment outcome research. Use of resources such as the PILOTS database (see p. 263) and the *Journal of Traumatic Stress* can help you keep abreast of these developments. In this way, you can be informed about emerging evidence that supports or fails to support the efficacy of particular treatment methods. At the same time, you can watch for developments and innovations in assessment of trauma and trauma responses that reflect improvements in measurement and that may aid you in treatment planning. In a field as "young" as traumatic stress, it is especially important to continually update your knowledge base.

SUMMARY

This chapter reviewed a variety of methods for treating trauma-related disorders. Treatments for adults that were described include general individual treatment approaches, individual treatments with specific theoretical orientations, individual treatments for specific trauma populations and diagnostic groups, and group treatments. Treatments for children were described, including general individual treatment approaches and individual treatments for specific trauma populations and diagnostic groups. Citations were provided for sources describing these treatment methods.

Chapter 11

Future Directions

Because systematic research focusing on traumatic experiences and their consequences began only relatively recently, development of measures of many aspects of trauma and trauma responses is still in progress. For some constructs, measures exist but still require further validation. For other constructs, measures have not yet been developed.

In the area of traumatic experiences, numerous brief screens have been designed, but very little information is available about their reliability and validity. More detailed structured interviews regarding traumatic experiences have also been developed, but these, too, have not been adequately validated to date. Progress is likely to be slow in this area, however, given the considerable methodological difficulties associated with validating measures of past experiences (see Chapter 8, p. 151).

While some trauma experience measures inquire about whether the trauma involved actual or threatened death or injury, no measures have yet been developed to specifically assess subjective characteristics of traumatic events, such as controllability, negative valence, and immediacy of threat. This type of measure might prove useful in furthering our understanding of the influences of these subjective trauma characteristics on trauma responses and, ultimately, in planning treatment for traumatized persons.

In the realm of posttraumatic response measurement, several well-validated brief scales are available to assess symptoms following a single traumatic event. Two brief measures that can be used to assess responses to multiple traumatic events have been designed, but only preliminary evidence has been collected to support their reliability and validity. Structured interviews for assessing posttraumatic stress responses following both single and multiple traumatic events are available, but the most current version of the latter has not yet been validated.

With the exception of the TSI and the TSCC, all of the available measures of posttraumatic stress symptoms are closely tied to the DSM criteria for PTSD. One advance in this area of measurement might be the development of measures that assess a wider variety of posttraumatic symptoms. Given the controversies over the adequacy of the DSM diagnostic criteria for PTSD (see pp. 166–170), broader measures of posttraumatic symptoms might foster further refinement of these criteria.

To date, validated measures of dissociative symptoms are available that can be used to screen for trauma-related dissociation in children, adolscents, and adults. These measures do seem to have certain limitations, however, in that they may not adequately assess the types of dissociative responses that occur following different types of traumatic experiences, and they include items assessing normative dissociation. A dissociation measure that assesses a wider range of pathological dissociative responses and that assesses *only* the more pathological forms of dissociation might prove more sensitive in detecting trauma-related dissociative symptoms.

Two structured interviews for dissociation have been developed, but both focus on assessment of symptoms of dissociative disorders and have been validated only for use in diagnosing these disorders. Validation of structured interviews of dissociative symptoms for use in assessing dissociative aspects of PTSD might make them useful for assessing trauma-related disorders other than dissociative disorders.

As conceptualization of posttraumatic responses progresses, further developments in measurement are likely to follow. For example, the conceptualization of posttraumatic symptoms described in Chapter 3 might lead to the development of a measure that systematically assesses reexperiencing and avoidance symptoms in all four domains of interest (cognitive, affective, behavioral, and physiological). On another front, if research on acute stress responses supports a well-defined acute stress disorder, a measure to specifically assess acute response to trauma might be developed and prove valuable.

In general, most child measures of trauma and trauma responses are at the beginning stages of development. Although many have been designed, almost all are in need of further validation across populations of children and across ages. A dissociation interview for children has not yet been developed. Such an interview might prove useful, but, in general, caution is advised with use of structured interviews with children (see Chapter 6, p. 118). Basic research on the presentation of trauma responses in children is also much needed and may lead to the development of PTSD and dissociative disorder criteria that are specific to children (Peterson, 1991). If that occurs, measures will be needed to assess the new criteria.

Other areas of measurement in need of further development include measurement of some secondary and associated trauma symptoms. Measures are needed that focus on aggressive behaviors toward oneself and others, identity disturbances, interpersonal relationships, and guilt and shame. Given the increasing interest in trauma-related disorders among mental health researchers and clinicians, rapid expansion in many areas of measurement of trauma and trauma responses can be expected in the years to come.

MEASURE PROFILES

Section A

Measures of Traumatic Experiences

SELF-REPORT INVENTORIES OF TRAUMATIC EXPERIENCES

Trauma Assessment for Adults (TAA)—Self-Report
(H. Resnick, C. Best, D. Kilpatrick, J. Freedy, & S. Falsetti)

Recommended Uses

Recommended for brief screening for trauma history in clinical or research settings.

Special Features

Includes detailed assessment of childhood sexual assault, including probes to assess threat, injury, and penetration to allow evaluation of severity of incidents.

General Descriptive Information

Events assessed: Wide range of potentially traumatic events (high magnitude stressors), including combat, accidents, disasters, serious illnesses, sexual assaults (childhood and adult), physical assaults (childhood and adult), assaults with weapons, witnessing death or serious injury, friend/family member killed/murdered.

Note. References that do not appear in the Measure Profiles can be found in the References section (pp. 265–303).

Number of items; time to administer: 17 items; 10–15 minutes, depending on number of traumatic experiences.

Response format: Yes/No and other aspects of events (see below).

Training required to administer: Not applicable (self-report).

Sample item: "Have you ever served in the military in a war zone or had military combat experience?"

Type of outcome measure provided: Count of stressor events; count of stressor events with threat or injury.

Aspects of traumas assessed: For each event endorsed, collects age first or only time, age last time, perception that subject would be killed or injured, age(s) for any physical injuries suffered.

Time frame assessed: Lifetime.

Development notes: Adapted from the Potential Stressful Events Interview (PSEI; Kilpatrick, Resnick, & Freedy, 1991).

Correspondence with DSM: Assesses DSM-IV Criterion A-1 element of threat of death/injury for all events and fear of death/injury, but does not assess DSM-IV Criterion A-2 element of experiencing fear (other than death or injury), helplessness, or horror.

Psychometric Information

Validation populations: None to date.

Reliability: None to date.

Validity: None to date.

Descriptive/psychometric information sources: None to date.

How to Obtain Scale

Contact Heidi Resnick, PhD, National Crime Victims Research and Treatment Center, Department of Psychiatry and Behavioral Sciences, 171 Ashley Avenue, Charleston, SC 29425-0742.

Trauma History Questionnaire
(B. Green)

Recommended Uses

Recommended for brief screening for trauma history in clinical or research settings.

Special Features

Has detailed items inquiring about specific potentially traumatic crime-related events.

General Descriptive Information

Events assessed: Wide range of potentially traumatic events (high magnitude stressors) includes mugging, being robbed, home broken into, accidents, disasters, "man-made" disasters, exposure to environmental hazards, other situations with threat of death/serious injury, witnessing death/serious injury, seeing/handling dead bodies, friend/family member killed/murdered, death of spouse or child, life-threatening illness, sudden serious injury/illness/death of someone close, combat, sexual assault, physical assault (with or without weapon).

Number of items; time to administer: 24 items; 5–15 minutes, depending on number of traumatic experiences.

Response format: Yes/No, number of times, and age.

Training required to administer: Not applicable (self-report).

Sample item: "Has anyone ever tried to take something directly from you by using force or the threat of force, such as a stick-up or mugging?"

Type of outcome measure provided: Total score can be calculated, omitting item 24, but examination of responses is recommended before scoring to screen out false positive responses (i.e., client says "Yes" to an item, but describes a subthreshhold event such as grandfather dying of a heart attack following a minor traffic accident).

Aspects of traumas assessed: For each event endorsed, collects number of times event occurred and approximate age at the time of the event.

Time frame assessed: Lifetime.

Development notes: Adapted from the high magnitude stressor events section of the PSEI interview designed by D. Kilpatrick and H. Resnick for the DSM-IV field trials for PTSD (Kilpatrick et al., 1991).

Correspondence with DSM: Assessment of DSM-IV Criterion A-1 element of threat of life/injury is possible for some events but not for all. No assessment of DSM-IV Criterion A-2 element of experiencing fear, helplessness, or horror.

Psychometric Information

Validation populations: Psychiatric outpatients, college students, and women with breast cancer.

Reliability: Test–retest reliability in a sample of 25 females showed high levels of consistency (r's in the .7–.9 range) in reporting of specific events such as being mugged, experiencing a natural disaster, and being attacked with a weapon. Test–retest reliabilities were less strong for "catchall" items such as "Other unwanted sex" (Green, unpublished data).

Validity: Some norms have been collected for events experienced by psychiatric outpatients and university students.

Descriptive/psychometric information sources: Green, B. L. (1996). Trauma History Questionnaire. In B. H. Stamm (Ed.), *Measurement of stress, trauma, and adaptation* (pp. 366–369). Lutherville, MD: Sidran Press.

How to Obtain Scale

Contact Bonnie L. Green, PhD, Department of Psychiatry, Georgetown University, 611 Kober Cogan Hall, Washington, DC 20007.

INTERVIEWS FOR TRAUMATIC EXPERIENCES

Childhood Trauma Interview
(L. Fink)

Recommended Uses

Recommended for collecting detailed information about childhood interpersonal traumatic experiences in clinical or research settings.

Special Features

This interview is somewhat unique in providing a means of quantifying the frequency, severity, and duration of a wide range of childhood interpersonal traumatic events.

General Descriptive Information

Events assessed: Childhood separation and loss, physical neglect, emotional abuse/assault, physical abuse/assault, witnessing violence, and sexual abuse/assault.

Number of items; time to administer: A total of 49 screening items with numerous probes for screening items endorsed (3–11 screening items for each of six categories of events); 20–40 minutes, depending on number of traumatic experiences.

Response format: Screening questions and probes include open- and closed-ended questions.

Training required to administer: Some clinical training required to administer.

Sample item: "Did either of your parents, or anyone else who took care of you die while you were growing up?" (For each separation/loss reported, probes inquire about ages during separation, who lived with, who separated from, reason for separation, nature of communication during separation.)

Type of outcome measure provided: Yields considerable qualitative information about traumatic experiences and quantitative scoring for frequency, severity, and duration of experiences is described by the authors (Fink, Bernstein, Handelsman, Foote, & Lovejoy, 1995).

Aspects of traumas assessed: Probes vary across categories of interpersonal trauma. They include queries about persons involved, nature of the event, age at time of event, frequency of event, threats during event, telling about event, nature of injuries sustained.

Time frame assessed: Childhood up to the age of 18.

Correspondence with DSM: Does not assess DSM-IV Criterion A-1 element of threat of death and threat of or actual injury of Criterion A-2 element of fear, helplessness, or horror.

Psychometric Information

Validation populations: Drug- or alcohol-dependent patients.

Reliability: Interrater reliability in one study was high with intraclass correlations for 83% (of 24 variables) ranging from .73 to 1.0, intraclass correlations for 79% above .80, and intraclass correlations for 63% above .90 (Fink et al., 1995).

Validity: Construct validity of the CTI is supported by moderate correlations (ranging from $r = .43$ to $.57$) between scores for severity of trauma and analogous factor scores from the Childhood Trauma Questionnaire, a self-report retrospective measure of intrafamilial childhood abuse and neglect (Fink et al., 1995). Further evidence for the validity of the CTI includes correlations between total exposure scores for each trauma category that are consistent with predicted relationships between these types of experiences.

Descriptive/psychometric information sources: Fink, L. A., Bernstein, D., Handelsman, L., Foote, J., & Lovejoy, M. (1995). Initial reliability and validity of the Childhood Trauma Interview: A new multidimensional measure of childhood interpersonal trauma. *American Journal of Psychiatry, 152,* 1329–1335.

How to Obtain Scale

Contact Laura Fink, PhD, c/o Josephine Dodge, Bronx VA Medical Center, Psychiatry Service 116A, 130 West Kingsbridge Road, Bronx, NY 10468.

Evaluation of Lifetime Stressors (ELS)
(K. Krinsley, F. Weathers, M. Vielhauer, E. Newman,
E. Walker, D. Kaloupek, L. Young, & R. Kimerling)

Recommended Uses

Recommended for collecting detailed information about potentially traumatic experiences in clinical or research settings.

Special Features

The ELS has a unique format in which a self-report questionnaire is used in conjunction with a follow-up semistructured interview. Questionnaire items that are endorsed are queried about in detail during the interview. Design of the questionnaire and interview emphasize clinical sensitivity while gathering extremely detailed information about the nature and dimensions of past traumatic events.

General Descriptive Information

Events assessed: Very wide range of potentially traumatic events; 28 different events include disasters, illnesses, accidents, street/criminal violence, combat, physical assault/abuse, sexual assault/abuse; also inquires about a range of experiences and symptoms in childhood and adulthood that are associated with trauma.

Number of items; time to administer: 56 questionnaire items with detailed inquiries about items endorsed; 10–20 minutes for the questionnaire, 1–3 or more hours for interview.

Response format: Questionnaire response choices are "Yes, this happened to me," "I'm not sure if this happened," "No, but this happened to someone I knew," and "No, this did not happen."

Training required to administer: Should be administered by trained clinicians only.

Sample item: (questionnaire item) "Have you ever either witnessed or experienced a robbery, mugging, or violent attack?" [Probes include "Tell me more about this," or "What did you see?" and queries about trauma type, severity of worst event, emotional responses of fear/helplessness/horror, perpetrator, age(s) at time(s) of event(s), number of events, fear of being killed, injury, weapons used.]

Type of outcome measure provided: Yields considerable qualitative information about traumatic experiences. No quantitative scoring has been proposed by the authors.

Aspects of traumas assessed: Probes for all traumatic event items are listed under "Sample Item" above. Probes for assessment of the two or three worst traumatic events include detailed ratings of fear/helplessness/horror, degree of injuries, degree of life threat, memory for the event, feelings of responsibility for the event, disclosure of the event, social support at time of event, treatment related to the event, general social support, documentation of event, and mastery of event.

Time frame assessed: Lifetime.

Correspondence with DSM: Assesses DSM-IV Criterion A-1 element of threat of death and threat of or actual injury for all events and experience of fear of death/injury and DSM-IV Criterion A-2 element of fear, helplessness, or horror.

Psychometric Information

Validation populations: Male veterans, female sexual abuse survivors.

Reliability: Global test–retest reliability coefficients for a sample of 76 male veterans ranged from $r = .40$ to 1.0 for the presence/absence of eight trauma types in childhood and adulthood (Krinsley, Gallagher, Weathers, Kaloupek, & Vielhauer, 1997).

Validity: None to date.

Descriptive/psychometric information sources: Krinsley, K. (1996). Psychometric review of the Evaluation of Lifetime Stressors (ELS) Questionnaire & Interview. In B. H. Stamm (Ed.), *Measurement of stress, trauma and adaptation* (pp. 160–162). Lutherville, MD: Sidran Press.

Krinsley, K. E., Gallagher, J. G., Weathers, F. W., Kaloupek, D. G., & Vielhauer, M. (1997). *Reliability and validity of the Evaluation of Lifetime Stressors questionnaire.* Unpublished manuscript.

How to Obtain Scale

Contact Karen Krinsley, PhD, National Center for PTSD (116B-2), Boston VA Medical Center, 150 South Huntington Avenue, Boston, MA 02130.

National Women's Study Event History
(D. Kilpatrick, H. Resnick, B. Saunders, & C. Best)

Recommended Uses

Recommended for collecting detailed information about potentially traumatic experiences in clinical or research settings.

Special Features

This interview includes detailed assessment of first, most recent, and worst sexual completed rape experiences and of a single molestation, attempted sexual assault, and physical assault experience. The interview also contains carefully worded prefaces to each section to orient the subject to the types of experiences that are of interest and to show the interviewer's sensitivity and knowledge.

General Descriptive Information

Events assessed: Range of potentially traumatic events (high magnitude stressors), including serious accidents, natural disasters, witnessing death/injury, friend or family member killed, completed rape, molestation, attempted sexual assault, and physical assault.

Number of items; time to administer: 17 screening items with numerous probes for most screening items endorsed; 15–30 minutes, depending on number of traumatic experiences.

Response format: Screening questions are Yes/No; probes include closed- and open-ended questions.

Training required to administer: Can be administered by trained interviewers.

Sample item: "During your lifetime, have any of the following types of things ever happened to you? A serious accident at work, in a car, or somewhere else?" (Probes include queries about number of events, age at first, fear of being injured or killed, actual injury, time of most recent event, fear of being injured or killed during first or most recent event, injuries during first or most recent event.)

Type of outcome measure provided: Yields considerable qualitative information about traumatic experiences. No quantitative scoring is described by the authors in published discussion of the interview.

Aspects of traumas assessed: Probes for assessment of first, most recent, and worst completed rape experiences and a single molestation, attempted sexual assault and physical assault experience include: age at time of event, familiarity with assailant, relationship to assailant, fear of death/injury, actual injury, use of drugs/alcohol by subject or assailant, whether incident was reported to police/authorities. Also see probes for other traumatic event items under "Sample Item" above.

Time frame assessed: Lifetime.

Development notes: Adapted from the Incident Report Interview (Kilpatrick, Saunders, Veronen, Best, & Von, 1987) and the Stressful and Traumatic Life Events interview (Kulka et al., 1990d).

Correspondence with DSM: Assesses DSM-IV Criterion A-1 element of threat of death and threat of or actual injury for all events and experience of fear of death/injury, but does not assess DSM-IV Criterion A-2 element of fear (other than of death/injury), helplessness, or horror.

Psychometric Information

Validation populations: Frequency of exposure to trauma has been gathered for a racially and demographically representative national sample of women between 18 and 34 years of age (Resnick, Kilpatrick, Dansky, Saunders, & Best, 1993).

Reliability: None to date.

Validity: Construct validity of the NWS Event History is supported by the finding that frequencies of exposure to traumatic events yielded by the interview is identical to those found using Norris's Traumatic Stress Schedule (Norris & Riad, 1996; Resnick, 1996a).

Descriptive/psychometric information sources: Resnick, H. (1996). Psychometric review of National Women's Study (NWS) Event History– PTSD Module. In B. H. Stamm (Ed.), *Measurement of stress, trauma, and adaptation* (pp. 214–217). Lutherville, MD: Sidran Press.

Resnick, H. S., Falsetti, S. A., Kilpatrick, D. G., & Freedy, J. R. (1996). Assessment of rape and other civilian trauma-related post-traumatic stress disorder: Emphasis on assessment of potentially traumatic events. In T. W. Miller (Ed.), *Stressful life events* (pp. 231–266). Madison: International Universities Press.

Resnick, H. S., Kilpatrick, D. G., Dansky, B. S., Saunders, B. E., & Best, C. L. (1993). Prevalence of civilian trauma and posttraumatic stress disorder on a representative sample of women. *Journal of Consulting and Clinical Psychology, 61,* 984–991.

How to Obtain Scale

Contact Dean Kilpatrick, PhD, National Crime Victims Research and Treatment Center, Department of Psychiatry and Behavioral Sciences, 171 Ashely Avenue, Charleston, SC 29425-0742.

Trauma Assessment for Adults (TAA)
(H. Resnick, C. Best, D. Kilpatrick, J. Freedy, & S. Falsetti)

Recommended Uses

Recommended for brief screening for trauma history in clinical or research settings.

Special Features

Includes detailed assessment of childhood sexual assault, including probes to assess threat, injury, and penetration to allow evaluation of severity of incidents.

General Descriptive Information

Events assessed: Wide range of potentially traumatic events (high-magnitude stressors), including combat, accidents, disasters, serious illnesses, sexual assaults (childhood and adult), physical assaults (childhood and adult), assaults with weapons, witnessing death or serious injury, friend/family member killed/murdered.

Number of items; time to administer: 13 items; 10–15 minutes, depending on number of traumatic experiences.

Response format: Yes/No and other aspects of events (see below).

Training required to administer: None specified.

Sample item: "During your life, have any of the following types of things happened to you? Military combat experience or military service in a war zone?"

Type of outcome measure provided: Count of stressor events; count of stressor events with threat or injury.

Aspects of traumas assessed: For each event endorsed, collects age first or only time, age last time, perception that subject would be killed or injured.

Time frame assessed: Lifetime.

Development notes: Adapted from the Potential Stressful Events Interview (Kilpatrick et al., 1991).

Correspondence with DSM: Assesses DSM-IV Criterion A-1 element of threat of death/injury for all events and fear of death/injury, but does not assess DSM-IV Criterion A-2 element of experiencing fear (other than death or injury), helplessness, or horror.

Psychometric Information

Validation populations: Adult mental health center clients.

Reliability: None to date.

Validity: Construct validity of the measure is supported by findings of rates of general trauma and crime exposure that were highly consistent with those of studies of this population using a different measure (Resnick, 1996b). In addition, a small study of archival data found that stressor events noted in the archival records were all identified with the TAA (Resnick, 1996b).

Descriptive/psychometric information sources: Resnick, H. S. (1996). Psychometric review of Trauma Assessment for Adults (TAA). In B. H. Stamm (Ed.), *Measurement of stress, trauma, and adaptation* (pp. 362–365). Lutherville, MD: Sidran Press.

Resnick, H. S., Falsetti, S. A., Kilpatrick, D. G., & Freedy, J. R. (1996). Assessment of rape and other civilian trauma-related post-traumatic stress disorder: Emphasis on assessment of potentially traumatic events. In T. W. Miller (Ed.), *Stressful life events* (pp. 231–266). Madison: International Universities Press.

How to Obtain Scale

Contact Heidi Resnick, PhD, National Crime Victims Research and Treatment Center, Department of Psychiatry and Behavioral Sciences, 171 Ashely Avenue, Charleston, SC 29425-0742.

Traumatic Stress Schedule
(F. Norris)

Recommended Uses

Recommended for brief screening for potentially traumatic experiences in clinical or research settings.

Special Features

Format of interview is very flexible with nine screening questions and very detailed probes for each question if endorsed. Probes assess dimensions of experiences including loss, scope, threat to life or physical integrity, blame, and familiarity.

General Descriptive Information

Events assessed: Range of potentially traumatic events (high magnitude stressors), including combat, robbery/mugging, physical assault, sexual assault, traffic accidents, sudden death of loved one, disasters, exposure to environmental hazards, other terrifying/shocking experiences, major life changes.

Number of items; time to administer: 10 screening items with 12 probes for each screening item endorsed; 5–30 minutes, depending on number of traumatic experiences.

Response format: Screening questions are Yes/No; probes include closed- and open-ended questions.

Training required to administer: Can be administered by lay interviewer.

Sample item: "In the past year, did anyone take something from you by force or threat of force, such as in a robbery, mugging, or hold-up?" (Probes include queries about persons involved, value of property, injuries, life threat, blame, time of event, description of event, similar past experiences, being reminded of event, intrusive thoughts, nightmares, behavioral avoidance.)

Type of outcome measure provided: Yields considerable qualitative information about traumatic experiences. No quantitative scoring is described in the initial published report on the schedule.

Aspects of traumas assessed: For each event endorsed, dimensions of experiences are assessed including loss, scope, threat to life or physical integrity, blame, familiarity, and some associated PTSD symptoms.

Time frame assessed: Published version specifies past year, but author suggests that schedule may be used to assess any specified time period.

Correspondence with DSM: Assesses DSM-IV Criterion A-1 element of threat of death for all events and fear of death but does not assess threat of serious injury to self/others or DSM-IV Criterion A-2 element of experiencing fear (other than of death), helplessness, or horror.

Psychometric Information

Validation populations: Frequency of exposure to trauma has been gathered for six southeastern U.S. cities (Norris & Riad, 1996).

Reliability: Test–retest reliability was reported for the TSS to be .88 across English and Spanish versions of the measure given 1 week apart (Norris & Perilla, 1996).

Validity: Construct validity of the TSS is supported by the finding that frequencies of exposure to traumatic events have been very stable across purposive and random samples from six southeastern cities. Furthermore, TSS estimates of the frequency of any trauma are identical to those found using the National Women's PTSD Module in a nationally representative sample of women (Norris & Riad, 1996).

Descriptive/psychometric information sources: Norris, F. H. (1990). Screening for traumatic stress: A scale of use in the general population. *Journal of Applied Social Psychology, 20,* 1704–1718. (Includes measure in its entirety.)

Norris, F. H. (1992). Epidemiology of trauma: Frequency and impact of different potentially traumatic events on different demographic groups. *Journal of Consulting and Clinical Psychology, 60,* 409–418.

Norris, F. H., & Perilla, J. L. (1996). The Revised Civilian Mississippi Scale for PTSD: Reliability, validity, and cross-language stability. *Journal of Traumatic Stress, 9,* 285–297.

How to Obtain Scale

Contact Fran Norris, PhD, Department of Psychology, Georgia State University, University Plaza, Atlanta, GA 30303.

Self-Report Measures of Responses to Trauma

Davidson Trauma Scale (DTS)
(J. Davidson)

Recommended Uses

Recommended for use in clinical or research settings to measure PTSD symptoms related to identified trauma.

Special Features

This measure is brief and easy to administer. It yields scores for both frequency and severity of PTSD symptoms. There is very strong evidence for this scale's reliability and validity and validation samples have included subjects with a wide variety of traumatic experiences.

General Descriptive Information

Symptoms assessed: Assesses DSM-III-R/DSM-IV symptoms for PTSD.

Number of items; time to complete: 17 items; takes 10–15 minutes to complete.

Response format: For each item, client rates frequency (from 0 = "Not at all" to 4 = "Every day") and severity (from 0 = "Not at all distressing" to 4 = "Extremely distressing").

Sample item: "Have you had painful images, memories, or thoughts about the event?"

Type of outcome measure provided: Scale yields frequency scores (ranging from 0 to 68), severity scores (ranging from 0 to 68), and total scores (ranging from 0 to 136) and can be used to make a preliminary determination about whether client's symptoms meet DSM criteria for PTSD.

Time frame assessed: Past week.

Correspondence with DSM: Assesses DSM-III-R and DSM-IV symptom criteria (B, C, and D) for PTSD.

Psychometric Information

Validation populations: Rape victims, war veterans, hurricane victims, and survivors of miscellaneous traumas.

Reliability: Evidence of internal consistency includes Cronbach's α values of .99 for total score, .97 for frequency items, and .98 for severity items (Davidson et al., in press). Evidence for consistency over time includes a 2-week test–retest reliability correlation for total score of .86.

Validity: Evidence for construct validity includes a sensitivity rate of .69 and a specificity rate of .95 when diagnosis of PTSD using a DTS cutoff score of 40 was compared to the results of the SCID (Davidson et al., in press). Convergent validity was supported by strong correlations between scores on the DTS and the CAPS ($r = .78$), the IES ($r = .64$), and the anxiety subscale of the Symptom Checklist 90—Revised (SCL-90-R) ($r = .65$).

Descriptive/psychometric information sources: Davidson, J. R. T., Book, S. W., Colket, J. T., Tupler, L. A., Roth, S., David, D., Hertzberg, M., Mellman, T., Beckham, J. C., Smith, R., Davison, R. M., Katz, R., & Feldman, M. (in press). Assessment of a new self-rating scale for post-traumatic stress disorder. *Psychological Medicine.*

How to Obtain Scale

Contact Mental Health Systems, Inc., 908 Niagara Falls Boulevard, North Tonawanda, NY 14120-2060; 800-456-3003.

Dissociative Experiences Scale (DES)
(E. Carlson & F. Putnam)

Recommended Uses

Recommended for measuring dissociation symptoms in clinical or research settings.

Special Features

This is a brief scale that inquires about the frequency of a wide range of pathological and normative dissociative experiences. It has been translated into 16 languages.

General Descriptive Information

Symptoms assessed: Items assess domains of dissociative amnesia, gaps in awareness, derealization, depersonalization, absorption, and imaginative involvement.

Number of items; time to complete: 28 items; takes about 5–10 minutes to complete.

Response format: For each item, client rates frequency by circling a number on an 11-point scale that ranges from 0 = "Never" to 100 = "Always" (by mutiples of 10).

Sample item: "Some people have the experience of feeling that other people, objects, and the world around them are not real. Circle a number to show what percentage of the time this happens to you."

Type of outcome measure provided: Total scale scores are the average of item scores and range from 0 to 100.

Time frame assessed: None specified.

Development notes: Adapted from previous version of the same scale that had a different response scale (Bernstein & Putnam, 1986).

Correspondence with DSM: Contains items that correspond to symptoms of dissociative disorders and PTSD but does not specifically assess DSM criteria for any disorder.

Psychometric Information

Validation populations: The scale has been used in over 250 published studies to date across a very wide range of populations including general population, psychiatric inpatients, psychiatric outpatients, university students, rape victims, disaster victims, persons with childhood abuse histories, war veterans, refugees, and people meeting DSM criteria for various diagnostic categories.

Reliability: Evidence of internal consistency includes a Cronbach's α value of .95 in one sample and split-half reliabilities of .83 and .93 in two other samples (Carlson & Putnam, 1993). Evidence for consistency over time includes reliability correlations over 4- to 8-week test–retest intervals ranging from .79 to .96 in various studies.

Validity: Evidence for construct validity includes findings of high scores in samples of subjects with trauma histories (Carlson & Putnam,

1993). The scale shows good convergent validity when correlated with measures of similar constructs. When DES scores were used to predict DID diagnosis using a cutoff score of 30, the DES showed a sensitivity rate of 74% and a specificity rate of 80%.

Descriptive/psychometric information sources: Bernstein, E. M., & Putnam, F. W. (1986). Development, reliability, and validity of a dissociation scale. *Journal of Nervous and Mental Disease, 174,* 727–735.

Carlson, E. B., & Armstrong, J. (1994). Diagnosis and assessment of dissociative disorders. In S. J. Lynn & J. W. Rhue (Ed.), *Dissociation: Theoretical, clinical, and research perspectives* (pp. 159–174). New York: Guilford Press.

Carlson, E. B., & Putnam, F. W. (1993). An update on the Dissociative Experiences Scale. *Dissociation, 6,* 16–27. (Includes measure in its entirety.)

Carlson, E. B., Putnam, F. W., Ross, C. A., Torem, M., Coons, P., Dill, D. L., Loewenstein, R. J., & Braun, B. G. (1993). Validity of the Dissociative Experiences Scale in screening for multiple personality disorder: A multicenter study. *American Journal of Psychiatry, 150*(7), 1030–1036.

Waller, N. G. (1996). The Dissociative Experiences Scale. In *Twelfth Mental Measurements Yearbook*. Lincoln, NE: Buros Institute of Mental Measurement.

How to Obtain Scale

Contact Sidran Foundation, 2328 West Joppa Road, Suit 15, Lutherville, MD 21093; 410-825-8888.

Impact of Event Scale–Revised (IES-R)
(D. Weiss & C. Marmar)

Recommended Uses

Recommended for use in clinical or research settings to screen for or measure PTSD symptoms related to a single identified traumatic event.

Special Features

This measure is very brief and easy to administer. It is a revised version of the oldest and most widely used measure of responses to traumatic stressors.

General Descriptive Information

Symptoms assessed: Assesses 14 of the 17 DSM-III-R/DSM-IV symptoms for PTSD.

Number of items; time to complete: 22 items; takes 5–10 minutes to complete.

Response format: Clients rate the degree of distress associated with each item (from 0 = "Not at all" to 4 = "Extremely").

Sample item: "Any reminders brought back feelings about it."

Type of outcome measure provided: Yields subscale scores for Intrusion, Avoidance, and Hyperarousal (each of which can range from 0–4).

Time frame assessed: Past 7 days.

Development notes: Adapted from the Impact of Event Scale (Horowitz, Wilner, & Alvarez, 1979).

Correspondence with DSM: Assesses 14 of the 17 DSM-III-R and DSM-IV symptom criteria (B, C, and D) for PTSD.

Psychometric Information

Validation populations: Earthquake survivors, emergency disaster workers (police, fire, emergency medical personnel, and highway department workers), Vietnam combat veterans, men and women who have been subject to violence, and women who have been sexually assaulted.

Reliability: Evidence of internal consistency includes Cronbach's α values for subscale scores ranging from .79 to .92 in various samples (Weiss & Marmar, 1996). Evidence for consistency over time includes 6-month test–retest reliability correlations for subscale scores that ranged from .89 to .94.

Validity: Evidence for construct validity includes strong correlations among the three subscale scores. Correlations between subscale scores in one study ranged from .74 to .87.

Descriptive/psychometric information sources: Weiss, D. S., & Marmar, C. R. (1996). The Impact of Event Scale—Revised. In J. Wilson & T. M. Keane (Eds.), *Assessing psychological trauma and PTSD* (pp. 399–411). New York: Guilford Press. (Includes measure in its entirety.)

How to Obtain Scale

Contact Daniel Weiss, PhD, Department of Psychiatry, University of California–San Francisco, Box F-0984, San Francisco, CA 94143-0984.

Modified PTSD Symptom Scale:
Self-Report Version (MPSS-SR)
(S. Falsetti, P. Resick, H. Resnick, & D. Kilpatrick)

Recommended Uses

Recommended for measuring PTSD symptoms in clinical or research settings. Especially useful for clients with histories of multiple traumatic events or for clients whose trauma history is unknown.

Special Features

This measure does not key symptoms to any single traumatic event. The scale inquires about each symptom in general and then asks what event the symptom is related to. Yields scores for both frequency and severity of PTSD symptoms.

General Descriptive Information

Symptoms assessed: Assesses DSM-III-R/DSM-IV symptoms for PTSD.

Number of items; time to complete: 17 items; takes 10–15 minutes to complete.

Response format: For each item, client rates frequency (from 0 = "Not at all" to 3 = "5 or more times per week") and severity (from A = "Not at all distressing" to D = "Extremely distressing"). Client also answers "About which event(s)?" for each item.

Sample item: "Have you had repeated upsetting thoughts that happened even when you didn't want them to?" "About which event(s)?"

Type of outcome measure provided: Scale yields frequency scores (ranging from 0 to 51), severity scores (ranging from 0 to 51), and total scores ranging from 0 to 102 and can be used to make a preliminary determination about whether client's symptoms meet DSM criteria for PTSD.

Time frame assessed: Past 2 weeks.

Development notes: Adapted from the PTSD Symptom Scale (Foa et al., 1993).

Correspondence with DSM: Assesses DSM-III-R and DSM-IV symptom Criteria (B, C, and D) for PTSD.

Psychometric Information

Validation populations: Psychiatric patients exposed to various traumatic experiences and a community sample.

Reliability: Evidence of internal consistency includes Cronbach's α values of .96 for the treatment sample and .97 for the community sample (Falsetti, Resnick, Resick, & Kilpatrick, 1993).

Validity: Evidence for construct validity includes a sensitivity rate of .93 for a treatment sample and .91 for a community sample when MPSS-SR results were compared to those of the Structured Clinical Interview for DSM-III-R (SCID) (Falsetti, Resick, Resnick, & Kilpatrick, 1992). The specificity of the scale was .62 in the treatment sample and .84 in the community sample. The moderate specificity rate indicates that the MPSS-SR is more likely to identify patients as meeting criteria for PTSD than is the SCID. This may be because the MPSS-SR allows clients to endorse symptoms relating to different traumatic experiences while the SCID asks only about symptoms relating to a single identified traumatic event.

Descriptive/psychometric information sources: Falsetti, S. A., Resick, P. A., Resnick, H. S., & Kilpatrick, D. (1992, November). *Post-traumatic stress disorder: The assessment of frequency and severity of symptoms in clinical and nonclinical samples.* Paper presented at the annual convention of the Association for Advancement of Behavior Therapy, Boston.

Falsetti, S. A., Resnick, H. S., Resick, P. A., & Kilpatrick, D. (1993). The Modified PTSD Symptom Scale: A brief self-report measure of posttraumatic stress disorder. *The Behavioral Therapist, 16,* 161–162.

How to Obtain Scale

Contact Sherry Falsetti, PhD, Medical University of South Carolina, Crime Victims Research and Treatment Center, Medical University of North Carolina, 171 Ashley Avenue, Charleston, SC 29425-0742.

Penn Inventory for Posttraumatic Stress Disorder
(M. Hammarberg)

Recommended Uses

Recommended for screening for PTSD in clinical or research settings. Can be used with clients with multiple traumatic experiences. May not discriminate clients with PTSD from others in samples with relatively few PTSD patients.

Special Features

This measure's response format is unique: It resembles that of the Beck Depression Inventory and asks clients to endorse the one statement of four that best describes their feelings. Symptoms described are not keyed to any particular traumatic event.

General Descriptive Information

Symptoms assessed: Items are generally based on DSM-III-R/DSM-IV symptoms for PTSD, but they do not assess all of the DSM symptoms. Some symptoms are assessed by more than one item (e.g., intrusive thoughts), and some symptoms are included that are not directly related to DSM criteria (e.g., self-knowledge).

Number of items; time to complete: 26 items; takes 5–15 minutes to complete.

Response format: For each item, clients circle a number next to the one statement of four that best describes their feelings. Scale scores for statements range from 0 to 3, reflecting the degree, frequency, or severity of the particular symptom.

Sample item: 0 = "I know someone nearby who really understands me"; 1 = "I'm not concerned whether anyone nearby really understands me"; 2 = "I'm worried because no one nearby really understands me"; 3 = "I'm very worried because no one nearby understands me at all."

Type of outcome measure provided: Scale yields total scores ranging from 0 to 78.

Time frame assessed: Past week.

Correspondence with DSM: Does not directly correspond to DSM symptom criteria for PTSD.

Psychometric Information

Validation populations: Combat veterans, Vietnam-era veterans, oil-rig disaster survivors.

Reliability: Evidence of internal consistency includes Cronbach's α values of .94 for total score in two samples (Hammarberg, 1992). Evidence for consistency over time includes a test–retest reliability correlation for total score of .96 with a test–retest period of 3 to 8 days.

Validity: Evidence for construct validity includes sensitivity rates ranging from .90 to .98 in three samples when Penn Inventory scores were compared to results of a structured clinical interview (Hammarberg, 1992). Specificity rates ranged from .61 to 1.0 for the same three samples. However, in a study of subjects with a lower prevalence rate of PTSD than the Hammarberg samples, specificity dropped to .33, indicating that the ability of the scale to discriminate PTSD patients from those with other psychiatric diagnoses may be limited in samples that have relatively few subjects with PTSD (Kutcher, Tremont, Burda, & Mellman, 1994). Convergent validity was supported by strong correlations between scores on the Penn Inventory and the Mississippi Scale for

Combat-Related PTSD $(r = .85)$ and the state anxiety subscale of the Spielberger State–Trait Anxiety Inventory (STAI) $(r =.77)$.

Descriptive/psychometric information sources: Hammarberg, M. (1992). Penn Inventory for posttraumatic stress disorder: Psychometric properties. *Psychological Assessment, 4,* 67–76. (Includes measure in its entirety.)

Hammarberg, M. (1996). Psychometric review of the Penn Inventory for Post Traumatic Stress Disorder. In B. H. Stamm (Ed.), *Measurement of stress, trauma, and adaptation* (pp. 231–235). Lutherville, MD: Sidran Press. (Includes measure in its entirety.)

How to Obtain Scale

Contact Melvyn Hammarberg, PhD, Department of Anthropology, University of Pennsylvania, 325 University Museum, 33rd and Spruce Street, Philadelphia, PA 19104-6398.

Posttraumatic Stress Diagnostic Scale (PDS)
(E. Foa)

Recommended Uses

Recommended for use in clinical or research settings to measure severity of PTSD symptoms related to a single identified traumatic event. Can also be used to make a preliminary DSM-IV diagnosis for PTSD.

Special Features

The PDS is unique in that it assesses all of the DSM-IV criteria for PTSD. In addition to measuring the severity of PTSD symptoms, this measure inquires about the experience of Criterion A traumatic events, about duration of symptoms, and about the effects of symptoms on daily functioning.

General Descriptive Information

Symptoms assessed: Assesses DSM-IV symptoms for PTSD.

Number of items; time to complete: 49 items; takes 10–15 minutes to complete.

Response format: For each item, client gives a severity rating that largely reflects frequency (from 0 = "Not at all or only one time" to 3 = "5 or more times a week/almost always").

Sample item: "Having upsetting thoughts or images about the traumatic event that came into your head when you didn't want them to."

Type of outcome measure provided: Scale yields total severity scores ranging from 0 to 51 that largely reflect the frequency of symptoms. PDS Profile Reports also provide a preliminary determination of DSM-IV PTSD diagnostic status, a count of the number of symptoms endorsed, a rating of symptom severity, and a rating of the level of impairment of functioning.

Time frame assessed: Past month (time frame can be adjusted for different uses).

Correspondence with DSM: Assesses all of the DSM-IV criteria for PTSD (A, B, C, D, E, and F).

Psychometric Information

Validation populations: Accident/fire, natural disaster, nonsexual assault, sexual assault, combat, sexual abuse, life-threatening illness.

Reliability: Evidence of internal consistency includes a Cronbach's α value of .92 for the total score and values ranging from .78 to .84 for cluster subscale scores (Foa, Cashman, Jaycox, & Perry, in press). Evidence for consistency over time includes a 2- to 3-week test–retest reliability correlation for total score of .83.

Validity: Evidence for construct validity includes a sensitivity rate of .89 and a specificity rate of .75 when PDS results were compared to those of the Structured Clinical Interview for DSM-III-R (SCID) (Foa et al., in press). Furthermore, convergent validity was supported by a correlation of .77 between PDS reexperiencing cluster scores and IES-R scores and a correlation of .69 PDS avoidance cluster scores and IES-R scores.

Descriptive/psychometric information sources: Foa, E. (1996). *Posttraumatic Diagnostic Scale manual.* Minneapolis, MN: National Computer Systems.
    Foa, E., Cashman, L., Jaycox, L., & Perry, K. (in press). The validation of a self-report measure of PTSD: The Posttraumatic Diagnostic Scale (PDS). *Psychological Assessment.*

How to Obtain Scale

Contact National Computer Systems (NCS), 5605 Green Circle Drive, Minnetonka, MN 55343; 800-627-7271 (ext. 5151).

Revised Civilian Mississippi Scale for PTSD (R-CMS)
(F. Norris & J. Perilla)

Recommended Uses

Recommended for use in clinical or research settings to measure PTSD symptoms related to a single identified traumatic event.

Special Features

This revised version of the civilian version of Mississippi PTSD Scale (Vreven, King, & King, 1995) uses a very simple response format that is particularly easy for some clients to understand. The scale is available and validated in both English and Spanish.

General Descriptive Information

Symptoms assessed: Items assess DSM-III-R/DSM-IV symptom criteria (B, C, and D) for PTSD along with a number of other symptoms associated with PTSD (e.g., guilt).

Number of items; time to complete: 30 items; takes 5–10 minutes to complete.

Response format: Client rates each item on a scale from 1 = "Not at all true" to 5 = "Extremely true." Items reflect the degree, frequency, or severity of the particular symptom.

Sample item: "If something happens that reminds me of the event, I become very distressed and upset."

Type of outcome measure provided: Scale yields total scores ranging from 30 to 150 (with five items requiring reverse scoring).

Time frame assessed: "Since the event."

Development notes: Adapted from the Mississippi Scale for Combat-Related PTSD (Keane, Caddell, & Taylor, 1988).

Correspondence with DSM: Contains items that correspond to DSM-III-R/DSM-IV symptom criteria (B, C, and D) for PTSD.

Psychometric Information

Validation populations: Two bilingual community samples, hurricane victims.

Reliability: Evidence of internal consistency includes Cronbach's α values of .86 and .88 for two samples completing the English version and .88 and .92 for two samples completing the Spanish version. Evidence for consistency across time and languages includes a 1-week test–retest reliability correlation for total score of .84 (Norris & Perilla, 1996).

Validity: Evidence for construct validity includes findings that hurricane victims scored higher on the R-CMS than did community sample subjects whose traumatic events were generally not as recent. Furthermore, scale scores were higher among those who experienced life threat or injury in relation to a traumatic event.

Descriptive/psychometric information sources: Norris, F. H., & Perilla, J. L. (1996). The Revised Civilian Mississippi Scale for PTSD: Reliability, validity, and cross-language stability. *Journal of Traumatic Stress, 9,* 285–298.

How to Obtain Scale

Contact Fran Norris, PhD, Department of Psychology, Georgia State University, University Plaza, Atlanta, GA 30303.

Screen for Posttraumatic Stress Symptoms (SPTSS)
(E. Carlson)

Recommended Uses

Recommended for screening for PTSD symptoms in clinical or research settings. Especially useful for clients with histories of multiple traumatic events or for clients whose trauma history is unknown.

Special Features

This measure is very brief and does not key symptoms to any single traumatic event. First person item wording is easy for clients to understand.

General Descriptive Information

Symptoms assessed: Assesses DSM-III-R/DSM-IV symptoms for PTSD.

Number of items; time to complete: 17 items; takes 5 minutes to complete.

Response format: For each item, client rates frequency from 0 = "Not at all" to 10 = "Always."

Sample item: "I get very upset when something reminds me of something bad that happened to me."

Type of outcome measure provided: Scale yields total score that is the average of the item scores and ranges from 0 to 10. Item scores can be used to make a preliminary determination about whether client's symptoms meet DSM criteria for PTSD.

Time frame assessed: Past 2 weeks.

Correspondence with DSM: Assesses DSM-III-R and DSM-IV symptom criteria (B, C, and D) for PTSD.

Psychometric Information

Validation populations: Psychiatric inpatients (some with exposure to traumatic experiences).

Reliability: Evidence of internal consistency includes a split-half reliability of .91 (Carlson, 1997). Preliminary test–retest results (for a small number of subjects) show good consistency over time ($r = .82$).

Validity: Evidence for construct validity includes a strong correlation between SPTSS scores and scores on the Structured Interview for PTSD (SI-PTSD) with $r = .67$ (Carlson, 1997). Other evidence for the concurrent validity of the SPTSS includes a sensitivity rate of .95 when endorsement of SPTSS items (at 5 or higher) were compared to SI-PTSD (Davidson, Smith, & Kudler, 1989) diagnoses (Carlson, 1997). Specificity levels were considerably lower (.57), indicating that the SPTSS is more likely to identify patients as possibly meeting criteria for PTSD than is the SI-PTSD. This finding may result, in part, from the fact that the SPTSS allows clients to endorse symptoms relating to different traumatic experiences, while the SI-PTSD asks only about symptoms relating to a single identified traumatic event.

Descriptive/psychometric information sources: Carlson, E. (1997). Validation of a brief scale to measure posttraumatic stress disorder symptoms following single or multiple traumas. (Unpublished manuscript.)

How to Obtain Scale

Contact Eve Carlson, PhD, Clinical Psychology Associates, 611 East Walworth Avenue, Delavan, WI 53115.

Trauma Symptom Inventory (TSI)
(J. Briere)

Recommended Uses

Recommended for measuring a variety of trauma-related symptoms in clinical or research settings.

Special Features

This measure has 10 clinical scales that assess a variety of symptom domains related to trauma, including several that are not measured by the brief self-report PTSD measures. The measure also includes three validity scales that may be useful in identifying response tendencies that would invalidate the test results.

General Descriptive Information

Symptoms assessed: Items assess domains of anxious arousal, depression, anger/irritability, intrusive experiences, defensive avoidance, dissociation, sexual concerns, dysfunctional sexual behavior, impaired self-reference, and tension-reduction behavior. Validity scales assess atypical responses, response level (very low reporting), and inconsistent reponses.

Number of items; time to complete: 100 items; takes about 20 minutes to complete.

Response format: For each item, client rates frequency (from 0 = "Never" to 3 = "Often").

Sample item: "Pushing painful memories out of your mind."

Type of outcome measure provided: Raw scale scores are converted to T scores for the 10 clinical scales and the three validity scales based on a normative sample. A computer scoring program is available from the test publisher.

Time frame assessed: "Last 6 months."

Correspondence with DSM: Contains items that correspond to DSM-III-R/DSM-IV symptom criteria (B, C, and D) for PTSD but does not specifically assess these criteria.

Psychometric Information

Validation populations: General population, psychiatric inpatients, psychiatric outpatients, university students, Navy recruits.

Reliability: Evidence of internal consistency includes mean Cronbach's α values for the 10 clinical scales of .84 to .87 across general population, clinical, university, and Navy recruit samples (Briere, 1995).

Validity: Evidence for construct validity includes findings that subjects who report past trauma scored higher on all 10 clinical scales than those who report no trauma (Briere, 1995). Evidence for convergent validity includes a strong correlation ($r = .69$) between TSI Defensive Avoidance scores and scores on the avoidance subscale of the IES (Horowitz et al., 1979). Similarly, there was a strong correlation ($r = .67$) between TSI Intrusive Experiences scores and scores on the instrusion subscale of the IES. Criterion validity was shown by a sensitivity rate of 92% and a specificity rate of 91% when weighted TSI scale scores were used to predict PTSD status established by joint scoring of the IES and the Los Angeles Symptom Checklist.

Descriptive/psychometric information sources: Briere, J. (1995). *Trauma Symptom Inventory professional manual.* Odessa, FL: Psychological Assessment Resources.

Briere, J. (1996). Psychometric review of Trauma Symptom Inventory (TSI). In B. H. Stamm (Ed.), *Measurement of stress, trauma, and adaptation* (pp. 381–383). Lutherville, MD: Sidran Press.

How to Obtain Scale

Contact Psychological Assessment Resources, Box 998, Odessa, FL 33556; 1-800-331-8378.

Section C

Structured Interviews for Posttraumatic and Dissociative Disorders

STRUCTURED INTERVIEWS FOR POSTTRAUMATIC STRESS DISORDER

Clinician-Administered PTSD Scale (CAPS)
(D. Blake, F. Weathers, L. Nagy, D. Kaloupek, D. Charney, & T. Keane)

Recommended Uses

Recommended for use in clinical or research settings to measure PTSD and ASD symptoms related to up to three identified traumatic events. Can also be used to make DSM-IV PTSD and ASD diagnoses.

Special Features

Two new versions of the CAPS are now available that assess DSM-IV PTSD and ASD criteria. These include the CAPS-DX, which gathers information to make a current or lifetime diagnosis of PTSD, and the CAPS-SX, which assesses symptoms over the past week. The CAPS has the advantages of being extremely thorough and detailed and the disadvantage of taking longer to administer than some other PTSD-structured interviews. Some of the unique elements that the measure allows you to assess include the impact of symptoms on social and occupational functioning, improvement in symptoms since a previous CAPS administration, overall response validity, overall PTSD severity, and five associated symptoms (see details below).

General Descriptive Information

Experiences and symptoms assessed: The most recent version assesses DSM-IV symptoms for PTSD, including Criteria A–F, the impact of symptoms on social and occupational functioning, improvement in symptoms since a previous CAPS administration, overall response validity, overall PTSD severity, and five associated symptoms (guilt over acts, survivor guilt, gaps in awareness, depersonalization, and derealization). As part of the assessment of Criterion A, a Life Events Checklist is used to determine experiences with 17 different traumatic events. The most recent version also assesses DSM-IV symptoms for ASD.

Number of items; time to complete: 30 items; takes 30–60 minutes to administer.

Response format: For each item, multiple standard questions are provided to elicit information about experiences or symptoms. For symptom items, the interviewer uses the client's answers to assign a frequency rating (e.g., from 0 = "Never" to 4 = "Daily or almost every day") and an intensity rating (e.g., from 0 = "None" to 4 = "Extreme, incapacitating distress"). For each item, the verbal ratings for intensity are tailored to that particular item.

Training required to administer: The CAPS was designed to be administered by clinicians and clinical researchers who have a working knowledge of PTSD but can also be administered by appropriately trained paraprofessionals (Blake et al., 1995).

Sample item: (For frequency rating of intrusive recollections) "Have you ever had unwanted memories of [event]? What were they like? What did you remember? [If not clear] Did they ever occur while you were awake, or only in dreams? [Exclude if memories occurred only during dreams.] How often have you had these memories in the past month?"

Type of outcome measure provided: CAPS responses can be used to determine whether a client's symptoms meet DSM-IV criteria for PTSD or ASD. Continuous ratings are also calculated for frequency and for intensity of symptoms (ranging from 0–68) and for severity (frequency + intensity; ranging from 0–136). Additional scoring options have been devised and are provided with the CAPS.

Time frame assessed: CAPS-DX: past month or worst month ever (if criteria are not met for current diagnosis). CAPS-SX: past week.

Correspondence with DSM: Assesses DSM-IV Criteria A–F for PTSD and Criteria A–G for ASD.

Psychometric Information

The psychometric information available for the CAPS was gathered using a previous version of the scale, though further validation will no doubt follow the revision of the CAPS. Until then, given that the changes made to the measure were relatively minor, it seems reasonable to assume that the psychometric properties of the CAPS-DX and CAPS-SX are similar to those of the original CAPS.

Validation populations: Combat veterans, motor vehicle accidents.

Reliability: Evidence of internal consistency includes an alpha of .94 for the 17 PTSD items. Consistency over time was determined by having two different interviewers administer the CAPS with a 2–3 day test–retest interval. For three different pairs of interviewers, reliability correlations for total score between the two administrations varied from .90 to .98.

Validity: Evidence for construct validity includes a sensitivity rate of .84 and a specificity rate of .95 when CAPS results were compared to those of the PTSD module of the SCID (Blake et al., 1995). Furthermore, convergent validity was established with an extremely high correlation of .91 between CAPS scores and scores on the Mississippi Scale for Combat-related PTSD.

Descriptive/psychometric information sources: Blake, D. D. (1994). Rationale and development of the clinician-administered PTSD scales. *PTSD Research Quarterly, 5,* 1–2.

Blake, D. D., Weathers, F. W., Nagy, L. M., Kaloupek, D. G., Gusman, F. D., Charney, D. S., & Keane, T. M. (1995). The development of a clinician-administered PTSD scale. *Journal of Traumatic Stress, 8,* 75–90.

Weathers, F. W., & Litz, B. T. (1994). Psychometric properties of the clinician-administered PTSD scales. *PTSD Research Quarterly, 5,* 2–6.

How to Obtain Scale

Contact Frank W. Weathers, PhD, National Center for PTSD, Boston VA Medical Center, 116B, 150 South Huntington Avenue, Boston, MA 02130.

PTSD Symptom Scale—Interview (PSS-I)
(E. Foa)

Recommended Uses

Recommended for use in clinical or research settings to measure PTSD symptoms related to a single identified traumatic event.

Special Features

This measure has the advantages of being relatively quick to administer and of having the option to have lay interviewers administer the measure after a fairly brief training session.

General Descriptive Information

Symptoms assessed: Assesses DSM-III-R/DSM-IV symptoms for PTSD.

Number of items; time to complete: 17 items; takes 20 minutes to administer.

Response format: For each item, the interviewer assigns a severity rating that largely reflects frequency (from 0 = "Not at all" to 3 = "Very much").

Training required to administer: Can be administered by a master-level interviewer after a few hours of training.

Sample item: "Have you had upsetting thoughts or images about the event that came into your head when you didn't want them to?"

Type of outcome measure provided: Scale yields total severity scores ranging from 0 to 51 that largely reflect the frequency of symptoms. Cluster severity scores can also be calculated for reexperiencing, avoidance, and arousal symptom clusters. Item responses can be used to make a determination about whether client's symptoms meet DSM Criteria B, C, and D for PTSD.

Time frame assessed: Past 2 weeks (time frame can be adjusted for different uses).

Correspondence with DSM: Assesses DSM-III-R and DSM-IV symptom criteria (B, C, and D) for PTSD.

Psychometric Information

Validation populations: Female sexual assault victims and female nonsexual assault victims.

Reliability: Evidence of internal consistency includes a Cronbach's α value of .85 for the total score and values ranging from .65 to .71 for cluster subscale scores (Foa, Riggs, Dancu, & Rothbaum, 1993). Evidence for consistency over time includes a 1-month test–retest reliability correlation for total score of .80.

Validity: Evidence for construct validity includes a sensitivity rate of .88 when PSS-SR results were compared to those of the PTSD module of the SCID (Foa et al., 1993). The specificity of the scale was .96. Furthermore, convergent validity was established with correlations ranging from .48 to .80 between PSS-I scores and scores on the Impact of Events intrusion scores, Impact of Events avoidance scores, the state portion of the State–Trait Anxiety Inventory, and the PSS-SR.

Descriptive/psychometric information sources: Foa, E. B., Riggs, D. S., Dancu, C. V., & Rothbaum, B. O. (1993). Reliability and validity of a brief instrument for assessing post-traumatic stress disorder. *Journal of Traumatic Stress, 6,* 459–474.

How to Obtain Scale

Contact Edna Foa, PhD, Medical College of Pennsylvania, Department of Psychiatry, 3200 Henry Avenue, Philadelphia, PA 19129-1137.

Structured Interview for PTSD (SI-PTSD)
(J. Davidson)

Recommended Uses

Recommended for use in clinical or research settings to measure PTSD symptoms related to a single identified traumatic event.

Special Features

This measure has the advantages of being fairly thorough but also relatively simple to administer and score.

General Descriptive Information

Symptoms assessed: Assesses DSM-III-R/DSM-IV symptoms for PTSD.

Number of items; time to complete: 17 items; takes 20–30 minutes to administer if initial screen questions are positive.

Response format: For each item, client gives a severity rating which largely reflects frequency (from 0 = "Not at all" to 4 = "Extremely severe: daily or produces so much impairment that patient cannot work or enter social situations").

Training required to administer: Can be administered by mental health professionals or by paraprofessionals after some training.

Sample item: "Have you experienced painful images or memories of combat or other trauma which you couldn't get out of your mind, even though you may have wanted to? Have these been recurrent?"

Type of outcome measure provided: Scale yields total scores ranging from 0 to 68 that largely reflect the frequency of symptoms. Some items focus more on frequency and some focus on intensity of symptoms. Scores are obtained for symptoms in the past 4 weeks and for "Worst ever" symptoms. Item responses can be used to make a determination about whether client's symptoms meet DSM Criteria B, C, and D for PTSD. It is important to note, however that the "Worst ever" for different symptoms may have occurred at different times. Without specifying a period of 1 month in which symptoms occurred, it is not possible to determine if the client met criteria for PTSD some time in the past.

Time frame assessed: Past 4 weeks.

Correspondence with DSM: Assesses DSM-III-R and DSM-IV symptom criteria (B, C, and D) for PTSD.

Psychometric Information

Validation populations: War veterans.

Reliability: Evidence of internal consistency includes a Cronbach's α of .94 for the total score (Davidson, Smith, & Kudler, 1989). Evidence for consistency over time includes a 2-week test–retest reliability correlation for total score of .71. The SI-PTSD has good interrater reliability with intraclass correlation coefficients of agreement for total scores of .97.

Validity: Evidence for construct validity includes a sensitivity rate of .96 when SI-PTSD results were compared to those of the PTSD module of the SCID (Davidson et al., 1989). The specificity of the scale was .80. Furthermore, convergent validity is supported by moderately high correlations between SI-PTSD scores and total scores on the IES ($r = .61$) and scores on the Hamilton Anxiety Scale ($r = .51$).

Descriptive/psychometric information sources: Davidson, J. R. T., Kudler, H. S., & Smith, R. D. (1990). Assessment and pharmacotherapy of posttraumatic stress disorder. In J. E. L. Giller (Ed.), *Biological assessment and treatment of posttraumatic stress disorder* (pp. 205–221). Washington, DC: American Psychiatric Press. (Includes measure in its entirety.)

Davidson, J., & Smith, R. (1990). Traumatic experiences in psychiatric outpatients. *Journal of Traumatic Stress, 3,* 459–475.

Davidson, J. R. T., Smith, R. D., & Kudler, H. S. (1989). Validity and reliability of the DSM-III criteria for posttraumatic stress disorder: Experience with a structured interview. *Journal of Nervous and Mental Disease, 177,* 336–341.

How to Obtain Scale

Contact Jonathan Davidson, MD, Department of Psychiatry, Box 3812, Duke University Medical Center, Durham, NC 27710-3812.

STRUCTURED INTERVIEWS
FOR DISSOCIATIVE DISORDERS

Clinical Mental Status Examination
for Complex Dissociative Symptoms
(R. Loewenstein)

Recommended Uses

Recommended for use in clinical or research settings to gather information about dissociative symptoms and to diagnose dissociative disorders.

Special Features

This semistructured interview can be used to inquire about a variety of symptoms associated with dissociative disorders. The interview begins with symptoms common to many trauma-related disorders (such as amnesia, dissociative intrusions, and autohypnotic phenomena) and proceeds to more specific dissociative disorder symptoms (such as perceptions of multiple identities).

General Descriptive Information

Symptoms and experiences assessed: Assesses symptoms in six domains including process symptoms (identity confusion and state changes), amnesia symptoms, autohypnotic symptoms, PTSD symptoms, somatoform symptoms, and affective symptoms.

Number of items; time to complete: 103 items (most are in the first four domains listed above); takes 30–60 minutes to administer (depending on the number of positive responses).

Response format: Most of the items are dichotomous ("Yes" or "No") questions. Respondents are encouraged to elaborate on all endorsed symptoms.

Training required to administer: This measure should be administered by a trained and experienced mental health professional.

Sample item: "Do you ever have blackouts? Blank spells? Memory lapses?"

Type of outcome measure provided: Answers to items may provide enough information to allow a clinician to determine whether a client meets DSM-IV diagnostic criteria for any dissociative disorders. No quantitative scoring system has been developed.

Time frame assessed: Lifetime.

Correspondence with DSM: Assesses DSM-IV criteria for the five dissociative disorders as well as most of DSM-IV PTSD criteria.

Psychometric Information

Validation populations: None to date.

Reliability: None to date.

Validity: None to date.

Descriptive/psychometric information sources: Loewenstein, R. J. (1991). An office mental status examination for complex chronic dissociative symptoms and multiple personality disorder. *Psychiatric Clinics of North America, 14,* 567–604. (Includes measure in its entirety.)

How to Obtain Scale

Contact Richard J. Loewenstein, MD, Department of Psychiatry, Sheppard Pratt Health System, 6501 North Charles Street, Baltimore, MD 21285-6815.

Dissociative Disorders Interview Schedule (DDIS)
(C. Ross)

Recommended Uses

Recommended for use in clinical or research settings to gather information about symptoms of dissociative disorders.

Special Features

This measure assesses a wide variety of domains related to dissociative disorders. It is fairly brief and simple to use and can be administered by a lay interviewer.

General Descriptive Information

Symptoms and experiences assessed: Assesses symptoms for dissociative disorders (DID, dissociative amnesia, dissociative fugue, depersonalization disorder, and dissociative disorder not otherwise specified), somatization disorder, borderline personality disorder, and major depressive disorder. Also inquires about some symptoms of schizophrenia, secondary features of dissociative identity disorder, substance abuse, extrasensory experiences, and childhood abuse experiences.

Number of items; time to complete: 128 items (fewer if screening questions elicit negative responses); takes 30–45 minutes to administer (depending on the number of positive responses to screen questions).

Response format: All DDIS items have categorical response options. Most of the items allow essentially dichotomous responding with "Yes,"

"No," or "Unsure" options. A few items offer response options with ranges of ages or frequency categories.

Training required to administer: This measure can be administered by mental health professionals or by lay interviewers.

Sample item: "Have you ever experienced inability to recall important personal information, particularly of a traumatic or stressful nature, that is too extensive to be explained by ordinary forgetting?"

Type of outcome measure provided: The DDIS inquires about symptoms that constitute criteria for the five dissociative disorders as well as somatization disorder, borderline personality disorder, and major depressive disorder. Answers to items may allow the clinician to determine whether a client meets DSM-IV diagnostic criteria for these disorders, but for the dissociative disorders, relatively few items directly assess symptom criteria. Also, dichotomous answers to criterion items may not provide enough information to make conclusive diagnoses without further information.

Time frame assessed: Lifetime.

Correspondence with DSM: Assesses DSM-IV criteria for the five dissociative disorders as well as somatization disorder, borderline personality disorder, and major depressive disorder.

Psychometric Information

Validation populations: Dissociative psychiatric patients, nondissociative psychiatric patients, general population subjects, patients in various DSM diagnostic categories.

Reliability: Evidence of consistency across raters includes an interrater reliability coefficient of .68 (Ross et al., 1989).

Validity: Construct validity of the DDIS is supported by a correlation between the secondary features of DID items and scores on the Dissociative Experiences Scale of .78. Good specificity and sensitivity are reported for the DDIS based on cumulative data from studies where DDIS diagnosis was compared to an independent clinical diagnosis (Ross, 1997).

Descriptive/psychometric information sources: Ross, C. A. (1997). *Dissociative Identity Disorder: Diagnosis, clinical features, and treatment of multiple personality* (2nd ed.). New York: Wiley.

Ross, C. A., Heber, S., Norton, G. R., Anderson, D., Anderson, G., & Barchet, P. (1989). The Dissociative Disorders Interview Schedule: A structured interview. *Dissociation, 2*(3), 169–189. (Includes measure in its entirety.)

How to Obtain Scale

Contact Colin Ross, MD, 1701 Gateway, Suite 349, Richardson, TX 75080.

Structured Clinical Interview for DSM-IV Dissociative Disorders–Revised (SCID-D-R)
(M. Steinberg)

Recommended Uses

Recommended for use in clinical or research settings to measure dissociation symptoms and to diagnose dissociative disorders.

Special Features

This measure is extremely thorough and detailed. It elicits detailed information about a range of dissociative experiences and allows clinicians to diagnose dissociative disorders. For each inquiry, there is a general screening question with detailed follow-up questions to explore the symptoms.

General Descriptive Information

Symptoms assessed: Assesses the severity of five core dissociative symptoms.

Number of items; time to complete: 277 items (fewer if screening questions elicit negative responses); takes 30–90 minutes to administer (depending on the number of positive responses to screen questions).

Response format: Many SCID-D items are free response items, while others require the interviewer to select the most accurate statement in a series, based on the client's responses to specific questions. For example, for many items, the interviewer indicates the frequency of a symptom with choices ranging from "Rarely (up to four isolated episodes)" to "Daily or weekly episodes."

Training required to administer: This measure is designed to be administered by a mental health professional who follows the procedures outlined in Steinberg (1994).

Sample item: "Have you ever felt as if there were large gaps in your memory? [If yes] Can you describe what that experience is like? What made you aware of these gaps? How often does that occur?"

Type of outcome measure provided: The SCID-D allows the clinician to determine whether a client meets DSM-IV diagnostic criteria for any of five dissociative disorders. Scoring for each diagnostic criterion relies on a combination of specific interview items.

Time frame assessed: Lifetime.

Correspondence with DSM: Assesses DSM-IV criteria for dissociative identity disorder, depersonalization disorder, dissociative fugue, dissociative amnesia, and dissociative disorder not otherwise specified.

Psychometric Information

Validation populations: Psychiatric outpatients.

Reliability: Evidence of consistency across raters includes a rate of agreement of 96% for the presence or absence of a dissociative disorder between two raters (Steinberg, Rounsaville, & Cicchetti, 1990).

Validity: Construct validity of the SCID-D is supported by analyses showing the ability of the measure to distinguish between patients with dissociative disorders, patients with nondissociative psychiatric disorders, and normal control subjects (Steinberg et al., 1990). Other analyses have shown close correspondence between scores on the Dissociative Experiences Scale and SCID-D diagnoses (Steinberg, Rounsaville, & Cicchetti, 1991).

Descriptive/psychometric information sources: Steinberg, M. (1994). *Interviewer's guide to the Structured Clinical Interview for DSM-IV Dissociative Disorders—Revised (SCID-D).* Washington, DC: American Psychiatric Press.

Steinberg, M. (1995). *Handbook for the assessment of dissociation: A clinical guide.* Washington, DC: American Psychiatric Press.

Steinberg, M., Rounsaville, B., & Cicchetti, D. (1990). The Structured Clinical Interview for DSM-III-R Dissociative Disorders: Preliminary report on a new diagnostic instrument. *American Journal of Psychiatry, 147,* 76–82.

How to Obtain Scale

Contact American Psychiatric Press, 1400 K Street, NW, Washington, DC 20005; 800-368-5777.

Measures of Trauma and Trauma Responses for Children

MEASURES OF TRAUMATIC EXPERIENCES

Dimensions of Stressful Events (DOSE)
(K. Fletcher)

Recommended Uses

Recommended for gathering qualitative information about dimensions of traumatic events in children that influence responses to trauma.

Special Features

This series of questions provides a systematic approach to gathering information about a wide variety of characteristics of a traumatic event. This information can be collected from the child and/or other informants and may be very valuable to treatment planning.

General Descriptive Information

Measure format: Interviewer completes based on information from child, caretakers, or other informants.

Targeted age group: Children and adolescents (ages not specified).

Events assessed: Inquires about a range of potentially traumatic events including actual or threatened physical injury, sexual abuse, witnessing violence, death, serious injury, or threat of injury/death. Most questions relate to characteristics of an identified traumatic event (see

Aspects of Traumas Assessed below) rather than assessing different types of traumatic events.

Number of items; time to administer: 25 general items; 24 additional items for sexually abused children; 15–30 minutes for administration to each informant.

Response format: Varies across items, included items with dichotomous choices and categorical choices (e.g., categories for who was injured, how much control child felt he had, certainty that abuse took place).

Training required to administer: Information should be gathered by experienced mental health professional.

Sample item: "Who were the direct victims or the stressful events?" (Check all that apply.)

Type of outcome measure provided: Possibilities for scoring are suggested by the authors, but there is no established scoring method.

Aspects of traumas assessed: Inquires about a very wide range of characteristics of traumatic events including persons affected, frequency, duration, source of event, preparedness for event, feelings of control over event, separation from family related to event, losses due to event, perceived causes of event. For sexually abused children, inquires about many aspects of abuse including seriousness of abuse, certainty, frequency, resistance, offender's use of rewards, restraint, threats, denial, and various postevent responses by caretakers.

Time frame assessed: Not specified; designed for inquiries relevant to a recent traumatic event.

Correspondence with DSM: Assesses DSM-IV Criterion A-1 (experiencing or witnessing actual injury or threat of death/injury) and Criterion A-2 (experiencing fear, helplessness, or horror).

Psychometric Information

Validation populations: Children in treatment who had been exposed to traumatic events; children from a community sample.

Reliability: None to date.

Validity: Evidence that supports construct validity includes significant associations between DOSE levels and PTSD diagnosis assigned from results of the When Bad Things Happen Scale, the Child PTSD Interview, and the Child PTSD Interview—Parent Form.

Descriptive/psychometric information sources: Fletcher, K. (1996). Psychometric review of Dimensions of Stressful Events (DOSE) Ratings

Scale. In B. H. Stamm (Ed.), *Measurement of stress, trauma, and adaptation* (pp. 144–151). Lutherville, MD: Sidran Press. (Includes measure in its entirety.)

How to Obtain Scale

Contact Kenneth E. Fletcher, PhD, Department of Psychiatry, University of Massachusetts Medical Center, 55, Lake Avenue North, Worcester, MA 01655.

Exposure Questions
(K. Nader)

Recommended Uses

Recommended for gathering information about dimensions of exposure to war and natural disaster in children in clinical or research settings.

Special Features

This measure provides a structure for gathering detailed information about the nature of traumatic experiences related to war or natural disaster and the child's response at the time of the event(s).

General Descriptive Information

Measure format: Structured interview format.

Targeted age group: Children aged 5–17.

Events assessed: Traumatic experiences related to war or natural disaster and coping behaviors employed by child since the event.

Number of items; time to administer: 16 items on war exposure with follow-up questions for most positive responses; 18 items on exposure to natural disaster with follow-up questions for most positive responses; 4 items on coping behaviors; 15–45 minutes for each section, depending on number of traumatic experiences.

Response format: Some items are open-ended. Most items, initial response choices are "Yes" or "No." Positive and "Unsure" responses are followed up with open-ended questions about what happened (see Aspects of Trauma Assessed below).

Training required to administer: A training manual accompanies the measure, and training in its use is recommended.

Sample item: War-related item: "Was anyone you know captured or killed during the event?" Disaster-related item: "Did you think/worry that you would be hurt during the event?" Coping item: "What has helped you feel better since the incident?"

Type of outcome measure provided: None. Provided qualitative information only.

Aspects of traumas assessed: Assesses a wide variety of dimensions of traumatic experiences including capture, injury, or death of others, witnessing death, injury, or rape, and threat of death or injury of self.

Time frame assessed: Specific identified incidents or time periods.

Correspondence with DSM: Assesses DSM-IV Criterion A-1 (experiencing or witnessing actual injury or threat of death/injury).

Psychometric Information

Validation populations: Kuwaiti children exposed to war, Yugoslavian refugee children.

Reliability: None to date.

Validity: In studies of Kuwaiti children and child refugees from the former Yugoslavia, exposure questions results were found to correspond to levels of posttraumatic symptoms measured by the *Child Posttraumatic Stress Reaction Index* (Nader & Fairbanks, 1994; Nader, Pynoos, Fairbanks, Al-Ajeel, & Al-Asfour, 1993).

Descriptive/psychometric information sources: Nader, K. (1993). *Instruction manual: Child PTS Reaction Index, Revised (CPTS-RI).* Unpublished manuscript.

Nader, K. (1997). Assessing trauma in children. In J. Wilson & T. M. Keane (Ed.), *Assessing psychological trauma and PTSD: A practitioner's handbook* (pp. 291–348). New York: Guilford Press.

Nader, K., & Fairbanks, L. (1994). The suppression of reexperiencing: Impulse control and somatic symptoms in children following traumatic exposure. *Anxiety, Stress, and Coping: An International Journal, 7,* 229–239.

Nader, K., Pynoos, R., Fairbanks, L., Al-Ajeel, M., & Al-Asfour, A. (1993). Acute post traumatic stress reactions among Kuwait children following the Gulf Crisis. *British Journal of Clinical Psychology, 32,* 407–416.

How to Obtain Scale

Contact Kathleen Nader, PhD, P.O. Box 2251, Laguna Hills, CA 92654.

Traumatic Events Screening Inventory (TESI)
(K. Rogers, J. Ford, R. Racusin, C. Ellis, J. Thomas, J. Schiffman, D. Ribbe, P. Cone, M. Lukovits, & J. Edwards)

Recommended Uses

Recommended for brief screening for trauma history in children in clinical or research settings.

Special Features

This measure can be administered as a semistructured interview to children (TESI-C) or to parents (TESI-P) allowing collection of information from both sources. It is also available in the form of a questionnaire for use with parents (TESI-P).

General Descriptive Information

Measure format: Comes in both semistructured interview and questionnaire formats.

Targeted age group: Children aged 4–18.

Events assessed: Wide range of potentially traumatic events including accidents, hospitalizations, physical or sexual abuse, natural disasters, community violence, witnessing domestic violence, and interpersonal losses due to severe illness or injury.

Number of items; time to administer: 15 items (TESI-C) and 19 items (TESI-P); 10–30 minutes, depending on number of traumatic experiences.

Response format: Initial response choices are "Yes," "No," "Not sure," "Refused," and "Questionable validity." Positive and "Not sure" responses are followed up with open-ended questions about what happened and closed-ended questions (see "Aspects of traumas assessed," below).

Training required to administer: All versions are designed to be administered only by qualified mental health professionals or advanced trainees supervised by a qualified mental health professional. The critical qualifications are licensure for independent practice in child assessment and psychotherapy and supervised experience in assessment of psychotherapy with child survivors of trauma and their families.

Sample item: TESI-C: "Have you ever *been in* a really bad accident, like a car accident, a fall, or a fire?" "How old were you when this happened?" "Were you hurt? (What was the hurt?)" "Did you go to the doctor or hospital?" "Was someone else hurt in the accident? (Who? What was the hurt? Did they go to the doctor or the hospital?)"

Type of outcome measure provided: Until studies of quantitative scoring algorithms are completed, authors suggest scoring each potential event using DSM-IV Criterion A.

Aspects of traumas assessed: For each event endorsed, collects age of onset, age of offset, frequency, relationship of others involved, consequences, and appraisals of objective physical threat and fear, helplessness, or horror.

Time frame assessed: Lifetime.

Correspondence with DSM: Assesses DSM-IV Criterion A-1 (experiencing or witnessing actual injury or threat of death/injury) and Criterion A-2 (experiencing fear, helplessness, or horror).

Psychometric Information

Validation populations: Child psychiatry and pediatric trauma patients.

Reliability: Evidence of consistency in scoring includes coefficients of agreement between two scorers of a videotaped interview of .85 for Criterion A-1 (clinician's appraisal) and .81 for Criterion A-2 (child's appraisal) (Ford et al., 1996).

Validity: Evidence of convergent validity includes correlations between TESI-C and TESI-P results for presence of a trauma ranging from .42 to .91 for eight different types of trauma (Ford et al., 1996).

Descriptive/psychometric information sources: Ford, J. P., Thomas, J., Rogers, K., Racusin, R., Ellis, C. G., Schiffman, J., Daviss, W. B., & Friedman, M. J. (1996). *Assessment of children's PTSD following abuse or accidental trauma.* Paper presented at the 12th annual meeting of the International Society for Traumatic Stress Studies, San Francisco.

National Center for PTSD/Dartmouth Child Trauma Research Group (1996). *Traumatic Events Screening Inventory, Version 8.3.* Hanover, NH: Dartmouth Hitchcock Medical Center.

Ribbe, D. (1996). Psychometric review of Traumatic Event Screening Instrument for Children (TESI-C). In B. H. Stamm (Ed.), *Measurement of stress, trauma, and adaptation* (pp. 386–387). Lutherville, MD: Sidran Press.

Ribbe, D. (1996). Psychometric review of Traumatic Event Screening Instrument for Parents (TESI-P). In B. H. Stamm (Ed.), *Measurement of stress, trauma, and adaptation* (pp. 388–389). Lutherville, MD: Sidran Press.

How to Obtain Scale

Contact Julian Ford, PhD, National Center for PTSD, VAMC 116D, 215 North Main Street, White River Junction, VT O5009-0001.

MEASURES OF TRAUMA RESPONSES

Adolescent Dissociative Experiences Scale (A-DES)
(J. Armstrong, F. Putnam, & E. Carlson)

Recommended Uses

Recommended for measuring dissociation symptoms in adolescents in clinical or research settings.

Special Features

This brief self-report scale offers a convenient way to assess the frequency of a wide range of pathological and normative dissociative experiences in adolescents.

General Descriptive Information

Measure format: Self-report.

Targeted age group: Children aged 11–18.

Symptoms assessed: Items assess four domains of dissociation including dissociative amnesia, absorption and imaginative involvement, passive influence, and derealization and depersonalization.

Number of items; time to complete: 30 items; takes about 10–15 minutes to complete.

Response format: For each item, client rates frequency by circling a number on an 11-point scale that ranges from 0 = "never" to 10 = "always."

Sample item: "I get so wrapped up in watching TV, reading, or playing video games that I don't have any idea what's going on around me."

Type of outcome measure provided: Total scale scores are the average of item scores and range from 0 to 10.

Time frame assessed: None specified.

Correspondence with DSM: Contains items that correspond to DSM criteria for dissociative disorders and PTSD but does not specifically assess DSM criteria for any disorder.

Psychometric Information

Validation populations: Junior and senior high school students, adolescent psychiatric inpatients, adolescent psychiatric outpatients.

Reliability: Evidence of internal consistency includes a Cronbach's α for total scores of .93 with α values for subscale scores ranging from .72 to .85 (Armstrong, Putnam, Carlson, Libero, & Smith, 1997). Evidence for consistency over time includes a 2-week test–retest correlation of $r = .77$.

Validity: Evidence for construct validity includes the finding that A-DES scores were significantly elevated in subjects who had experienced childhood abuse compared to those who had not (Armstrong et al., in press). Some evidence of convergent validity is provided by the finding of a strong correlation between scores on the A-DES and the DES in college students ($r = .77$). In addition, A-DES scores were found to differ significantly across diagnostic groups with adolescents with dissociative disorder diagnoses scoring higher than adolescents with any other diagnosis.

Descriptive/psychometric information sources: Armstrong, J., Putnam, F. W., Carlson, E., Libero, D., & Smith, S. (1997). The Adolescent Dissociative Experiences Scale. *Journal of Nervous and Mental Disease.* (Includes measure in its entirety.)

How to Obtain Scale

Contact Judith Armstrong, PhD, Suite 402, 501 Santa Monica Boulevard, Santa Monica, CA 90401.

Childhood PTSD Interview (CPTSDI)–Child Form
(K. Fletcher)

Recommended Uses

Recommended for use in clinical or research settings to measure PTSD symptoms and make a PTSD diagnosis in children related to single- or multiple-identified traumatic events.

Special Features

This measure offers a way to collect information about DSM-IV PTSD symptoms in a structured interview format and to collect information about a range of additional symptoms that may be associated with traumatic experiences. Parallel versions of the interview for child and parent allow the clinician to assess the convergence of the child's and parent's reports.

General Descriptive Information

Measure format: Structured interview.

Targeted age group: Children and adolescents (no ages specified).

Symptoms assessed: Assesses DSM-III-R and DSM-IV symptom criteria (A-1, B, C, and D) for PTSD and a range of symptoms that may be associated with trauma including anxiety, depression, omens, survivor guilt, self-blame, fantasy denial, self-destructive behavior/thoughts, dissociation, antisocial behavior, risk-taking, and changed eating habits.

Number of items; time to complete: 93 items with follow-up questions for many positive responses; takes 30–45 minutes to administer.

Response format: For each item, child or parent answers "Yes" or "No." Some child form items and all parent form items also allow a "Don't know" response. Some positive responses are followed by open-ended questions to elicit details.

Sample item: Child form: "Do you sometimes think about [the event/s] when you don't want to?" Parent form: "Does your child think about [the event/s] even when he/she doesn't want to?"

Type of outcome measure provided: A scoring scheme is built into the interview to allow DSM-III-R or DSM-IV diagnosis of PTSD to be made based on item responses. Total scores can also be calculated for child and parent forms by counting the number of symptoms endorsed.

Time frame assessed: None specified.

Correspondence with DSM: Assesses DSM-III-R and DSM-IV symptom Criteria A-1, B, C, and D for PTSD. All criteria assessed by more than one item.

Psychometric Information

Validation populations: Children in treatment who had been exposed to traumatic events; children from a community sample.

Reliability: Evidence of internal consistency for the child form includes a Cronbach's α value of .91 for the total score and α values ranging from .52 to .80 for DSM-IV Criteria A–D (Fletcher, 1996b [in "Descriptive/psychometric information sources"]). Evidence of internal consistency for the parent form includes a Cronbach's α of .94 for the total score and α values ranging from .60 to .86 for DSM-IV Criteria A–D.

Validity: Evidence for construct validity of both child and adult forms of the interview includes convergent validity with other measures of PTSD symptoms. Correlations ranged from .60 and .87 between the CPTSDI—Child Form and the WBTH scale, the CPTSDI—Parent Form, and the

PRCRS (Fletcher, 1996b [in "Descriptive/psychometric information sources"]). Scores on the CPTSDI scale were also significantly associated with scores on a measure of the dimensions of potentially traumatic events (the DOSE) (r =.77) and with the PTSD subscale of the CBC (r = .52). In addition, CPTSDI scores were higher for children in the clinical sample who had been exposed to traumatic stressors than in community sample children. Evidence for convergent validity of the parent form includes correlations ranging from .59 and .93 between the CPTSDI—Parent Form and the WBTH scale, the CPTSDI—Child Form, and the PRCRS (Fletcher, 1996b [in Descriptive/psychometric information sources]). Scores on the CPTSDI scale were also significantly associated with scores on a measure of the dimensions of potentially traumatic events (the DOSE) (r = .66) and with the PTSD subscale of the CBC (r = .78). In addition, CPTSDI—Parent Form scores were higher for children in the clinical sample who had been exposed to traumatic stressors than in community sample children.

Descriptive/psychometric information sources: Fletcher, K. E. (1996a). Psychometric review of the Childhood PTSD Interview. In B. H. Stamm (Ed.), *Measurement of stress, trauma, and adaptation* (pp. 87–89). Lutherville, MD: Sidran Press.

Fletcher, K. E. (1996b). Psychometric review of the Child PTSD Interview—Parent Form. In B. H. Stamm (Ed.), *Measurement of stress, trauma, and adaptation* (pp. 90–92). Lutherville, MD: Sidran Press.

Fletcher, K. E. (1996c, November). *Measuring school-aged children's PTSD: Preliminary psychometrics of four new measures.* Paper presented at the 12th annual meeting of the International Society for Traumatic Stress Studies, San Francisco.

How to Obtain Scale

Contact Kenneth E. Fletcher, PhD, Department of Psychiatry, University of Massachusetts Medical Center, 55 Lake Avenue North, Worcester, MA 01655.

Child PTS Reaction Index (CPTS-RI)
(C. Frederick, R. Pynoos, & K. Nader)

Recommended Uses

Recommended for use in clinical or research settings to measure PTSD symptoms in children related to a single identified traumatic event.

Special Features

This measure is relatively brief and easy to administer. An instruction manual and additional questions about trauma-related changes and exposure to particular traumatic stressors (see Exposure Questions profile on p. 243) are also available. A Parent Questionnaire is also available that corresponds to the CPTS-RI but has not yet been validated (Nader, 1994).

General Descriptive Information

Measure format: Interviewer administered scale.

Targeted age group: Children aged 6–17.

Symptoms assessed: Assesses most of the DSM-III-R/DSM-IV symptoms for PTSD plus guilt, impulse control, somatic symptoms, and regressive behaviors. Additional questions assess changes in play, newly developed fears, expectations about the future, and changes in relationships.

Number of items; time to complete: 20 items; takes 20–45 minutes to complete including additional questions (listed above).

Response format: For each item, client gives a rating that largely reflects frequency (from "None" to "Most of the time").

Sample item: "Do you ever get scared, afraid, or upset when you think about (event)?"

Type of outcome measure provided: Scale yields total scores ranging from 0 to 80 that reflect the frequency of symptoms. Categories of degree of disorder (from doubtful to very severe) can be assigned based on the total scale score.

Time frame assessed: Past month.

Correspondence with DSM: Assesses 11 of the 17 DSM-IV symptom criteria (B, C, and D) for PTSD. Some criteria assessed by more than one item.

Psychometric Information

Validation populations: Children exposed to violence and children exposed to disasters.

Reliability: Evidence of internal consistency includes a Cronbach's α value of .78 for the total score (Nader, 1996a [in "Descriptive/psychometric information sources"]). Evidence for interrater reliability includes correlations for total score of .94 and .97 in two studies.

Validity: Evidence for construct validity includes findings in one study of progressively greater frequency of being assigned a PTSD diagnosis across degree of disorder categories. For example, in one study, 44% of subjects who were rated as showing "moderate" degree of distress according to CPTS-RI scores met DSM-III-R criteria for PTSD compared to 92% of those rated "very severe." In studies of Kuwaiti children and child refugees from the former Yugoslavia, CPTS-SR results were found to correspond to levels of exposure to trauma measured by the Exposure Questions (Nader & Fairbanks, 1994; Nader et al., 1993).

Descriptive/psychometric information sources: Nader, K. (1996a). Assessing trauma in children. In J. Wilson & T. M. Keane (Eds.), *Assessing psychological trauma and PTSD* (pp. 291–348). New York: Guilford Press.

Nader, K. (1996b). Psychometric review of Child PTS Reaction Index (CPTS-RI). In B. H. Stamm (Ed.), *Measurement of stress, trauma, and adaptation* (pp. 83–86). Lutherville, MD: Sidran Press.

How to Obtain Scale

Scale can be obtained from any of the authors. Scale and instruction manual can be obtained from Kathleen Nader, PhD, P.O. Box 2251, Laguna Hills, CA 92654.

Clinician-Administered PTSD Scale for Children and Adolescents for DSM-IV (CAPS-CA)
(K. Nader, J. Kriegler, D. Blake, R. Pynoos, E. Newman, & F. Weathers)

Recommended Uses

Recommended for use in clinical or research settings to measure children's and adolescents' PTSD symptoms related to up to three identified traumatic events. Can also be used to make PTSD diagnoses in children and adolescents.

Special Features

Two versions of the CAPS-CA are now available that assess DSM-IV PTSD criteria. These include the a current or lifetime diagnostic version (Form 1) and a 1-week version (Form 2), which assesses symptoms over the past week. The CAPS-CA has the advantages of being extremely thorough and detailed and offerring a continuous measure of posttraumatic symptoms and the disadvantage of taking longer to administer than some other PTSD structured interviews. Some of the unique elements that the measure allows you to assess include the impact of symptoms on functioning, improvement in symptoms since a previous CAPS-CA administration, overall response validity, overall PTSD severity, and five associated symptoms (see details below). Other unique features include iconic representations of positive symptoms, practice questions, a standard procedure for identifying the 1-month time frame for current symptoms.

General Descriptive Information

Measure format: Structured interview.

Targeted age group: Children aged 7–18 years.

Experiences and symptoms assessed: The CAPS-CA assesses DSM-IV symptoms for PTSD, including Criteria A–F, the impact of symptoms on social, scholastic, and developmental functioning, improvement in symptoms since a previous CAPS administration, overall response validity, overall PTSD severity, and eight associated symptoms (guilt over acts, survivor guilt, shame, gaps in awareness, derealization, depersonalization, changes in attachment, and trauma-specific fears). As part of the assessment of Criterion A, a Life Events Checklist is used to help the interviewer determine experiences with 17 different traumatic events.

Number of items; time to complete: 33 items; takes 30–120 minutes to administer.

Response format: For each item, multiple standard questions are provided to elicit information about experiences or symptoms. For symptom items, the interviewer uses the client's answers to assign a frequency rating (from 0 = "None of the time" to 4 = "Most of the time, daily or almost every day") and an intensity rating (from 0 = "Not at all, none" to 4 = "A whole lot, extreme, drastic attempts at avoidance, unable to continue activities, or excessive involvement in certain activities as avoidant strategy"). For each item, the verbal ratings for intensity are tailored to that particular item.

Training required to administer: The CAPS was designed to be administered by clinicians and clinical researchers who have a working knowledge of PTSD and experience interviewing children.

Sample item: (For frequency ranging) "Did you think about [event] even when you didn't want to? Did you see pictures in your head (mind) or hear the sounds in your head (mind) from [event]? What were they like? (Did you cover your eyes or ears to block things you saw or heard in your head? What were you trying to block out?) How many times did that happen in the past month [lifetime worst month]?"

Type of outcome measure provided: CAPS responses can be used to make a determination about whether client's symptoms meet DSM-IV Criteria A–F for PTSD. Continuous ratings are also calculated for frequency and for intensity of symptoms (ranging from 0–68) and for severity (frequency + intensity; ranging from 0–134).

Time frame assessed: Form 1: past month or worst month ever (if criteria are not met for current diagnosis). Form 2: past week.

Correspondence with DSM: Assesses DSM-IV symptom criteria (A–F) for PTSD.

Psychometric Information

Validation populations: None to date.

Reliability: None available to date.

Validity: None available to date.

Descriptive/psychometric information sources: Newman, E., & Ribbe, D. (1996). Psychometric review of the Clinician Administered PTSD Scale for Children. In B. H. Stamm (Ed.), *Measurement of stress, trauma, and adaptation* (pp. 106–114). Lutherville, MD: Sidran Press.

How to Obtain Scale

Contact Elana Newman, PhD, University of Tulsa, Department of Psychology, Lorton Hall, 600 South College Avenue, Tulsa, OK 74104-3189.

Posttraumatic Symptom Inventory for Children (PTSIC)
(M. Eisen)

Recommended Uses

Recommended for use in clinical or research settings to measure PTSD symptoms in young children related to single or multiple traumatic events.

Special Features

This measure is brief and easy to administer. It allows clinicians to assess symptoms related to multiple traumatic events and can be used with children as young as 4 years.

General Descriptive Information

Measure format: Interviewer administered scale.

Targeted age group: Children aged 4–8.

Symptoms/events assessed: Assesses DSM-IV symptoms for PTSD. Also includes a checklist to screen for 11 traumatic events.

Number of items; time to complete: 30 items; takes 15–20 minutes to complete.

Response format: For each item, client gives a rating that largely reflects frequency where 0 = "never," 1 = "some," and 2 = "lots."

Sample item: "Do you think about bad things that happened to you even when you don't want to?" "Do you think about what happened almost everyday or do you just think about it sometimes?"

Type of outcome measure provided: Scale yields total scores ranging from 0 to 60 that reflect the frequency of symptoms. DSM-IV diagnosis for PTSD can be assigned based on endorsement of items for each criterion.

Time frame assessed: None specified.

Correspondence with DSM: Assesses DSM-IV symptom criteria (B, C, and D) for PTSD. Most criteria (15 of 17) are assessed by two items.

Psychometric Information

Validation populations: Children being assessed for maltreatment.

Reliability: Evidence of internal consistency includes a Cronbach's α value of .91 for total score (Eisen & Carlson, 1997). Evidence for consistency of scores over time includes a 2-week test–retest reliability correlation of .97.

Validity: Evidence for convergent validity includes a correlation of .64 with the total score of the TSCC and a correlation of .53 with the A-DES (Eisen & Carlson, 1997).

Descriptive/psychometric information sources: Eisen, M., & Carlson, E. B. (1997). *Development, reliability, and validity of a brief PTSD measure for young children.* Unpublished manuscript.

How to Obtain Scale

Contact Mitchell Eisen, PhD, Department of Psychology, California State University at Los Angeles, 5151 State University Drive, Los Angeles, CA 90032-8200.

Trauma Symptom Checklist for Children (TSCC)
(J. Briere)

Recommended Uses

Recommended for use in clinical or research settings to measure a variety of trauma-related symptoms in children related to single or multiple identified traumatic events.

Special Features

This self-report measure for children is fairly brief and assesses a variety of symptoms that have been found to be related to traumatic experiences. Unlike most other child measures, it contains two validity scales. Since it does not key symptoms to a particular event, it can be used to quantify symptoms related to single or multiple traumatic events including physical abuse, sexual abuse, neglect, witnessing violence, accidents, and disasters.

General Descriptive Information

Measure format: Self-report.

Targeted age group: Children ages 8–16 (manual also contains norms for 17-year-olds).

Symptoms assessed: Assesses some DSM-IV symptom criteria for PTSD including cognitive avoidance, numbing, nightmares, and intrusive thinking. Also assesses a wide range of symptoms that may be associated with trauma such as anxiety, depression, anger, dissociation, and sexual concerns. Validity scales assess underresponse (very low reporting) and hyperresponse (unusually high reporting).

Number of items; time to complete: 54 items; takes 10–20 minutes to complete.

Response format: For each item, child chooses a rating of "Never," "Sometimes," "Lots of times," or "Almost all of the time" to indicate how often each symptom happens to them.

Sample item: Bad dreams or nightmares.

Type of outcome measure provided: Scale scores (raw and T) are calculated for six clinical scales: anxiety, depression, anger, posttraumatic stress, dissociation (including overt dissociation and fantasy dissociation subscales), and sexual concerns (including sexual preoccupation and sexual distress subscales). Scale scores are also calculated for two validity scales: underresponse and hyperresponse. A computer scoring program is available from the test publisher.

Time frame assessed: None specified.

Correspondence with DSM: Does not correspond to DSM-IV diagnostic criteria for any disorder.

Psychometric Information

Validation populations: General population, children exposed to traumatic events, sexually abused children, children in treatment following sexual abuse.

Reliability: Evidence of internal consistency includes Cronbach's α values ranging from .77 to .89 for the six clinical scales and from .66 to .85 for the two validity scales (Briere, 1996a [in "Descriptive/psychometric information sources"]).

Validity: Evidence for construct validity includes convergent validity with other measures of symptoms in children (Briere, 1996a [in "Descriptive/psychometric information sources"]). The six clinical subscale scores were highly correlated with scores on the CBC—youth reports of internalization (with r's ranging from .51 to .82). The TSCC posttraumatic stress scale scores have been found to be strongly related to the intrusive thoughts scale of the Child Impact of Events Scale—Revised. Further evidence of construct validity includes findings from several studies of an association between elevated scores on specific TSCC clinical scales and exposure to violence, sexual abuse, and other traumatic events. In one study, posttraumatic stress, dissociation, and anxiety scale scores were related to the experience of traumatic events involving life threat, and anger and depression scores were negatively related to clinician ratings of parental support following disclosure of abuse.

Descriptive/psychometric information sources: Briere, J. (1996a). *Trauma Symptom Checklist for Children professional manual.* Odessa, FL: Psychological Assessment Resources.

Briere, J. (1996b). Psychometric review of Trauma Symptom Checklist for Children (TSCC). In B. H. Stamm (Ed.), *Measurement of stress, trauma, and adaptation* (pp. 378–380). Lutherville, MD: Sidran Press.

How to Obtain Scale

Contact Psychological Assessment Resources, Box 998, Odessa, FL 33556; 800-331-8378.

When Bad Things Happen Scale (WBTH)
(K. Fletcher)

Recommended Uses

Recommended for use in clinical or research settings to measure PTSD symptoms in children related to single or multiple identified traumatic events.

Special Features

This measure is unique in that it is truly a self-report measure for children. It can be administered to children who have at least a 3rd-grade reading level. Although the measures are fairly long, briefer versions are being developed.

General Descriptive Information

Measure format: Self-report.

Targeted age group: Children (with at least a 3rd-grade reading level).

Symptoms assessed: Assesses DSM-III-R and DSM-IV symptom criteria (A-1, B, C, and D) for PTSD. Also assesses a wide range of symptoms that may be associated with trauma such as anxiety, depression, omens, survivor guilt, self-blame, fantasy denial, self-destructive behavior/thoughts, dissociation, antisocial behavior, risk taking, and changed eating habits.

Number of items; time to complete: 95 items; takes 10–20 minutes to complete.

Response format: For each item, child chooses a rating of "Never," "Some," or "Lots."

Sample item: "Do you think about the bad thing now even when you do not want to?"

Type of outcome measure provided: Total scores can be calculated that reflect severity of PTSD symptoms. A scoring scheme is also provided to allow DSM-III-R or DSM-IV diagnosis of PTSD to be made based on item scores.

Time frame assessed: None specified.

Correspondence with DSM: Assesses DSM-III-R and DSM-IV symptom criteria (A-1, B, C, and D) for PTSD. All criteria assessed by more than one item.

Psychometric Information

Validation populations: Children in treatment who had been exposed to traumatic events, children from a community sample.

Reliability: Evidence of internal consistency includes a Cronbach's α value of .92 for the total score (Fletcher, 1996b [in "Descriptive/psychometric information sources"]). Cronbach's α values for DSM-IV Criteria A–D ranged from .70 to .89.

Validity: Evidence for construct validity includes convergent validity with other measures of PTSD symptoms. Correlations ranged from .54 and .87 between the WBTH scale and the CPTSDI-C, the CPTSDI-P, and the Parent Report of the CRS (Fletcher, 1996b [in "Descriptive/psychometric information sources"]). Scores on the WBTH scale were also significantly associated with scores on a measure of the dimensions of potentially traumatic events (the DOSE) ($r = 70$) and with the PTSD subscale of the CBC ($r = .54$). In addition, WBTH scores were higher for children in the clinical sample who had been exposed to traumatic stressors than in community sample children.

Descriptive/psychometric information sources: Fletcher, K. E. (1996a). Psychometric review of the When Bad Things Happen Scale (WBTH). In B. H. Stamm (Ed.), *Measurement of stress, trauma, and adaptation* (pp. 435–437). Lutherville, MD: Sidran Press.

Fletcher, K. E. (1996b, November). *Measuring school-aged children's PTSD: Preliminary psychometrics of four new measures*. Paper presented at the 12th annual meeting of the International Society for Traumatic Stress Studies, San Francisco.

How to Obtain Scale

Contact Kenneth E. Fletcher, PhD, Department of Psychiatry, University of Massachusetts Medical Center, 55 Lake Avenue North, Worcester, MA 01655.

MEASURES ADMINISTERED TO PARENT

Child Dissociative Checklist (CDC)
(F. Putnam)

Recommended Uses

Recommended for measuring dissociation symptoms in children in clinical or research settings.

Special Features

This is a brief scale that obtains reports of a parent, guardian, teacher, or other observer about the presence of a wide range of dissociative symptoms and symptoms that may reflect dissociation. This measure can be especially useful for gathering information about children who are too young to make accurate verbal reports.

General Descriptive Information

Measure format: Parent or observer self-report.

Targeted age group: Children aged 5–12.

Symptoms assessed: Items assess domains of dissociative amnesia, rapid shifts in demeanor, cognitive abilities or behavior, spontaneous trance states, hallucinations, identity alterations, and aggressive and sexual behaviors.

Number of items; time to complete: 20 items; takes about 5–10 minutes to complete.

Response format: For each item, observer rates each symptom or behavior as 0 = "Not true," 1 = "Somewhat or sometimes true," or 2 = "Very true."

Sample item: Child does not remember or denies traumatic or painful experiences that are known to have occurred.

Type of outcome measure provided: Total scale scores are the average of item scores and range from 0 to 40.

Time frame assessed: Past 12 months or as specified by clinician.

Development notes: The CDC was developed based on childhood MPD (now DID) predictor lists developed by Putnam. An earlier version of the CDC contained the first 16 of the 20 items in the most current version.

Correspondence with DSM: Contains items that correspond to symptoms of dissociative disorders but does not specifically assess DSM criteria for any disorder.

Psychometric Information

Validation populations: Normal control children, sexually abused children, children with dissociative disorder diagnoses, inpatient children, outpatient children.

Reliability: Evidence of internal consistency includes Cronbach's α values of .78 and .95 in two studies (Putnam & Peterson, 1994). Evidence for consistency of scores over time includes test–retest reliability correlations between first and second administrations of .69 and .73 for two studies.

Validity: Evidence for construct validity includes findings of higher scores for subjects with dissociative disorders than for subjects with other disorders (Putnam & Peterson, 1994). Subjects with a diagnosis of MPD (now DID) scored higher than subjects with other dissociative diagnoses. Sexually abused children also were found to score higher on the CDC than normal control children. The scale shows evidence of convergent validity when correlated with clinician ratings of dissociation symptoms ($r = .33$).

Descriptive/psychometric information sources: Putnam, F. W., Helmers, K., & Trickett, P. K. (1993). Development, reliability, and validity of a child dissociation scale. *Child Abuse and Neglect, 17,* 731–741. (Includes measure in its entirety.)

Putnam, F. W., & Peterson, G. (1994). Further validation of the Child Dissociative Checklist. *Dissociation, 7,* 204–211.

How to Obtain Scale

Contact Frank Putnam, MD, Unit on Developmental Traumatology, National Institute of Mental Health, Building 15K, 9000 Rockville Pike, Bethesda, MD 20892.

Childhood PTSD Interview (CPTSDI)–Parent Form
(K. Fletcher)

See profile for Childhood PTSD Interview on pp. 248–250.

Child PTSD Reaction Index:
Parent Questionnaire (CPTS-RI)
(K. Nader)

See profile for Child PTS Reaction Index on pp. 250–251.

Parent Report of Child's Reaction to Stress (PR-CRS)
(K. Fletcher)

Recommended Uses

Recommended for use in clinical or research settings to measure PTSD symptoms in children related to single- or multiple-identified traumatic events.

Special Features

Because it is a self-report measure, this is a convenient way to obtain parents' perceptions about their child's reaction to a single or multiple traumatic events. It is fairly long, but a briefer version is under development.

General Descriptive Information

Measure format: Self-report (by parent).

Targeted age group: Children (no ages specified).

Symptoms assessed: Assesses DSM-III-R and DSM-IV symptoms for PTSD and a range of symptoms that may be associated with trauma including anxiety, depression, omens, survivor guilt, self-blame, fantasy denial, self-destructive behavior/thoughts, dissociation, antisocial behavior, risk taking, and changed eating habits.

Number of items; time to complete: 79 items; takes 30–45 minutes to complete

Response format: Varies across items. Most items offer a range of choices indicating either frequency of symptoms (from "Never" to "Always"), changes in symptoms (from "Much easier" to "Much harder" or from "Much less" to "Much more"), and severity of symptoms (from "Very little" to "Extremely").

Sample item: "Does your child seem to have a hard time putting the event or events out of his or her mind?"

Type of outcome measure provided: Total scores can be calculated that reflect severity of PTSD symptoms. A scoring scheme is also provided to allow DSM-III-R or DSM-IV diagnosis of PTSD to be made based on item scores.

Time frame assessed: None specified.

Correspondence with DSM: Assesses DSM-III-R and DSM-IV Criterion A-1 and symptom criteria (B, C, and D) for PTSD. All criteria assessed by more than one item.

Psychometric Information

Validation populations: Children in treatment who have been exposed to traumatic events; children from a community sample.

Reliability: Evidence of internal consistency includes a Cronbach's α value of .89 for the total score (Fletcher, 1996b [in "Descriptive/psychometric information sources"]). Cronbach's α values for DSM-IV Criteria A–D ranged from .70 to .86.

Validity: Evidence for construct validity includes convergent validity with other measures of PTSD symptoms. Correlations ranged from .54 and .93 between the PR-CRS and the CPTSDI, the CPTSDI-Parent Form, and the WBTH scale (Fletcher, 1996b [in "Descriptive/psychometric information sources"]). Scores on the PR-CRS scale were also significantly associated with scores on a measure of the dimensions of potentially traumatic events (the DOSE) $(r = .54)$ and with the PTSD subscale of the Child Behavior Checklist $(r = .82)$. In addition, PR-CRS scores were higher for children in the clinical sample who had been exposed to traumatic stressors than in community sample children.

Descriptive/psychometric information sources: Fletcher, K. E. (1996a). Psychometric review of the Parent Report of the Child's Reaction to Stress. In B. H. Stamm (Ed.), *Measurement of stress, trauma, and adaptation* (pp. 225–227). Lutherville, MD: Sidran Press.

Fletcher, K. E. (1996b, November). *Measuring school-aged children's PTSD: Preliminary psychometrics of four new measures.* Paper presented at the 12th annual meeting of the International Society for Traumatic Stress Studies, San Francisco.

How to Obtain Scale

Contact Kenneth E. Fletcher, PhD, Department of Psychiatry, University of Massachusetts Medical Center, 55 Lake Avenue North, Worcester, MA 01655.

Appendix

Resources on Trauma and Trauma-Related Disorders

INTERNATIONAL SOCIETY FOR TRAUMATIC STRESS STUDIES

The ISTSS is a professional society that promotes and provides a forum for disseminating theory, research, clinical interventions, and public policy formulations related to traumatic stress. Membership benefits include the ISTSS newsletter Traumatic Stress Points, subscriptions to *Journal of Traumatic Stress,* the *PTSD Research Quarterly,* a membership directory, and reduced fees at yearly conferences. Contact: ISTSS, 60 Revere Drive, Suite 500, Northbrook, IL 60062; 847-480-9028; e-mail: istss@istss.com; Internet: http://www.istss.com

PILOTS DATABASE

This electronic database of traumatic stress literature is available through the National Center for PTSD, White River Junction. A guide to use of the database is available in Lerner, F. (1996). Searching the traumatic stress literature. In E. B. Carlson (Ed.), *Trauma research methodology* (pp. 1–21). Lutherville, MD: Sidran Press. The PILOTS database can be accessed through the Internet and can be searched for literature on diagnosis and treatment of traumatic disorders. For more information, contact: National Center for PTSD (116D), VA Medical Center, White River Junction, VT 05009; 802-296-5132; e-mail: ptsd@dartmouth.edu; Internet: http://www.dartmouth.edu/dms/ptsd/

NATIONAL CENTER FOR PTSD RESEARCH QUARTERLY

This publication provides up-to-date topical reviews and reports on traumatic stress research. It is published by the National Center for PTSD Central Office and provided free of charge as a benefit of membership in the ISTSS. Current and back issues can also be downloaded electronically and individuals can purchase a subscription to the *Quarterly*. For information contact the National Center for PTSD (address given above).

NATIONAL CENTER FOR PTSD CLINICAL QUARTERLY

This publication provides up-to-date clinical reviews and reports relating to traumatic stress. Individuals can purchase a subscription for to the *Quarterly* by contacting Superintendent of Documents, P.O. Box 371954, Pittsburgh, PA 15250-7954; 202-512-1800. Specify Order-Processing Code 5737.

JOURNAL OF TRAUMATIC STRESS

This is the official journal of the ISTSS. It publishes a wide range of research and theory relating to PTSD. The journal is provided free of charge as a membership benefit of the ISTSS. Journal articles can also be obtained from university libraries throughout the country, and yearly subscriptions to the journal are available. Contact Subscription Department, Plenum Publishing Corporation, 233 Spring Street, New York, NY 10013; 212-620-8468.

SIDRAN FOUNDATION

Sidran Foundation is a nonprofit foundation devoted to advocacy, education, and research in support of people with severe psychiatric disabilities. The current focus of the Foundation is the development of programs, projects, and publications for survivors of catastrophic trauma and those who live and work with them. For more information contact Sidran Foundation, 2328 West Joppa Road, Suite 15, Lutherville, MD 21093; 410-825-8888; e-mail: Sidran@access.digex.net; Internet: http://www.access.digex.net/sidran

References

Aber, J. L., & Allen, J. P. (1987). The effects of maltreatment on young children's socioemotional development: An attachment perspective. *Developmental Psychology, 23*, 406–414.

Aber, J. L., & Zigler, E. (1981). Developmental considerations in the definition of child maltreatment. In R. Rizley & D. Cicchetti (Eds.), *New directions for child development: Developmental perspectives on child maltreatment* (pp. 1–29). San Francisco: Jossey-Bass.

Abramson, L. Y., Seligman, M. E. P., & Teasdale, J. D. (1978). Learned helplessness in humans: Critique and reformulation. *Journal of Abnormal Psychology, 87*, 49–74.

Abueg, F. R., & Chun, K. M. (1996). Traumatization stress among Asians and Asian Americans. In A. J. Marsella, M. J. Friedman, E. T. Gerrity, & R. M. Scurfield (Eds.), *Ethnocultural aspects of posttraumatic stress disorder: Issues, research, and clinical applications* (pp. 285–299). Washington, DC: American Psychological Association.

Abueg, F. R., & Fairbank, J. A. (1992). Behavioral treatment of posttraumatic stress disorder and co-occurring substance abuse. In P. A. Saigh (Ed.), *Posttraumatic stress disorder: Behavioral assessment and treatment* (pp. 111–146). Elmsford, NY: Maxwell Press.

Alexander, P. C. (1992). Application of attachment theory to the study of sexual abuse. *Journal of Consulting and Clinical Psychology, 60*, 185–195.

Alexander, P. C. (1993). The differential effects of abuse characteristics and attachment in the prediction of long-term effects of sexual abuse. *Journal of Interpersonal Violence, 8*, 346–362.

Alexander, P. C., & Lupfer, S. L. (1987). Family characteristics and long-term consequences associated with sexual abuse. *Archives of Sexual Behavior, 16*, 235–245.

Allen, I. M. (1996). PTSD among African Americans. In A. J. Marsella, M. J. Friedman, E. T. Gerrity, & R. M. Scurfield (Eds.), *Ethnocultural aspects of posttraumatic stress disorder: Issues, research, and clinical applications* (pp. 209–238). Washington, DC: American Psychological Association.

Allen, J. G. (1995a). *Coping with trauma: A guide to self-understanding.* Washington, DC: American Psychiatric Press.

Allen, J. G. (1995b). The spectrum of accuracy in memory of childhood trauma. *Harvard Review of Psychiatry, 3,* 84–95.

Allen, J. G., & Coyne, L. (1995). Dissociation and vulnerability to psychotic experience: The Dissociative Experiences Scale and the MMPI-2. *Journal of Nervous and Mental Disease, 183,* 615–622.

Allen, J. G., & Smith, W. H. (1993). Diagnosing dissociative disorders. *Bulletin of the Menninger Clinic, 57,* 328–343.

Allen, J. G., & Smith, W. H. (Eds.). (1995). *Diagnosis and treatment of dissociative disorders.* Northvale, NJ: Jason Aronson.

Allen, S. N. (1994). Psychological assessment of post-traumatic stress disorder. *Psychiatric Clinics of North America, 17,* 327–349.

American Professional Society on the Abuse of Children. (1995a). *Photographic documentation of child abuse.* Chicago: Author.

American Professional Society on the Abuse of Children. (1995b). *Psychosocial evaluation of suspected sexual abuse in young children.* Chicago: Author.

American Professional Society on the Abuse of Children. (1995c). *Use of anatomical dolls in child abuse assessments.* Chicago: Author.

American Psychiatric Association. (1987). *Diagnostic and statistical manual of mental disorders* (3rd ed., rev.). Washington, DC: Author.

American Psychiatric Association. (1994). *Diagnostic and statistical manual of mental disorders* (4th ed.). Washington, DC: Author.

Anastasi, A. (1988). *Psychological testing.* New York: Macmillan.

Andersen, H. S., Christensen, A. K., & Petersen, G. O. (1994). Post-traumatic stress reactions amongst rescue workers after a major railway accident. *Anxiety Research, 4,* 245–251.

Anderson, K. M., & Manuel, G. (1994). Gender differences in reported stress response to the Loma Prieta earthquake. *Sex Roles, 30,* 725–733.

Armstrong, J. (1995). Psychological assessment. In J. L. Spira (Ed.), *Treating dissociative identity disorder* (pp. 3–37). San Francisco: Jossey-Bass.

Armstrong, J., Putnam, F. W., Carlson, E., Libero, D., & Smith, S. (1997). Development and validation of a measure of adolescent dissociation: The Adolescent Dissociative Experiences Scale. *Journal of Nervous and Mental Disease.*

Armstrong, J. G., & Loewenstein, R. J. (1990). Characteristics of patients with multiple personality and dissociative disorders on psychological testing. *Journal of Nervous and Mental Disease, 178,* 448–454.

Arthur, R. J. (1982). Psychiatric syndromes in prisoner of war and concentration camp survivors. In C. T. Freeman & R. A. Faguet (Eds.), *Extraordinary disorders of human behavior* (pp. 47–63). New York: Plenum Press.

Atlas, J. A., Wolfson, M. A., & Lipschitz, D. S. (1995). Dissociation and somatization in adolescent inpatients with and without history of abuse. *Psychological Reports, 76,* 1101–1102.

Atlas, J. A., & Hiott, J. (1994). Dissociative experiences in a group of adolescents with history of abuse. *Perceptual and Motor Skills, 78,* 121–122.

August, L., & Gianola, B. (1987). Symptoms of war trauma induced psychiatric disorders: Southeast Asian refugees and Vietnam veterans. *International Migration Review, 21,* 820–831.

Banaji, M. R., & Hardin, C. (1994). Affect and memory in retrospective reports. In N. Schwarz & S. Sudman (Eds.), *Autobiographical memory and the validity of retrospective reports* (pp. 71–86). New York: Springer-Verlag.

Barach, P. M., & Comstock, C. M. (1996). Psychodynamic psychotherapy of dissociative identity disorder. In L. K. Michelson & W. J. Ray (Eds.), *Handbook of dissociation: Theoretical, empirical, and clinical perspectives* (pp. 413–430). New York: Plenum Press.

Basoglu, M., Paker, M., Paker, O., Ozmen, E., Isaac, M., Incesu, C., Sahin, D., & Sarimurat, N. (1994). Psychological effects of torture: A comparison study of tortured with nontortured political activists in Turkey. *American Journal of Psychiatry, 151,* 76–81.

Beck, A. T., & Steer, R. A. (1993). *Beck Depression Inventory manual.* San Antonio, TX: Psychological Corporation.

Beckham, J. C., Roodman, A. A., Barefoot, J. C., Haney, T. L., Helms, M. J., Fairbank, J. A., Hertzberg, M. A., & Kudler, H. S. (1996). Interpersonal and self-reported hostility among combat veterans with and without posttraumatic stress disorder. *Journal of Traumatic Stress, 9,* 335–342.

Beitchman, J. H., Zucker, K. J., Hood, J. E., & DaCosta, G. A. (1991). A review of the short-term effects of child sexual abuse. *Child Abuse and Neglect, 15,* 537–556.

Beitchman, J. H., Zucker, K. J., Hood, J. E., DaCosta, G. A., Akman, D., & Cassavia, E. (1992). A review of the long-term effects of child sexual abuse. *Child Abuse and Neglect, 16,* 101–118.

Belsey, E. M., Greer, H. S., Lal, S., Lewis, S. C., & Beard, R. W. (1977). Predictive factors in emotional response to abortion: King's termination study—IV. *Social Science and Medicine, 11,* 71–82.

Berliner, L., & Williams, L. M. (1994). Memories of child sexual abuse: A response to Lindsay and Read. *Applied Cognitive Psychology, 8,* 379–387.

Bernstein, E. M., & Putnam, F. W. (1986). Development, reliability, and validity of a dissociation scale. *Journal of Nervous and Mental Disease, 174,* 727–735.

Bertilson, H. S. (1991). Aggression. In V. J. Derlega, B. A. Winstead, & W. H. Jones (Eds.), *Personality: Contemporary theory and research* (pp. 457–480). Chicago: Nelson-Hall.

Bifulco, A., Brown, G. W., & Adler, Z. (1991). Early sexual abuse and clinical depression in adult life. *British Journal of Psychiatry, 159,* 115–122.

Blake, D. D. (1994). Rationale and development of the clinician-administered PTSD scales. *PTSD Research Quarterly, 5,* 1–6.

Blake, D. D., Weathers, F. W., Nagy, L. M., Kaloupek, D. G., Charney, D. S., & Keane, T. M. (1996). *The Clinician-Administered PTSD Scale (CAPS).* Boston: National Center for PTSD, Boston VA Medical Center.

Blake, D. D., Weathers, F. W., Nagy, L. M., Kaloupek, D. G., Gusman, F. D., Charney, D. S., & Keane, T. M. (1995). The development of a clinician-admininstered PTSD scale. *Journal of Traumatic Stress, 8,* 75–90.

Blanchard, E. B., Hickling, E. J., Taylor, A. E., & Loos, W. R. (1995). Psychiatric comorbidity associated with motor vehicle accidents. *Journal of Nervous and Mental Disease, 183,* 495–504.

Blank, A. S. (1993). The longitudinal course of posttraumatic stress disorder. In J. R. T. Davidson & E. B. Foa (Eds.), *Posttraumatic stress disorder: DSM-IV and beyond* (pp. 3–22). Washington, DC: American Psychiatric Press.

Blank, A. S. (1994). Clinical detection, diagnosis, and differential diagnosis of post-traumatic stress disorder. *Psychiatric Clinics of North America, 17,* 351–384.

Boehnlein, J. K. (1987). Clinical relevance of grief and mourning among Cambodian refugees. *Social Science and Medicine, 25,* 765–772.

Boudewyn, A. C., & Liem, J. H. (1995). Childhood sexual abuse as a precursor to depression and self-destructive behavior in adulthood. *Journal of Traumatic Stress, 8,* 445–459.

Boudewyns, P., & Hyer, L. (1990). Physiological response to combat memories and preliminary treatment outcome in Vietnam veteran PTSD patients treated with direct therapeutic exposure. *Behavior Therapy, 21,* 63–87.

Bowen, G. R., & Lambert, J. A. (1986). Systematic desensitization therapy with post-traumatic stress disorder cases. In C. R. Figley (Ed.), *Trauma and its wake* (pp. 280–291). New York: Brunner/Mazel.

Bradburn, N. M., Rips, L. J., & Shevell, S. K. (1987). Answering autobiographical questions: The impact of memory and inference on surveys. *Science, 236,* 157–161.

Brand, E. F., King, C. A., Olson, E., Ghaziuddin, N., & Naylor, M. (1996). Depressed adolescents with a history of sexual abuse: Diagnostic comorbidity and suicidality. *Journal of the American Academy of Child and Adolescent Psychiatry, 35,* 34–41.

Branscomb, L. (1991). Dissociation in combat-related post-traumatic stress disorder. *Dissociation, 4*(1), 13–20.

Bremner, J. D., Southwick, S., Brett, E., Fontana, A., Rosenheck, R., & Charney, D. S. (1992). Dissociation and posttraumatic stress disorder in Vietnam combat veterans. *American Journal of Psychiatry, 149,* 328–332.

Bremner, J. D., Southwick, S. M., Johnson, D. R., Yehuda, R., & Charney, D. S. (1993). Childhood physical abuse and combat-related posttraumatic stress disorder in Vietnam veterans. American Journal of Psychiatry, *150*(2), 235–239.

Breslau, N. (1987). Inquiring about the bizarre: False positives in Diagnostic Interview Schedule for Children (DISC) ascertainment of obsessions, compulsions, and psychotic symptoms. *Journal of the American Academy of Child and Adolescent Psychiatry, 26,* 639–644.

Breslau, N., & Davis, G. C. (1987). Posttraumatic stress disorder: The etiologic specificity of wartime stressors. *American Journal of Psychiatry, 144,* 578–583.

Breslau, N., Davis, G. C., Andreski, P., & Peterson, E. (1991). Traumatic events and posttraumatic stress disorder in an urban population of young adults. *Archives of General Psychiatry, 48,* 216–222.

Brett, E. A. (1993). Psychoanalytic contributions to a theory of traumatic stress. In J. P. Wilson & B. Raphael (Eds.), *International handbook of traumatic stress syndromes* (pp. 61–68). New York: Plenum Press.

Brett, E. A. (1996). The classification of posttraumatic stress disorder. In B. A. van der Kolk, A. C. McFarlane, & L. Weisaeth (Eds.), *Traumatic stress: The effects of overwhelming experience on mind, body, and society* (pp. 117–128). New York: Guilford Press.

Brewin, C. R., Andrews, B., & Gotlib, I. H. (1993). Psychopathology and early experience: A reappraisal of retrospective reports. *Psychological Bulletin, 113,* 82–98.

Briere, J. (1988). The long-term clinical correlates of childhood sexual victimization. *Annals of the New York Academy of Sciences, 528,* 327–334.

Briere, J. (1992). *Child abuse trauma: Theory and treatment of the lasting effects.* Newbury Park, CA: Sage.

Briere, J. (1995). *Trauma Symptom Inventory professional manual.* Odessa, FL: Psychological Assessment Resources.

Briere, J. (1996a). Psychological assessment of child abuse effects in adults. In J. Wilson & T. M. Keane (Eds.), *Assessing psychological trauma and PTSD* (pp. 43–68). New York: Guilford Press.

Briere, J. (1996b). A self-trauma model for treating adult survivors of severe child abuse. In J. Briere, L. Berliner, J. A. Bulkley, C. Jenny, & T. Reid (Eds.), *The APSAC handbook on child maltreatment* (pp. 140–157). Chicago: APSAC.

Briere, J. (1996c). *Therapy for adults molested as children* (2nd ed.). New York: Springer.

Briere, J. (1996d). *Trauma Symptom Checklist for Children, professional manual.* Odessa, FL: Psychological Assessment Resources.

Briere, J. (1997). *Psychological assessment of adult posttraumatic states.* Washington, DC: American Psychological Association Books.

Briere, J., & Conte, J. (1993). Self-reported amnesia for abuse in adults molested as children. *Journal of Traumatic Stress, 6,* 21–31.

Briere, J., & Elliott, D. M. (1993). Sexual abuse, family environment, and psychological symptoms: On the validity of statistical control. *Journal of Consulting and Clinical Psychology, 61,* 284–288.

Briere, J., & Runtz, M. (1987). Post sexual abuse trauma. *Journal of Interpersonal Violence, 2,* 367–379.

Briere, J., & Runtz, M. (1988). Multivariate correlates of childhood psychological and physical maltreatment among university women. *Child Abuse and Neglect, 12,* 331–341.

Briere, J., & Zaidi, L. Y. (1989). Sexual abuse histories and sequelae in female psychiatric emergency room patients. *American Journal of Psychiatry, 146,* 1602–1606.

Brom, D., Kleber, R. J., & Defares, P. B. (1989). Brief psychotherapy for PTSD. *Journal of Consulting and Clinical Psychology, 57,* 607–612.

Browne, A., & Finkelhor, D. (1986). Impact of child sexual abuse: A review of the research. *Psychological Bulletin, 99,* 66–77.

Bryant, R. A., & Harvey, A. G. (1996). Initial posttraumatic stress responses following motor vehicle accidents. *Journal of Traumatic Stress, 9,* 223–234.

Bryer, J. B., Nelson, B. A., Miller, J. B., & Krol, P. A. (1987). Childhood sexual and physical abuse as factors in adult psychiatric illness. *American Journal of Psychiatry, 144,* 1426–1430.

Bunch, J. (1972). Recent bereavement in relation to suicide. *Journal of Psychosomatic Research, 16,* 361–366.

Burgess, A. W., Hartman, C. R., & McCormack, A. (1987). Abused to abuser: Antecedents of socially deviant behavior. *American Journal of Psychiatry, 144,* 1431–1436.

Butcher, J. N., Dahlstrom, W. G., Graham, J. R., Tellegen, A., & Kaemmer, B. (1989). *Minnesota Multiphasic Personality Inventory—2 (MMPI-2): Manual for administration and scoring.* Minneapolis: University of Minnesota Press.

Buydens-Branchey, L., Noumair, D., & Branchey, M. (1990). Duration and intensity of combat exposure and posttraumatic stress disorder in Vietnam veterans. *Journal of Nervous and Mental Disease, 178,* 582–587.

Cardeña, E. (1994). The domain of dissociation. In S. J. Lynn & J. W. Rhue (Eds.), *Dissociation: Theoretical, clinical, and research perspectives* (pp. 15–31). New York: Guilford Press.

Cardeña, E., & Speigel, D. (1993). Dissociative reactions to the Bay Area Earthquake. *The American Journal of Psychiatry, 150,* 474–478.

Cardeña, E., & Spiegel, D. (1996). Diagnostic issues, criteria, and comorbidity of dissociative disorders. In L. K. Michelson & W. J. Ray (Eds.), *Handbook of dissociation: Theoretical, empirical, and clinical perspectives* (pp. 227–250). New York: Plenum Press.

Carlson, E. B. (1997). *Validation of a brief scale to measure posttraumatic stress disorder symptoms following single or multiple traumas.* Unpublished manuscript.

Carlson, E. B., & Armstrong, J. (1994). Diagnosis and assessment of dissociative disorders. In S. J. Lynn & J. W. Rhue (Eds.), *Dissociation: Theoretical, clinical, and research perspectives* (pp. 159–174). New York: Guilford Press.

Carlson, E. B., Armstrong, J., & Loewenstein, R. (1997). Reported amnesia for childhood abuse and other traumatic events in psychiatric inpatients. In D. Read & S. Lindsay (Eds.), *Recollections of trauma: Scientific research and clinical practice.* New York: Plenum Press.

Carlson, E. B., Armstrong, J., Loewenstein, R., & Roth, D. (1997). Relationships between traumatic experiences and symptoms of posttraumatic stress, dissociation, and amnesia. In J. D. Bremner (Ed.), *Trauma, memory, and dissociation.* Washington, DC: American Psychiatric Press.

Carlson, E. B., Furby, L., Armstrong, J. A., & Shlaes, J. (1997). A conceptual framework for the long-term psychological effects of traumatic childhood abuse. *Child Maltreatment.*

Carlson, E. B., & Putnam, F. W. (1993). An update on the Dissociative Experiences Scale. *Dissociation, 6,* 16–27.

Carlson, E. B., & Rosser-Hogan, R. (1991). Trauma experiences, posttraumatic stress, dissociation, and depression in Cambodian refugees. *American Journal of Psychiatry, 148,* 1548–1551.

Carlson, E. B., & Rosser-Hogan, R. (1993). Mental health status of Cambodian refugees ten years after leaving home. *American Journal of Orthopsychiatry, 63,* 223–231.

Carlson, E. B., & Rosser-Hogan, R. (1994). Cross-cultural response to trauma: A study of traumatic experiences and posttraumatic stress symptoms in Cambodian refugees. *Journal of Traumatic Stress, 7,* 43–58.

Carlson, G. A., Kashani, J. H., & de Fatima Thomas, M. (1987). Comparison of two structured interviews on a psychiatrically hospitalized population of children. *Journal of the American Academy of Child and Adolescent Psychiatry, 26,* 645–648.

Carroll, E. M., & Foy, D. W. (1992). Assessment and treatment of combat-related post-traumatic stress disorder in a medical center setting. In D. W. Foy (Ed.), *Treating PTSD: Cognitive-behavioral strategies* (pp. 39–68). New York: Guilford Press.

Chemtob, C., & Roitblat, H. L. (1994). Anger, impulsivity, and anger control in combat-related posttraumatic stress disorder. *Journal of Consulting and Clinical Psychology, 62*(2), 827–832.

Chemtob, C., Roitblat, H. L., Hamada, R. S., Carlson, J. G., & Twentyman, C. T. (1988). A cognitive action theory of post-traumatic stress disorder. *Journal of Anxiety Disorders, 2,* 253–275.

Christianson, S., & Loftus, E. F. (1987). Memory for traumatic events. *Applied Cognitive Psychology, 1,* 225–239.

Christianson, S.-A. (1992). Emotional stress and eyewitness memory: A critical review. *Psychological Bulletin, 112*(2), 284–309.

Chu, J. A., & Dill, D. L. (1990). Dissociative symptoms in relation to childhood physical and sexual abuse. *American Journal of Psychiatry, 147,* 887–892.

Cicchetti, D. (1989). How research on child maltreatment has informed the study of child development. In D. Cicchetti & V. Carlson (Eds.), *Child maltreatment* (pp. 377–431). Cambridge, MA: Cambridge University Press.

Cicchetti, D., & Barnett, D. (1991). Attachment organization in maltreated preschoolers. *Development and Psychopathology, 3,* 397–411.

Cicchetti, D., & Howes, P. W. (1991). Developmental psychopathology in the context of the family: Illustrations from the study of child maltreatment. *Canadian Journal of Behavioural Science, 23,* 257–281.

Cicchetti, D., & Rizley, R. (1981). Developmental perspectives on the etiology, intergenerational transmission, and sequelae of child maltreatment. In R. Rizley & D. Cicchetti (Eds.), *New directions for child development: Developmental perspectives on child maltreatment* (pp. 31–55). San Francisco: Jossey-Bass.

Cicchetti, D., Rogosch, F. A., Lynch, M., & Holt, K. D. (1993). Resilience in maltreated children: Processes leading to adaptive outcome. *Development and Psychopathology, 5,* 629–647.

Classen, C., Koopman, C., & Spiegel, D. (1993). Trauma and dissociation. *Bulletin of the Menninger Clinic, 57,* 178–194.

Cole, P. M., & Putnam, F. W. (1992). Effect of incest on self and social functioning: A developmental psychopathology perspective. *Journal of Consulting and Clinical Psychology, 60,* 174–184.

Conte, J. R., & Schuerman, J. R. (1987). Factors associated with an increased impact of child sexual abuse. *Child Abuse and Neglect, 11,* 201–211.

Cooper, N. A., & Clum, G. A. (1989). Imaginal flooding as a supplementary treatment for PTSD in combat veterans: A controlled study. *Behavior Therapy, 20,* 381–391.

Courtois, C. (1988). *Healing the incest wound: Adult survivors in therapy.* New York: Norton.

Craine, L. A., Henson, C. E., Colliver, J. A., & MacLean, D. G. (1988). Prevalence of a history of sexual abuse among female psychiatric patients in a state hospital system. *Hospital and Community Psychiatry, 39,* 300–304.

Creamer, M., Burgess, P., & Pattison, P. (1992). Reaction to trauma: A cognitive processing model. *Journal of Abnormal Psychology, 101,* 452–459.

Crittenden, P. M., & Ainsworth, M. D. S. (1989). Child maltreatment and attachment theory. In D. Cicchetti & V. Carlson (Eds.), *Child maltreatment: Theory and research on the causes and consequences of child abuse and neglect* (pp. 432–463). New York: Cambridge University.

Crocq, M.-A., Macher, J.-P., Barros-Beck, J., Rosenberg, S. J., & Duval, F. (1993). Posttraumatic stress disorder in World War II prisoners of war from Alsace-Lorraine who survived captivity in the USSR. In J. P. Wilson & B. Raphael (Eds.), *International handbook of traumatic stress syndromes* (pp. 253–261). New York: Plenum Press.

Dahl, S. (1989). Acute response to rape—a PTSD variant. *Acta Psychiatrica Scandinavica Supplementum, 355,* 56–62.

Dalenberg, C. (1996). Fantastic elements in child disclosure of abuse. *APSAC Advisor, 9*(1), 5–10.

Dalenberg, C. (in press-a). Accuracy, timing, and circumstances of disclosure in therapy of recovered and continuous memories of abuse. *Psychiatry and the Law.*

Dalenberg, C. (in press-b). Ethical issues in the assessment and treatment of child abuse victims. In S. Bucky (Ed.), *The comprehensive textbook of ethics and law in the practice of psychology.* New York: Plenum Press.

Dalenberg, C., & Carlson, E. B. (in press). Ethical issues in the treatment of recovered memory trauma victims and patients with false memories of trauma. In S. Bucky (Ed.), *The comprehensive textbook of ethics and law in the practice of psychology.* New York: Plenum Press.

Dalenberg, C., & Jacobs, D. (1994). Attributional analysis of child sexual abuse episodes: Empirical and clinical issues. *Journal of Child Sexual Abuse, 3,* 37–50.

Damon, A., Damon, S. T., Reed, R. B., & Valadian, I. (1969). Age at menarche of mothers and daughters, with a note on accuracy of recall. *Human Biology, 41,* 161–175.

Dancu, C. V., Riggs, D. S., Hearst-Ikeda, D., Shoyer, G., & Foa, E. B. (1996). Dissociative experiences and posttraumatic stress disorder among female victims of criminal assault and rape. *Journal of Traumatic Stress, 9,* 253–267.

Daniella, D., Mellman, T. A., Mendoza, L. M., Kulick-Bell, R., Ironson, G., & Schneiderman, N. (1996). Psychiatric comorbidity following Hurricane Andrew. *Journal of Traumatic Stress, 9,* 607–612.

Davidson, J., & Smith, R. (1990). Traumatic experiences in psychiatric outpatients. *Journal of Traumatic Stress, 3,* 459–475.

Davidson, J. R. T., Book, S. W., Colket, J. T., Tupler, L. A., Roth, S., David, D., Hertzberg, M., Mellman, T., Beckham, J. C., Smith, R., Davison, R. M., Katz, R., & Feldman, M. (in press). Assessment of a new self-rating scale for post-traumatic stress disorder. *Psychological Medicine.*

Davidson, J. R. T., & Foa, E. B. (1991). Diagnostic issues in posttraumatic stress disorder: Considerations for the DSM-IV. *Journal of Abnormal Psychology, 100,* 346–355.

Davidson, J. R. T., Smith, R. D., & Kudler, H. S. (1989). Validity and reliability of the DSM-III criteria for posttraumatic stress disorder: Experience with a structured interview. *Journal of Nervous and Mental Disease, 177,* 336–341.

Davidson, J. R. T., & van der Kolk, B. A. (1996). The psychopharmacological treatment of postraumatic stress disorder. In B. A. van der Kolk, A. C. McFarlane, & L. Weisaeth (Eds.), *Traumatic stress: The effects of overwhelming experience on mind, body, and society* (pp. 510–524). New York: Guilford Press.

Davidson, R. J. (1992a). Anterior cerebral asymmetry and the nature of emotion. *Brain and Cognition, 20,* 125–151.

Davidson, R. J. (1992b). Emotion and affective style: Hemispheric substrates. *Psychological Science, 3,* 39–43.

Davies, J., & Frawley, M. (1994). *Treating the adult survivor of childhood sexual abuse: A psychoanalytic perspective.* New York: Basic Books.

De Loos, W. S. (1990). Psychosomatic manifestations of chronic posttraumatic stress disorder. In M. E. Wolf & A. D. Mosnaim (Eds.), *Posttraumatic stress disorder: Etiology, phenomenology, and treatment* (pp. 94–104). Washington, DC: American Psychiatric Press.

Deblinger, E. & Heflin, A. (1996). *Treating sexually abused children and their offending parents.* Thousand Oaks, CA: Sage.

Derogatis, L. R. (1983). *SCL-90-R: Administration, scoring and procedures manual-II.* Towson, MD: Clinical Psychometric Research.

deVries, M. W. (1996). Trauma in cultural perspective. In B. A. van der Kolk, A. C. McFarlane, & L. Weisaeth (Eds.), *Traumatic stress: The effects of overwhelming experience on mind, body, and society* (pp. 398–413). New York: Guilford Press.

Dienstbier, R. A. (1989). Arousal and physiological toughness: Implications for mental and physical health. *Psychological Review, 96,* 84–100.

Dinicola, V. F. (1996). Ethnocultural aspects of PTSD and related disorders among children and adolescents. In A. J. Marsella, M. J. Friedman, E. T. Gerrity, & R. M. Scurfield (Eds.), *Ethnocultural aspects of posttraumatic stress disorder: Issues, research, and clinical applications* (pp. 389–414). Washington, DC: American Psychological Association.

Draguns, J. G. (1996). Ethnocultural considerations in the treatment of PTSD: Therapy and service delivery. In A. J. Marsella, M. J. Friedman, E. T. Gerrity, & R. M. Scurfield (Eds.), *Ethnocultural aspects of posttraumatic stress disorder: Issues, research, and clinical applications* (pp. 459–482). Washington, DC: American Psychological Association.

Dutton, M. A. (1992). Assessment and treatment of post-traumatic stress disorder among battered women. In D. W. Foy (Ed.), *Treating PTSD: Cognitive-behavioral strategies* (pp. 69–98). New York: Guilford Press.

Dutton, M. A. (1994). Post-traumatic therapy with domestic violence survivors. In M. B. Williams & J. F. Sommer (Eds.), *Handbook of posttraumatic therapy* (pp. 146–161). Westport, CT: Greenwood Press.

Egeland, B., Jacobvitz, D., & Sroufe, L. A. (1988). Breaking the cycle of abuse. *Child Development, 59,* 1080–1088.

Eisen, M., & Carlson, E. B. (1997). *Development, reliability, and validity of a brief PTSD measure for young children.* Unpublished manuscript.

Elliott, D. M., & Briere, J. (1995). Posttraumatic stress associated with delayed recall of sexual abuse: A general population study. *Journal of Traumatic Stress, 8,* 629–647.

Erikson, E. H. (1963). *Childhood and society.* New York: Norton.

Everly, G. S. (1990). Post-traumatic stress disorder as a disorder of arousal. *Psychology and Health, 4,* 135–145.

Everson, M., & Boat, B. (1994). Putting the anatomical doll controversy in perspective: An examination of the major uses and criticisms of the dolls in child sexual abuse evaluations. *Child Abuse and Neglect, 18,* 113–129.

Eysenck, H. (1983). Stress, disease, and personality: The innoculation effect. In C. Cooper (Ed.), *Stress research* (pp. 121–146). New York: Wiley.

Falk, B., Hersen, M., & Van Hasselt, V. B. (1994). Assessment of post-traumatic stress disorder in older adults: A critical review. *Clinical Psychology Review, 14,* 383–415.

Falsetti, S. A., Resick, P. A., Resnick, H. S., & Kilpatrick, D. (1992, November). *Post-traumatic stress disorder: The assessment of frequency and severity of symptoms in clinical and nonclinical samples.* Paper presented at the annual convention of the Association for Advancement of Behavior Therapy, Boston.

Falsetti, S. A., & Resnick, H. S. (1994). Helping the victims of violent crimes. In J. R. Freedy & S. E. Hobfoll (Eds.), *Traumatic stress: From theory to practice.* New York: Plenum Press.

Falsetti, S. A., Resnick, H. S., Resick, P. A., & Kilpatrick, D. (1993). The Modified PTSD Symptom Scale: A brief self-report measure of posttraumatic stress disorder. *The Behavior Therapist, 16,* 161–162.

Finch, A. J., & Daugherty, T. K. (1993). Issues in the assessment of posttraumatic stress disorder in children. In C. F. Saylor (Ed.), *Children and disasters* (pp. 45–66). New York: Plenum Press.

Fine, C. G. (1993). A tactical integrationalist perspective on the treatment of multiple personality disorder. In R. P. Kluft & C. Fine (Eds.), *Clinical perspectives on multiple personality disorder* (pp. 135–153). Washington, DC: American Psychiatric Press.

Fine, C. G. (1996). A cognitively-based treatment model for DSM-IV dissociative identity disorder. In L. K. Michelson & W. J. Ray (Eds.), *Handbook of dissociation: Theoretical, empirical, and clinical perspectives* (pp. 401–412). New York: Plenum Press.

Fink, L. A., Bernstein, D., Handelsman, L., Foote, J., & Lovejoy, M. (1995).

Initial reliability and validity of the Childhood Trauma Interview: A new multidimensional measure of childhood interpersonal trauma. *American Journal of Psychiatry, 152,* 1329–1335.

Finkelhor, D. (1990). Early and long-term effects of child sexual abuse: An update. *Professional Psychology: Research and Practice, 21,* 325–330.

Finkelhor, D., & Berliner, L. (1995). Research on the treatment of sexually abused children: A review and recommendations. *Journal of the American Academy of Child and Adolescent Psychiatry, 34,* 1408–1423.

Fivush, R., & Schwarzmueller, A. (1995). Say it once again: Effects of repeated questions on children's event recall. *Journal of Traumatic Stress, 8,* 555–580.

Flannery, R. B. (1987). From victim to survivor: A stress management approach in the treatment of learned helplessness. In B. van der Kolk (Ed.), *Psychological trauma* (pp. 217–232). Washington, DC: American Psychiatric Press.

Fletcher, K. E. (1996a). Childhood posttraumatic stress disorder. In E. J. Mash & R. A. Barkley (Eds.), *Child psychopathology* (pp. 242–276). New York: Guilford Press.

Fletcher, K. E. (1996b, November). *Measuring school-aged children's PTSD: Preliminary psychometrics of four new measures.* Paper presented at the 12th annual meeting of the International Society for Traumatic Stress Studies, San Francisco.

Foa, D. B., & Kozak, M. J. (1986). Emotional processing of fear: Exposure to corrective information. *Psychological Bulletin, 99,* 20–35.

Foa, E., Cashman, L., Jaycox, L., & Perry, K. (in press). The validation of a self-report measure of PTSD: The Posttraumatic Diagnostic Scale (PDS). *Psychological Assessment.*

Foa, E., & Riggs, D. S. (1993). Posttraumatic stress disorder and rape. In J. M. Oldham, M. B. Riba, & A. Tasman (Eds.), *Review of psychiatry* (pp. 273–303). Washington, DC: American Psychiatric Press.

Foa, E. B., Molnar, C., & Cashman, L. (1995). Change in rape narratives during exposure to therapy for posttraumatic stress disorder. *Journal of Traumatic Stress, 8,* 675–690.

Foa, E. B., Riggs, D. S., Dancu, C. V., & Rothbaum, B. O. (1993). Reliability and validity of a brief instrument for assessing post-traumatic stress disorder. *Journal of Traumatic Stress, 6,* 459–474.

Foa, E. B., Rothbaum, B. O., Riggs, D. S., & Murdock, T. B. (1991). Treatment of posttraumatic stress disorder in rape victims: A comparison between cognitive–behavioral procedures and counseling. *Journal of Consulting and Clinical Psychology, 59,* 715–723.

Foa, E. B., Steketee, G., & Rothbaum, B. O. (1989). Behavioral/cognitive conceptualiztions of posttraumatic stress disorder. *Behavior Therapy, 20,* 155–176.

Foa, E. B., Zinbarg, R., & Rothbaum, B. O. (1992). Uncontrollability and unpredictability in post-traumatic stress disorder: An animal model. *Psychological Bulletin, 112*(2), 218–238.

Follette, V. M., Polusny, M. A., Bechtle, A. E., & Naugle, A. E. (1996).

Cumulative trauma: The impact of child sexual abuse, adult sexual assault, and spouse abuse. *Journal of Traumatic Stress, 9,* 25–35.

Ford, J. P., Thomas, J., Rogers, K., Racusin, R., Ellis, C. G., Schiffman, J., Daviss, W. B., & Friedman, M. J. (1996). *Assessment of children's PTSD following abuse or accidental trauma.* Paper presented at the 12th annual meeting of the International Society for Traumatic Stress Studies, San Francisco.

Foreman, C. (1994). Immediate post-disaster treatment of trauma. In M. B. Williams & J. F. Sommer (Eds.), *Handbook of posttraumatic therapy* (pp. 267–282). Westport, CT: Greenwood Press.

Foy, D. W. (Ed.). (1992). *Treating PTSD: Cognitive-behavioral strategies.* New York: Guilford Press.

Frankel, F. H. (1994). Dissociation in hysteria and hypnosis: A concept aggrandized. In S. J. Lynn & J. W. Rhue (Eds.), *Dissociation: Theoretical, clinical, and research perspectives* (pp. 80–93). New York: Guilford Press.

Freyd, J. J. (1996). *Betrayal trauma: The logic of forgetting.* Cambridge, MA: Harvard University Press.

Friedman, M. J. (1993). Biological and pharmacological approaches to treatment. In J. P. Wilson & B. Raphael (Eds.), *International handbook of traumatic stress syndromes* (pp. 785–794). New York: Plenum Press.

Friedman, M. J. (1994). Biological and pharmacological aspects of the treatment of PTSD. In M. B. Williams & J. F. Sommer (Eds.), *Handbook of posttraumatic therapy* (pp. 495–509). Westport, CT: Greenwood Press.

Friedman, M. J., & Schnurr, P. P. (1995). The relationship between trauma, post-traumatic stress disorder, and physical health. In M. J. Friedman, D. S. Charney, & A. Y. Deutch (Eds.), *Neurobiological and clinical consequences of stress: From normal adaptation to posttraumatic stress disorder* (pp. 507–524). Philadelphia: Lippincott-Raven.

Frisch, M. B., & MacKenzie, C. J. (1991). A comparison of formerly and chronically battered women on cognitive and situational dimensions. *Psychotherapy, 28,* 339–344.

Gerrity, E. T., & Solomon, S. D. (1996). The treatment of PTSD and related stress disorders: Current research and clinical knowledge. In A. J. Marsella, M. J. Friedman, E. T. Gerrity, & R. M. Scurfield (Eds.), *Ethnocultural aspects of posttraumatic stress disorder: Issues, research, and clinical applications* (pp. 87–102). Washington, DC: American Psychological Association.

Gil, E. (1988). *Treatment of adult survivors of childhood abuse.* Rockville, MD: Launch Press.

Giolas, M. H., & Sanders, B. (1992). Pain and suffering as a function of dissociation level and instructional set. *Dissociation, 5,* 205–209.

Glover, H., Ohlde, C., Silver, S., Packard, P., Goodnick, P., & Hamlin, C. L. (1994). The numbing scale: Psychometric properties, a preliminary report. *Anxiety, 1,* 70–79.

Goenjian, A. K., Pynoos, R. S., Steinberg, A. M., Najarian, L. M., Asarnow, J. R., Karayan, I., Ghurabi, M., & Fairbanks, L. A. (1995). Psychiatric comorbidity in children after the 1988 earthquake in Armenia. *Journal* of the American Academy of Child and Adolescent Psychiatry, 34, 1174–1184.

Gold, E. (1986). Long term effects of sexual victimization in childhood: An attributional approach. *Journal of Consulting and Clinical Psychology, 54,* 471–475.

Goodwin, J. M., Cheeves, K., & Connell, V. (1990). Borderline and other severe symptoms in adult survivors of incestuous abuse. *Psychiatric Annals, 20,* 22–32.

Grayston, A. D., De Luca, R. V., & Boyes, D. A. (1992). Self-esteem, anxiety, and loneliness in preadolescent girls who have experienced sexual abuse. *Child Psychiatry and Human Development, 22,* 277–286.

Green, A. H. (1978). Self-destructive behavior in battered children. *American Journal of Psychiatry, 135,* 579–582.

Green, B. (1994). Psychosocial research in traumatic stress: An update. *Journal of Traumatic Stress, 7,* 341–362.

Green, B. L. (1993). Identifying survivors at risk: Trauma and stressors across events. In J. P. Wilson & B. Raphael (Eds.), *International handbook of traumatic stress syndromes* (pp. 135–144). New York: Plenum Press.

Green, B. L. (1995). Recent research findings on the diagnosis of posttraumatic stress disorder: Prevalence, course, comorbidity, and risk. In R. Simon (Ed.), *Posttraumatic stress disorder in litigation* (pp. 13–29). Washington, DC: American Psychiatric Press.

Green, B. L., Epstein, S. A., Krupnick, J. L., & Rowland, J. H. (1996). Trauma and medical illness: Assessing trauma-related disorders in medical settings. In J. Wilson & T. M. Keane (Eds.), *Assessing psychological trauma and PTSD* (pp. 160–191). New York: Guilford Press.

Green, B. L., Grace, M. C., Lindy, J. D., Glese, G. C., & Leonard, A. (1990). Risk factors for PTSD and other diagnoses in a general sample of Vietnam veterans. *American Journal of Psychiatry, 147,* 729–733.

Green, B. L., & Wolfe, J. (Eds.) (1995). Research on traumatic memory [Special issue]. *Journal of Traumatic Stress, 8.*

Greenwald, R. (1994). Eye movement desensitization and reprocessing (EMDR): An overview. *Journal of Contemporary Psychotherapy, 24,* 15–34.

Gusman, F. D., Stewart, J., Young, B. H., Riney, S. J., Abueg, F. R., & Blake, D. D. (1996). A multicultural developmental approach for treating trauma. In A. J. Marsella, M. J. Friedman, E. T. Gerrity, & R. M. Scurfield (Eds.), *Ethnocultural aspects of posttraumatic stress disorder: Issues, research, and clinical applications* (pp. 439–457). Washington, DC: American Psychological Association.

Hammarberg, M. (1992). Penn Inventory for Posttraumatic Stress Disorder: Psychometric properties. *Psychological Assessment, 4,* 67–76.

Harber, K. D., & Pennebaker, J. W. (1992). Overcoming traumatic memories. In S. Christianson (Ed.), *The handbook of emotion and memory: Research and theory* (pp. 359–387). Hillsdale, NJ: Erlbaum.

Hartman, C. R., & Burgess, A. W. (1993). Treatment of victims of rape trauma. In J. P. Wilson & B. Raphael (Eds.), *International handbook of traumatic stress syndromes* (pp. 507–516). New York: Plenum Press.

Hartman, M., Finn, S. E., & Leon, G. R. (1987). Sexual abuse experiences in a clinical population: Comparisons of familial and nonfamilial abuse. *Psychotherapy, 24,* 154–159.

Harvey, J., & Herman, J. L. (1994). Amnesia, partial amnesia, and delayed recall among survivors of childhood trauma. *Consciousness and Cognition, 3,* 295–306.

Harvey, J., Orbuch, T., Chwalisz, K., & Garwood, G. (1991). Coping with sexual assault: The role of account making and confiding. *Journal of Traumatic Stress, 4,* 515–532.

Harvey, J. H., Stein, S. K., & Scott, P. K. (1995). Fifty years of grief: Accounts and reported psychological reactions of Normandy invasion veterans. *Journal of Narrative and Life History, 5,* 315–332.

Hauff, E., & Vaglum, P. (1994). Chronic posttraumatic stress disorder in Vietnamese refugees: A prospective community study of prevalence, course, psychopathology, and stressors. *Journal of Nervous and Mental Disease, 82,* 85–90.

Hendrix, C. C., Jurich, A. P., & Schumm, W. R. (1994). Validation of the Impact of Event Scale on a sample of American Vietnam veterans. *Psychological Reports, 75,* 321–322.

Herbert, J. D., & Mueser, K. T. (1992). Eye movement desensitization: A critique of the evidence. *Journal of Behavior Therapy and Experimental Psychiatry, 23,* 169–174.

Herman, J. (1993). Sequelae of prolonged and repeated trauma: Evidence for a complex posttraumatic syndrome (DESNOS). In J. R. T. Davidson & E. B. Foa (Eds.), *Posttraumatic stress disorder: DSM-IV and beyond* (pp. 207–212). Washington, DC: American Psychiatric Press.

Herman, J., & Lawrence, L. R. (1993). Group therapy and self-help groups for adult survivors of childhood incest. In J. P. Wilson & B. Raphael (Eds.), *International handbook of traumatic stress syndromes* (pp. 440–452). New York: Plenum Press.

Herman, J., Russell, D., & Trocki, K. (1986). Long-term effects of incestuous abuse in childhood. *American Journal of Psychiatry, 143,* 1293–1296.

Herman, J. L. (1992). *Trauma and recovery.* New York: Basic Books.

Herman, J. L., Perry, J. C., & van der Kolk, B. A. (1989). Childhood trauma in borderline personality disorder. *American Journal of Psychiatry, 146,* 490–495.

Herman, J. L., & Schatzow, E. (1987). Recovery and verification of memories of childhood sexual trauma. *Psychoanalytic Psychology, 4,* 1–14.

Herrenkohl, R. C., & Herrenkohl, E. C. (1981). Some antecedents and developmental consequences of child maltreatment. In R. Rizley & D. Cicchetti (Eds.), *New directions for child development: Developmental perspectives on child maltreatment* (pp. 31–56). San Francisco: Jossey-Bass.

Herrenkohl, R. C., Herrenkohl, E. C., Egolf, B. P., & Wu, P. (1991). The developmental consequences of child abuse: The Lehigh longitudinal study. In R. H. Starr & D. A. Wolfe (Eds.), *The effects of child abuse and neglect: Issues and research* (pp. 57–81). New York: Guilford Press.

Hilgard, E. R. (1986). *Divided consciousness: Multiple controls in human thought and action* (3rd ed.). New York: John Wiley.

Horevitz, R. (1994). Dissociation and multiple personality: Conflicts and controversies. In S. J. Lynn & J. W. Rhue (Eds.), *Dissociation: Theoretical, clinical, and research perspectives* (pp. 434–461). New York: Guilford Press.

Horevitz, R., & Loewenstein, R. J. (1994). The rational treatment of multiple personality disorder. In S. J. Lynn & J. W. Rhue (Eds.), *Dissociation: Theoretical, clinical, and research perspectives* (pp. 268–316). New York: Guilford Press.

Hornstein, N. L. (1996). Dissociative disorders in children and adolescents. In L. K. Michelson & W. J. Ray (Eds.), *Handbook of dissociation: Theoretical, empirical, and clinical perspectives* (pp. 139–159). New York: Plenum Press.

Hornstein, N. L., & Putnam, F. W. (1992). Clinical phenomenology of child and adolescent dissociative disorders. *Journal of the American Academy of Child and Adolescent Psychiatry, 31,* 1077–1085.

Hornstein, N. L., & Tyson, S. (1992). Inpatient treatment of children with multiple personality disorder. *Psychiatric Clinics of North America, 14,* 631–648.

Horowitz, M. (1993). Stress-response syndromes: A review of posttraumatic stress and adjustment disorders. In J. P. Wilson & B. Raphael (Eds.), *International handbook of traumatic stress syndromes* (pp. 49–60). New York: Plenum Press.

Horowitz, M. J. (1976). *Stress response syndromes.* Northvale, NJ: Jason Aronson.

Horowitz, M. J. (1986). *Stress response syndromes* (2nd ed.). Northvale, NJ: Jason Aronson.

Horowitz, M. J. (1991). Person schemas. In M. J. Horowitz (Ed.), *Person schemas and maladaptive interpersonal patterns* (pp. 13–31). Chicago: University of Chicago Press.

Horowitz, M. J., Wilner, N., & Alvarez, W. (1979). Impact of Event Scale: A measure of subjective stress. *Psychosomatic Medicine, 41,* 209–218.

Hough, R. L., Canino, G. J., Abueg, F. R., & Gusman, F. D. (1996). PTSD and related stress disorders among Hispanics. In A. J. Marsella, M. J. Friedman, E. T. Gerrity, & R. M. Scurfield (Eds.), *Ethnocultural aspects of posttraumatic stress disorder: Issues, research, and clinical applications* (pp. 301–338). Washington, DC: American Psychological Association.

Hovens, J. E. J. M., Op den Velde, W., Falger, P. R. J., Schouten, E. G. W., De Groen, J. H. M., & Van Duijn, H. (1992). Anxiety, depression and anger in Dutch resistance veterans. *Psychotherapy and Psychosomatics, 57,* 172–179.

Hubbard, J., Realmuto, G. M., Northwood, A. K., & Masten, A. S. (1995). Comorbidity of psychiatric diagnoses with posttraumatic stress disorder in survivors of childhood traumas. *Journal of the American Academy of Child and Adolescent Psychiatry, 34,* 1167–1173.

Hunter, E. J. (1993). The Vietnam prisoner of war experience. In J. P. Wilson & B. Raphael (Eds.), *International handbook of traumatic stress syndromes* (pp. 297–303). New York: Plenum Press.

Hyer, L., McCranie, E. W., & Peralme, L. (1993). Psychotherapeutic treatment of chronic PTSD. *PTSD Research Quarterly, 4,* 1–6.

Hyer, L. A., Albrecht, J. W., Boudewyns, P. A., Woods, M. G., & Brandsma, J. (1993). Dissociative experiences of Vietnam veterans with chronic post-traumatic stress disorder. *Psychological Reports, 73,* 519–530.

Irwin, H. J. (1994). Proneness to dissociation and traumatic childhood events. *Journal of Nervous and Mental Disease, 182,* 456–460.

Jacobson, A. J. (1989). Physical and sexual assault histories among psychiatric outpatients. *American Journal of Psychiatry, 146,* 755–758.

Jacobson, A. J., Koehler, J. E., & Jones-Brown, C. (1987). The failure of routine assessment to detect histories of assault experienced by psychiatric patients. *Hospital and Community Psychiatry, 38,* 386–389.

Jacobson, A. J., & Richardson, B. (1987). Assault experiences of 100 psychiatric inpatients: Evidence of the need for routine inquiry. *American Journal of Psychiatry, 144,* 908–913.

James, B. (1989). *Treating traumatized children.* Lexington, MA: Lexington Books.

James, B. (1994). Long-term treatment for children with severe trauma history. In M. B. Williams & J. F. Sommer (Eds.), *Handbook of posttraumatic therapy* (pp. 51–68). Westport, CT: Greenwood Press.

Janoff-Bulman, R. (1992). *Toward a new psychology of trauma.* New York: Free Press.

Jehu, D. (1989). Mood disturbances among women clients sexually abused in childhood. *Journal of Interpersonal Violence, 4,* 164–184.

Jensen, J. A. (1994). An investigation of eye movement desensitization and reprocessing (EMD/R) as a treatment for posttraumatic stress disorder (PTSD) symptoms of Vietnam combat veterans. *Behavior Therapy, 25,* 311–325.

Joseph, S. A., Brewin, C. R., Yule, W., & Williams, R. M. (1993). Causal attributions and posttraumatic stress in adolescents. *Journal of Child Psychology and Psychiatry and Allied Disciplines, 34,* 247–253.

Joseph, S. A., Hodgkinson, P. E., Yule, W., & Williams, R. M. (1993). Guilt and distress 30 months after the capsize of the Herald of Free Enterprise. *Personality and Individual Differences, 14,* 271–273.

Joseph, S. A., Yule, W., & Williams, R. M. (1994). The Herald of Free Enterprise disaster: The relationship of intrusion and avoidance to subsequent depression and anxiety. *Behaviour Research and Therapy, 32,* 115–117.

Joseph, S. A., Yule, W., & Williams, R. M. (1995). Emotional processing in survivors of the Jupiter cruise ship disaster. *Behaviour Research and Therapy, 33,* 187–192.

Justice, B., & Calvert, A. (1990). Family environment factors associated with child abuse. *Psychological Reports, 66,* 458.

Kaloupek, D. G., & Bremner, J. D. (1996). Psychophysiological measures and methods in trauma research. In E. B. Carlson (Ed.), *Trauma research methodology* (pp. 82–104). Lutherville, MD: Sidran Press.

Katz, S., Schonfeld, D. J., Carter, A. S., Leventhal, J. M., & Cicchetti, D. V. (1995). The accuracy of children's reports with anatomically correct dolls. *Developmental and Behavioral Pediatrics, 16,* 71–76.

Kaufman, J., & Zigler, E. (1987). Do abused children become abusive parents? *American Journal of Orthopsychiatry, 57,* 186–192.

Keane, T. M. (1995). Guidelines for the forensic psychological assessment of posttraumatic stress disorder claimants. In R. Simon (Ed.), *Posttraumatic stress disorder in litigation* (pp. 99–115). Washington, DC: American Psychiatric Press.

Keane, T. M., Caddell, J. M., & Taylor, K. L. (1988). Mississippi Scale for Combat-related Posttraumatic Stress Disorder: Three studies in reliability and validity. *Journal of Consulting and Clinical Psychology, 56,* 85–90.

Keane, T. M., Fairbank, J. A., Caddell, J. M., & Zimering, R. T. (1989). Implosive (flooding) therapy reduces symptoms of PTSD in Vietnam combat veterans. *Behavior Therapy, 20,* 245–260.

Keane, T. M., & Kaloupek, D. G. (1982). Imaginal flooding in the treatment of posttraumatic stress disorder. *Journal of Consulting and Clinical Psychology, 50,* 138–140.

Keane, T. M., Kaloupek, D. G., & Weathers, F. W. (1996). Ethnocultural considerations in the assessment of PTSD. In A. J. Marsella, M. J. Friedman, E. T. Gerrity, & R. M. Scurfield (Eds.), *Ethnocultural aspects of posttraumatic stress disorder: Issues, research, and clinical applications* (pp. 183–205). Washington, DC: American Psychological Association.

Keane, T. M., Litz, B. T., & Blake, D. D. (1990). Post-traumatic stress disorder in adulthood. In M. Hersen & C. G. Last (Eds.), *Handbook of child and adult psychopathology: A longitudinal perspective* (pp. 275–291). New York: Pergamon Press.

Keane, T. M., Newman, E., & Orsillo, S. M. (1996). Assessment of military-related posttraumatic stress disorder. In J. Wilson & T. M. Keane (Eds.), *Assessing psychological trauma and PTSD* (pp. 267–290). New York: Guilford Press.

Keane, T. M., Scott, W. O., Chavoya, G. A., Lamparski, D. M., & Fairbank, J. A. (1985). Social support in Vietnam veterans with posttraumatic stress disorder: A comparative analysis. *Journal of Consulting and Clinical Psychology, 53,* 95–102.

Keane, T. M., & Wolfe, J. (1990). Comorbidity in post-traumatic stress disorder: An analysis of community and clinical studies. *Journal of Applied Social Psychology, 20,* 1776–1788.

Keane, T. M., Zimering, R. T., & Caddell, J. M. (1985). A behavioral formulation of posttraumatic stress disorder in Vietnam veterans. *Behavior Therapist, 8,* 9–12.

Kendall-Tackett, K. A., Williams, L. M., & Finkelhor, D. (1993). Impact of sexual abuse on children: A review and synthesis of recent empirical studies. *Psychological Bulletin, 113,* 164–180.

Kilpatrick, D., Veronen, L., & Best, C. (1985). Factors predicting psychological distress among rape victims. In C. Figley (Ed.), *Trauma and its wake* (pp. 113–141). New York: Brunner/Mazel.

Kilpatrick, D. G., & Best, C. L. (1984). Some cautionary remarks in treating sexual abuse victims with implosion. *Behavior Therapy, 15,* 421–423.

Kilpatrick, D. G., & Resnick, H. S. (1993). PTSD associated with exposure to criminal victimization in clinical and community populations. In J. R. T. Davidson & E. B. Foa (Eds.), *Posttraumatic stress disorder: DSM-IV and beyond* (pp. 113–143). Washington, DC: American Psychiatric Press.

Kilpatrick, D. G., Resnick, H. S., & Freedy, J. R. (1991). *The Potential Stressful Events Interview.* Unpublished instrument, Crime Victims Research and Treatment Center, Medical University of South Carolina, Charleston, SC.

Kilpatrick, D. G., Saunders, B. E., Amick-McMullan, A., Best, C. L., Veronen, L. J., & Resnick, H. S. (1989). Victim and crime factors associated with the development of crime-related post-traumatic stress disorder. *Behavior Therapy, 20,* 199–214.

Kilpatrick, D. G., Saunders, B. E., Veronen, L. J., Best, C. L., & Von, J. M. (1987). Criminal victimization: Lifetime prevalence, reporting to police, and psychological impact. *Crime and Delinquency, 33,* 479–489.

Kinzie, J. D. (1993). Posttraumatic effects and their treatment among Southeast Asian refugees. In J. P. Wilson & B. Raphael (Eds.), *International handbook of traumatic stress syndromes* (pp. 311–319). New York: Plenum Press.

Kirby, J. S., Chu, J. A., & Dill, D. L. (1993). Correlates of dissociative symptomatology in patients with physical and sexual abuse histories. *Comprehensive Psychiatry, 34,* 258–263.

Kirmayer, L. J. (1996). Confusion of the senses: Implications of ethnocultural variations in somatoform and dissociative disorders for PTSD. In A. J. Marsella, M. J. Friedman, E. T. Gerrity, & R. M. Scurfield (Eds.), *Ethnocultural aspects of posttraumatic stress disorder: Issues, research, and clinical applications* (pp. 131–163). Washington, DC: American Psychological Association.

Kiser, L., Heston, J., Millsap, P., & Pruitt, D. (1991). Physical and sexual abuse in childhood: Relationship with posttraumatic stress disorder. *Journal of the American Academy of Child and Adolescent Psychiatry, 30,* 776–783.

Kleinknecht, R. (1994). Acquisition of blood, injury, and needle fears and phobias. *Behaviour Research and Therapy, 32,* 817–823.

Kluft, R. P. (1986). Treating children who have multiple personality disorder. In B. G. Braun (Ed.), *Treatment of multiple personality disorder* (pp. 81–105). Washington, DC: American Psychiatric Press.

Kluft, R. P. (1993). Basic principles in conducting the psychotherapy of multiple personality disorder. In R. P. Kluft & C. Fine (Eds.), *Clinical perspectives on multiple personality disorder* (pp. 19–50). Washington, DC: American Psychiatric Press.

Kluft, R. P. (1996a). Dissociative identity disorder. In L. K. Michelson & W. J. Ray (Eds.), *Handbook of dissociation: Theoretical, empirical, and clinical perspectives* (pp. 337–366). New York: Plenum Press.

Kluft, R. P. (1996b). Outpatient treatment of dissociative identity disorder and allied forms of dissociative disorder not otherwise specified in children and adolescents. *Child and Adolescent Psychiatric Clinics of North America, 5,* 471–494.

Kluft, R. P., & Fine, C. (Eds.). (1993). *Clinical perspectives on multiple personality disorder.* Washington, DC: American Psychiatric Press.

Knight, J. A. (1996). Neuropsychological assessment in posttraumatic stress disorder. In J. Wilson & T. M. Keane (Eds.), *Assessing psychological trauma and PTSD* (pp. 448–492). New York: Guilford Press.

Kobayashi, J., Sales, B., Beckers, J., & Figueredo, A. (1995). Perceived parental deviance, parent–child bonding, child abuse, and child sexual aggression. *Sexual Abuse: Journal of Research and Treatment, 7,* 25–44.

Koocher, G. P., Goodman, G. S., White, S., Friedrich, W. N., Sivan, A. B., & Reynolds, C. R. (1995). Psychological science and the use of anatomically detailed dolls in child sexual abuse assessments. Final report of the American Psychological Association Anatomical Doll Task Force. *Psychological Bulletin, 118,* 2.

Koopman, C., Classen, C., Cardeña, E., & Spiegel, D. (1995). When disaster strikes, acute stress disorder may follow. *Journal of Traumatic Stress, 8,* 29–46.

Koopman, C., Classen, C., & Spiegel, D. (1994). Predictors of posttraumatic stress symptoms among survivors of the Oakland/Berkeley, California, firestorm. *American Journal of Psychiatry, 151,* 888–894.

Koss, M. P., Gidycz, C. A., & Wisniewski, N. (1987). The scope of rape: Incidence and prevalence of sexual aggression and victimization in a national sample of higher education students. *Journal of Consulting and Clinical Psychology, 55,* 162–170.

Koverola, C., Pound, J., Heger, A., & Lytle, C. (1993). Relationship of child sexual abuse to depression. *Child Abuse and Neglect, 17,* 393–400.

Kramer, T. L., Lindy, J. D., Green, B. L., Grace, M. C., & Leonard, A. C. (1994). The comorbidity of post-traumatic stress disorder and suicidality in Vietnam veterans. *Suicide and Life-Threatening Behavior, 24,* 58–67.

Krinsley, K. E., Gallagher, J. G., Weathers, F. W., Kaloupek, D. G., & Vielhauer, M. (1997). *Reliability and validity of the Evaluation of Lifetime Stressors questionnaire.* Unpublished manuscript.

Krippner, S. (1994). Cross-cultural treatment perspectives on dissociative disorders. In S. J. Lynn & J. W. Rhue (Eds.), *Dissociation: Theoretical, clinical, and research perspectives* (pp. 338–361). New York: Guilford Press.

Kroll, J., Habenicht, M., Mackenzie, T., Yang, M., Sokha, C., Vang, T., Nguyen, T., Ly, M., Phommasouvanh, B., Nguyen, H., Vang, Y., Souvannasoth, L., & Cabugao, R. (1989). Depression and posttraumatic stress disorder in Southeast Asian refugees. *American Journal of Psychiatry, 146,* 1592–1597.

Kubany, E. S., Abueg, F. R., Owens, J. A., Brennan, J. M., Kaplan, A. S., & Watson, S. B. (1995). Initial examination of a multidimensional model of trauma-related guilt: Applications to combat veterans and battered women. *Journal of Psychopathology and Behavioral Assessment, 17,* 353–376.

Kulka, R. A., Schlenger, W. E., Fairbank, J. A., Hough, R. L., Jordan, B. K., Marmar, C. R., & Weiss, D. S. (1990a). Evidence of posttraumatic stress disorder. In *Trauma and the Vietnam War generation* (pp. 50–72). New York: Brunner/Mazel.

Kulka, R. A., Schlenger, W. E., Fairbank, J. A., Hough, R. L., Jordan, B. K., Marmar, C. R., & Weiss, D. S. (1990b). The prevalence of other postwar readjustment problems. In *Trauma and the Vietnam War generation* (pp. 139–188). New York: Brunner/Mazel.

Kulka, R. A., Schlenger, W. E., Fairbank, J. A., Hough, R. L., Jordan, B. K., Marmar, C. R., & Weiss, D. S. (1990c). The prevalence of physical health problems. In *Trauma and the Vietnam War generation* (pp. 189–199). New York: Brunner/Mazel.

Kulka, R. A., Schlenger, W. E., Fairbank, J. A., Hough, R. L., Jordan, B. K., Marmar, C. R., & Weiss, D. S. (1990d). *Trauma and the Vietnam War generation.* New York: Brunner/Mazel.

Kutcher, G., Tremont, M., Burda, P., & Mellman, T. (1994, November). *The effectiveness of PTSD self-report measures with an inpatient veteran population.* Paper presented at the annual meeting of the International Society for Traumatic Stress Studies, Chicago.

Lasko, N. B., Gurvits, T. V., Kuhne, A. A., Orr, S. P., & Pitman, R. K. (1994). Aggression and its correlates in Vietnam veterans with and without chronic posttraumatic stress disorder. *Comprehensive Psychiatry, 35,* 373–381.

Layman, M. J., Gidycz, C. A., & Lynn, S. J. (1996). Unacknowledged versus acknowledged rape victims: Situational factors and posttraumatic stress. *Journal of Abnormal Psychology, 105,* 124–131.

LeDoux, J., Romanski, L., & Xagorans, A. (1989). Indelibility of subcortical emotional memories. *Journal of Cognitive Neuroscience, 1,* 238–243.

Lee, E., & Lu, F. (1989). Assessment and treatment of Asian-American survivors of mass violence. *Journal of Traumatic Stress, 2,* 93–120.

Leserman, J., Toomey, T. C., & Drossman, D. A. (1995). Medical consequences of sexual and physical abuse in women. *Humane Medicine, 11,* 23–28.

Levin, P., & Reis, B. (1996). Use of the Rorschach in assessing trauma. In J. Wilson & T. M. Keane (Eds.), *Assessing psychological trauma and PTSD* (pp. 529–543). New York: Guilford Press.

Lewis, D. O. (1992). From abuse to violence: Psychophysiological consequences of maltreatment. *Journal of the American Academy of Child and Adolescent Psychiatry, 31,* 383–391.

Lewis, D. O. (1996). Diagnostic evaluation of the child with dissociative identity disorder/multiple personality disorder. *Child and Adolescent Psychiatric Clinics of North America, 5,* 303–331.

Lin, K.-M., Poland, R. E., Anderson, D., & Lesser, I. M. (1996). Ethnopsychopharmacology and the treatment of PTSD. In A. J. Marsella, M. J. Friedman, E. T. Gerrity, & R. M. Scurfield (Eds.), *Ethnocultural aspects of posttraumatic stress disorder: Issues, research, and clinical applications* (pp. 505–526). Washington, DC: American Psychological Association.

Lindsay, D. S., & Read, J. D. (1993). Psychotherapy and memory of child sexual abuse: A cognitive perspective. *Applied Cognitive Psychology, 8,* 281–338.

Lindy, J. D. (1993). Focal psychoanalytic psychotherapy of posttraumatic stress disorder. In J. P. Wilson & B. Raphael (Eds.), *International handbook of traumatic stress syndromes* (pp. 803–809). New York: Plenum Press.

Lindy, J. D. (1996). Psychoanalytic psychotherapy of postraumatic stress disorder: The nature of the therapeutic relationship. In B. A. van der Kolk, A. C. McFarlane, & L. Weisaeth (Eds.), *Traumatic stress: The effects of overwhelming experience on mind, body, and society* (pp. 525–536). New York: Guilford Press.

Lipovsky, J. A. (1992). Assessment and treatment of post-traumatic stress disorder child survivors of sexual assault. In D. W. Foy (Ed.), *Treating PTSD: Cognitive-behavioral strategies* (pp. 127–164). New York: Guilford Press.

Litz, B. T. (1992). Emotional numbing in combat-related post-traumatic stress disorder: A critical review and reformulation. *Clinical Psychology Review, 12,* 417–432.

Litz, B. T., & Keane, T. M. (1989). Information processing in anxiety disorders: Application to the understanding of post-traumatic stress disorder. *Clinical Psychology Review, 9,* 243–257.

Litz, B. T., & Weathers, F. W. (1994). The diagnosis and assessment of post-traumatic stress disorder in adults. In M. B. Williams & J. F. Sommer (Eds.), *Handbook of posttraumatic therapy* (pp. 19–37). Westport, CT: Greenwood Press.

Loewenstein, R. J. (1991). Psychogenic amnesia and psychogenic fugue: A comprehensive review. In A. Tasman & S. M. Goldfinger (Eds.), *American Psychiatric Press review of psychiatry* (pp. 189–221). Washington, DC: American Psychiatric Press.

Loewenstein, R. J. (1993). Posttraumatic and dissociative aspects of transference and countertransference in the treatment of multiple personality disorder. In R. P. Kluft & C. Fine (Eds.), *Clinical perspectives on multiple personality disorder* (pp. 19–50). Washington, DC: American Psychiatric Press.

Loewenstein, R. J. (1996). Dissociative amnesia and dissociative fugue. In L. K. Michelson & W. J. Ray (Eds.), *Handbook of dissociation: Theoretical, empirical, and clinical perspectives* (pp. 307–336). New York: Plenum Press.

Loftus, E., Polonsky, S., & Fullilove, M. T. (1994). Memories of childhood sexual abuse. *Psychology of Women Quarterly, 18,* 67–84.

Lohr, J. M., Kleinknecht, R. A., Tolin, D. F., & Barrett, R. H. (1995). The empirical status of the clinical application of eye movement desensitization and reprocessing. *Journal of Behavior Therapy and Experimental Psychiatry, 26,* 285–302.

Lorenz, K. (1966). *On aggression.* New York: Harcourt Brace Jovanovich.

Lu, F. G., Lim, R. F., & Mezzich, J. E. (1995). Issues in the assessment and diagnosis of culturally diverse individuals. In J. M. Oldham & M. B. Riba (Eds.), *Review of psychiatry* (pp. 477–510). Washington, DC: American Psychiatric Press.

Luthar, S., & Zigler, E. (1991). Vulnerability and competence: A review of research on resilience in childhood. *American Journal of Orthopsychiatry, 61,* 6–22.

Lynch, M., & Cicchetti, D. (1991). Patterns of relatedness in maltreated and nonmaltreated children: Connections among multiple representational models. *Development and Psychopathology, 3,* 207–226.

Lynn, S. J., Myers, B., & Malinoski, P. (1997). Hypnosis, pseudomemories, and clinical guidelines. In D. Read & S. Lindsay (Eds.), *Recollections of trauma: Scientific research and clinical practice.* New York: Plenum Press.

Lynn, S. J., & Rhue, J. W. (Eds.). (1994). *Dissociation: Theoretical, clinical, and research perspectives.* New York: Guilford Press.

Lyons, J. A., & Keane, T. M. (1992). Keane PTSD scale: MMPI and MMPI-2 update. *Journal of Traumatic Stress, 5,* 111–117.

MacKenzie, S. G., & Lippman, A. (1989). An investigation of report bias in a case-control study of pregnancy outcome. *American Journal of Epidemiology, 129,* 65–75.

Maier, S. F. (1984). Learned helplessness and animal models of depression. *Progress in Neuropsychopharmacology and Biological Psychiatry, 8,* 435–446.

Malinosky-Rummell, R., & Hoier, T. (1991). Validating measures of dissociation in sexually abused and nonabused children. *Behavioral Assessment, 13,* 341–357.

Malt, U. A. (1994). Traumatic effects of accidents. In R. J. Ursano, C. S. Fullerton, & B. G. McCaughey (Eds.), *Individual and community responses to trauma and disaster: The structure of human chaos* (pp. 103–135). Cambridge: Cambridge University Press.

Manson, S. M. (1996). Cross-cultural and multiethnic assessment of trauma. In J. Wilson & T. M. Keane (Eds.), *Assessing psychological trauma and PTSD* (pp. 239–266). New York: Guilford Press.

Manson, S. M., Beals, J., O'Nell, T., Piasecki, J., Bechtold, D., Keane, E. M., & Jones, M. (1996). Wounded spirits, ailing hearts: PTSD and related disorders among American Indians. In A. J. Marsella, M. J. Friedman, E. T. Gerrity, & R. M. Scurfield (Eds.), *Ethnocultural aspects of posttraumatic stress disorder: Issues, research, and clinical applications* (pp. 255–283). Washington, DC: American Psychological Association.

March, J. S. (1993). What constitutes a stressor? The "Criterion A" Issue. In J. R. T. Davidson & E. B. Foa (Eds.), *Posttraumatic stress disorder: DSM-IV and beyond* (pp. 37–54). Washington, DC: American Psychiatric Press.

Marmar, C. R., Foy, D., Kagan, B., & Pynoos, R. S. (1993). An integrated approach for treating posttraumatic stress. In J. M. Oldham, M. B. Riba, & A. Tasman (Eds.), *Review of psychiatry* (pp. 239–272). Washington, DC: American Psychiatric Press.

Marmar, C. R., & Freeman, M. (1991). Brief dynamic psychotherapy of treating posttraumatic stress disorder. *Psychiatric Annals, 21,* 405–414.

Marmar, C. R., Weiss, D. S., Metzler, T. J., Ronfeldt, H. M., & Foreman, C. (1996). Stress responses of emergency services personnel to the Loma Prieta earthquake Interstate 880 freeway collapse and control traumatic incidents. *Journal of Traumatic Stress, 9,* 63–85.

Marmar, C. R., Weiss, D. S., & Pynoos, R. S. (1995). Dynamic psychotherapy of post-traumatic stress disorder. In M. J. Friedman, D. S. Charney, & A. Y. Deutch (Eds.), *Neurobiological and clinical consequences of stress: From normal adaptation to post-traumatic stress disorder* (pp. 495–506). Philadelphia: Lippincott-Raven.

Marsella, A. J., Friedman, M. J., Gerrity, E. T., & Scurfield, R. M. (Eds.). (1996). *Ethnocultural aspects of posttraumatic stress disorder: Issues, research, and clinical applications.* Washington, DC: American Psychological Association.

Marsella, A. J., Friedman, M. J., & Spain, E. H. (1996). Ethnocultural aspects of

PTSD: An overview of issues and research directions. In A. J. Marsella, M. J. Friedman, E. T. Gerrity, & R. M. Scurfield (Eds.), *Ethnocultural aspects of posttraumatic stress disorder: Issues, research, and clinical applications* (pp. 105–129). Washington, DC: American Psychological Association.

Marsella, A. S., & Kameoka, V. A. (1989). Ethnocultural issues in the assessment of psychopathology. In S. Wetzler (Ed.), *Measuring mental illness: Psychometric assessment for clinicians* (pp. 229–256). Washington, DC: American Psychiatric Press.

Mayou, R., Bryant, B., & Duthie, R. (1993). Psychiatric consequences of road traffic accidents. *British Medical Journal, 307,* 647–651.

McCann, I. L., & Pearlman, L. A. (1990). *Psychological trauma and the adult survivor.* New York: Brunner/Mazel.

McFall, M. E., Mackay, P. W., & Donovan, D. M. (1991). Combat-related PTSD and psychosocial adjustment problems among substance abusing veterans. *Journal of Nervous and Mental Disease, 179,* 33–38.

McFall, M. E., Murburg, M. M., Ko, G. N., & Veith, R. C. (1990). Autonomic responses to stress in Vietnam combat veterans with posttraumatic stress disorder. *Biological Psychiatry, 27,* 1165–1175.

McFarlane, A. C. (1990). Vulnerability to posttraumatic stress disorder. In M. E. Wolf & A. D. Mosnaim (Eds.), *Posttraumatic stress disorder: Etiology, phenomenology, and treatment.* Washington, DC: American Psychiatric Press.

McFarlane, A. C. (1992). Avoidance and intrusion in posttraumatic stress disorder. *Journal of Nervous and Mental Disease, 180,* 439–445.

McFarlane, A. C., Atchison, M., Rafalowicz, E., & Papay, P. (1994). Physical symptoms in post-traumatic stress disorder. *Journal of Psychosomatic Research, 38,* 715–726.

McFarlane, A. C., & de Girolamo, G. (1996). The nature of traumatic stressors and the epidemiology of posttraumatic reactions. In B. A. van der Kolk, A. C. McFarlane, & L. Weisaeth (Eds.), *Traumatic stress: The effects of overwhelming experience on mind, body, and society* (pp. 129–154). New York: Guilford Press.

McFarlane, A. C., & Yehuda, R. (1996). Resilience, vulnerability, and the course of posttraumatic reactions. In B. A. van der Kolk, A. C. McFarlane, & L. Weisaeth (Eds.), *Traumatic stress: The effects of overwhelming experience on mind, body, and society* (pp. 155–181). New York: Guilford Press.

McLeer, S., Callaghan, M., Henry, D., & Wallen, J. (1994). Psychiatric disorders in sexually abused children. *Journal of the American Academy of Child and Adolescent Psychiatry, 33,* 313–319.

McLeer, S., Deblinger, E., Henry, D., & Orvaschel, H. (1992). Sexually abused children at high risk for post-traumatic stress disorder. *Journal of the American Academy of Child and Adolescent Psychiatry, 31,* 875–879.

McMahon, P. P., & Fagan, J. (1993). Play therapy with children with multiple personality disorder. In R. P. Kluft & C. Fine (Eds.), *Clinical perspectives on multiple personality disorder* (pp. 253–277). Washington, DC: American Psychiatric Press.

McNally, R. (1995). Cognitive processing of trauma-relevant information in PTSD. *PTSD Research Quarterly, 6,* 1–6.

McNally, R. J. (1991). Assessment of posttraumatic stress disorder in children. *Psychological Assessment, 3,* 531–537.

McNally, R. J. (1993). Stressors that produce posttraumatic stress disorder in children. In J. R. T. Davidson & E. B. Foa (Eds.), *Posttraumatic stress disorder: DSM-IV and beyond* (pp. 57–74). Washington, DC: American Psychiatric Press.

McNally, R. J., Eells, T. D., Fridhandler, B., Stinson, C. H., & Horowitz, M. J. (1993). Self-representation in post-traumatic stress disorder: A cognitive perspective. In Z. V. Segal & S. J. Blatt (Eds.), *The self in emotional distress: Cognitive and psychodynamic perspectives* (pp. 71–99). New York: Guilford Press.

McNally, R. J., & Saigh, P. A. (1993). On the distinction between traumatic simple phobia and posttraumatic stress disorder. In J. R. T. Davidson & E. B. Foa (Eds.), *Posttraumatic stress disorder: DSM-IV and beyond* (pp. 207–212). Washington, DC: American Psychiatric Press.

Meichenbaum, D. (1994). *A clinical handbook/practical therapist manual for assessing and treating adults with post-traumatic stress disorder.* Waterloo, Ontario: Institute Press.

Mellman, T. A., Kulick-Bell, R., Ashlock, L. E., & Nolan, B. (1995). Sleep events among veterans with combat-related posttraumatic stress disorder. *American Journal of Psychiatry, 152,* 110–115.

Mennen, F., & Meadow, D. (1994). Depression, anxiety, and self-esteem in sexually abused children. *Families in Society, 75,* 74–81.

Mennen, F. E., & Meadow, D. (1992). Process to recovery: In support of long-term groups for sexual abuse survivors. *International Journal of Group Psychotherapy, 42,* 29–44.

Michelson, L. K., & Ray, W. J. (Eds.). (1996). *Handbook of dissociation: Theoretical, empirical, and clinical perspectives.* New York: Plenum Press.

Miller, T., Jenkins, C., Kaplan, G., & Salonen, J. (1995). Are all hostility scales alike? Factor structure and covariation among measures of hostility. *Journal of Applied Social Psychology, 25,* 1142–1168.

Millon, T. (1994). *Millon Clinical Multiaxial Inventory III.* Minneapolis, MN: National Computer Systems.

Mineka, S., & Kilhstrom, J. F. (1978). Unpredictable and uncontrollable events: A new perspective on experimental neurosis. *Journal of Abnormal Psychology, 87,* 256–271.

Mineka, S. M. (1979). The role of fear in theories of avoidance learning, flooding, and extinction. *Psychological Bulletin, 86,* 985–1010.

Mischel, W. (1973). Toward a cognitive social learning reconceptualization of personality. *Psychological Review, 80,* 252–283.

Monane, M., Leichter, D., & Lewis, D. O. (1984). Physical abuse in psychiatrically hospitalized children and adolescents. *Journal of the American Academy of Child Psychiatry, 23,* 653–658.

Moss, M., Frank, E., & Anderson, B. (1990). The effects of marital status and partner support on rape trauma. *American Journal of Orthopsychiatry, 60,* 379–391.

Mullen, P. E., Martin, J. L., Anderson, J. C., Romans, S. E., & Herbison, G. P.

(1994). The effect of child sexual abuse on social, interpersonal, and sexual function in adult life. *British Journal of Psychiatry, 165,* 35–47.

Murphy, S. M., Amick-McMullan, A. E., Kilpatrick, D. G., Haskett, M. E., Veronen, L. J., Best, C. L., & Saunders, B. E. (1988). Rape victims' self-esteem: A longitudinal analysis. *Journal of Interpersonal Violence, 3,* 355–370.

Murphy, S. M., Kilpatrick, D. G., Amick-McMullan, A. E., & Veronen, L. J. (1988). Current psychological functioning of child sexual abuse survivors: A community study. *Journal of Interpersonal Violence, 3,* 55–79.

Nader, K. (1994). *Child Post-traumatic Stress Reaction Index: Parent Questionnaire.* Unpublished manuscript.

Nader, K. (1996). Assessing traumatic experiences in children. In J. Wilson & T. M. Keane (Eds.), *Assessing psychological trauma and PTSD* (pp. 291–348). New York: Guilford Press.

Nader, K., & Fairbanks, L. (1994). The suppression of reexperiencing: Impulse control and somatic symptoms in children following traumatic exposure. *Anxiety, Stress, and Coping: An International Journal, 7,* 229–239.

Nader, K., Pynoos, R., Fairbanks, L., Al-Ajeel, M., & Al-Asfour, A. (1993). Acute post traumatic stress reactions among Kuwait children following the Gulf Crisis. *British Journal of Clinical Psychology, 32,* 407–416.

Nash, M. R., Hulsey, T. L., Sexton, M. C., Harralson, T. L., & Lambert, W. (1993). Long-term sequelae of childhood sexual abuse: Perceived family environment, psychopathology, and dissociation. *Journal of Consulting and Clinical Psychology, 61*(2), 276–283.

Neal, A., & Turner, S. (1991). Anxiety disorders research with African Americans: Current status. *Psychological Bulletin, 109*(3), 400–410.

Newman, E., Kaloupek, D. G., & Keane, T. M. (1996). Assessment of PTSD in clinical and research settings. In B. A. van der Kolk, A. C. McFarlane, & L. Weisaeth (Eds.), *Traumatic stress: The effects of overwhelming experience on mind, body, and society* (pp. 242–275). New York: Guilford Press.

Nezu, A. M., & Carnevale, G. J. (1987). Interpersonal problem solving and coping reactions of Vietnam veterans with posttraumatic stress disorder. *Journal of Abnormal Psychology, 96,* 155–157.

Norris, F., & Murrell, S. (1988). Prior experience as a moderator of disaster impact on anxiety symptoms in older adults. *American Journal of Community Psychology, 16,* 665–683.

Norris, F. H. (1992). Epidemiology of trauma: Frequency and impact of different potentially traumatic events on different demographic groups. *Journal of Consulting and Clinical Psychology, 60,* 409–418.

Norris, F. H., & Perilla, J. L. (1996). The Revised Civilian Mississippi Scale for PTSD: Reliability, validity, and cross-language stability. *Journal of Traumatic Stress, 9,* 285–298.

Norris, F. H., & Riad, J. K. (1996). Standardized self-report measures of civilian trauma and PTSD. In J. Wilson & T. M. Keane (Eds.), *Assessing psychological trauma and PTSD* (pp. 7–42). New York: Guilford Press.

Ochberg, F. M. (1993). Posttraumatic therapy. In J. P. Wilson & B. Raphael (Eds.), *International handbook of traumatic stress syndromes* (pp. 773–783). New York: Plenum Press.

Op den Velde, W., Falger, P. R. J., Hovens, J. E. J. M., De Groen, J. H. M., Lasschuit, L. J., Van Duijn, H., & Schouten, E. G. W. (1993). Posttraumatic stress disorder in Dutch Resistance veterans from World War II. In J. P. Wilson & B. Raphael (Eds.), *International handbook of traumatic stress syndromes* (pp. 219–230). New York: Plenum Press.

Orava, T. A., McLeod, P. J., & Sharpe, D. (1996). Perceptions of control, depressive symptomatology, and self-esteem of women in transition from abusive relationships. *Journal of Family Violence, 11*, 167–186.

Orne, M. T., & Bauer-Manley, N. (1991). Disorders of self: Myths, metaphors, and the demand characteristics of treatment. In J. Strauss & G. Goethals (Eds.), *The self: Interdiscinplinary approaches* (pp. 93–106). New York: Springer-Verlag.

Ornstein, P. A. (1995). Children's long-term retention of salient personal experiences. *Journal of Traumatic Stress, 8*, 581–605.

Orr, S. P., Claiborn, J. M., Altmann, B., Forgue, D. F., de Jong, J. B., Pitman, R. K., & Herz, L. R. (1990). Psychometric profile of posttraumatic stress disorder, anxious, and healthy Vietnam veterans: Correlations with psychophysiologic responses. *Journal of Consulting and Clinical Psychology, 58*, 329–335.

Orr, S. P., & Kaloupek, D. G. (1996). Psychophysiological assessment of posttraumatic stress disorder. In J. Wilson & T. M. Keane (Eds.), *Assessing psychological trauma and PTSD* (pp. 69–97). New York: Guilford Press.

Orr, S. P., Pitman, R. K., Lasko, N. B., & Herz, L. R. (1993). Psychophysiological assessment of posttraumatic stress disorder imagery in World War II and Korean combat veterans. *Journal of Abnormal Psychology, 102*, 152–159.

Orsillo, S. M., Heimberg, R. G., Juster, H. R., & Garrett, J. C. (1996). Social phobia and PTSD in Vietnam veterans. *Journal of Traumatic Stress, 9*, 235–252.

Orsillo, S. M., Weathers, F. W., Litz, B. T., Steinberg, H. R., Huska, J. A., & Keane, T. M. (1996). Current and lifetime psychiatric disorders among veterans with war zone-related posttraumatic stress disorder. *Journal of Nervous and Mental Disease, 184*, 307–313.

Panel on Research on Child Abuse and Neglect (1993). *Understanding child abuse and neglect.* Washington, DC: National Academy Press.

Parker, S., & Parker, H. (1991). Female victims of child sexual abuse: Adult adjustment. *Journal of Family Violence, 6*, 183–197.

Pearlman, L., & Saakvitne, K. (1995). *Trauma and the therapist.* New York: Norton.

Pearlman, L. A., & McCann, I. L. (1994). Integrating structured and unstructured approaches to taking a trauma history. In M. B. Williams & J. F. Sommer (Eds.), *Handbook of posttraumatic therapy* (pp. 38–48). Westport, CT: Greenwood Press.

Pelcovitz, D., Kaplan, S., Goldenberg, B., & Mandel, F. (1994). Post-traumatic stress disorder in physically abused adolescents. *Journal of the American Academy of Child and Adolescent Psychiatry, 33*, 305–312.

Pennebaker (1988). Disclosure of traumas and immune function: Health implications for psychotherapy. *Journal of Consulting and Clinical Psychology, 56*, 239–245.

Perry, B. (1997). Incubated terror: Neurodevelopmental factors in the "cycle of violence." In J. D. Osofsky (Ed.), *Children in a violent society* (pp. 124–149). New York: Guilford Press.

Perry, S., Difede, J., Musngi, G., Frances, A. J., & Jacobsberg, L. (1992). Predictors of posttraumatic stress disorder after burn injury. *American Journal of Psychiatry, 149,* 931–935.

Peterson, G. (1990). Diagnosis of childhood multiple personality disorder. *Dissociation, 3,* 3–9.

Peterson, G. (1991). Children coping with trauma: Diagnosis of "Dissociative Identity Disorder." *Dissociation, 4,* 152–164.

Pezdek, K., & Banks, W. P. (Eds.). (1996). *The recovered memory/false memory debate.* Orlando, FL: Academic Press.

Pitman, R. K., Altman, B., Greenwald, E., Longpre, R. E., Macklin, M. L., Poire, R. E., & Steketee, G. (1991). Psychiatric complications during flooding therapy for posttraumatic stress disorder. *Journal of Clinical Psychiatry, 52,* 17–20.

Pitman, R. K., Orr, S. P., Forgue, D. F., Altman, B., de Jong, J. B., & Herz, L. R. (1990). Psychophysiologic responses to combat imagery of Vietnam veterans with posttraumatic stress disorder versus other anxiety disorders. *Journal of Abnormal Psychology, 99,* 49–54.

Pitman, R. K., Sparr, L. F., Saunders, L. S., & McFarlane, A. C. (1996). Legal issues in posttraumatic stress disorder. In B. A. van der Kolk, A. C. McFarlane, & L. Weisaeth (Eds.), *Traumatic stress: The effects of overwhelming experience on mind, body, and society* (pp. 398–413). New York: Guilford Press.

Pitman, R. K., van der Kolk, B. A., Orr, S. P., & Greenberg, M. S. (1990). Naloxone-reversible analgesia response to combat-related stimuli in posttraumatic stress disorder: A pilot study. *Archives of General Psychiatry, 47,* 541–544.

Pollock, V. E., Briere, J., Schneider, L., Knop, J., Mednick, S., & Goodwin, D. W. (1990). Childhood antecedents of antisocial behavior: Parental alcoholism and physical abusiveness. *American Journal of Psychiatry, 147,* 1290–1293.

Pope, K. S. (1996). Memory, abuse, and science: Questioning claims about the false memory syndrome epidemic. *American Psychologist, 51,* 957–974.

Pope, K. S., & Brown, L. S. (1996). *Recovered memories of abuse: Assessment, therapy, and forensics.* Washington, DC: American Psychological Association.

Prins, A., Kaloupek, D. G., & Keane, T. M. (1995). Psychophysiological evidence for autonomic arousal and startle in traumatized adult populations. In M. J. Friedman, D. S. Charney, & A. Y. Deutch (Eds.), *Neurobiological and clinical consequences of stress: From normal adaptation to posttraumatic stress disorder* (pp. 291–314). Philadelphia: Lippincott-Raven.

Putnam, F. W. (1985). Dissociation as a response to extreme trauma. In R. Kluft (Ed.), *Childhood antecedents of multiple personality* (pp. 65–97). Washington, DC: American Psychiatric Association.

Putnam, F. W. (1989). *Diagnosis and treatment of multiple personality disorder.* New York: Guilford Press.

Putnam, F. W. (1990). Disturbances of "self" in victims of childhood sexual abuse. In R. P. Kluft (Ed.), *Incest-related syndromes of adult psychopathology* (pp. 113–131). Washington, DC: American Psychiatric Press.

Putnam, F. W. (1991a). Dissociative disorders in children and adolescents: A developmental perspective. *Psychiatric Clinics of North America, 14,* 519–531.

Putnam, F. W. (1991b). Recent research on multiple personality disorder. *Psychiatric Clinics of North America, 14,* 489–502.

Putnam, F. W. (1994). Dissociative disorders in children and adolescents. In S. J. Lynn & J. W. Rhue (Eds.), *Dissociation: Theoretical, clinical, and research perspectives* (pp. 175–189). New York: Guilford Press.

Putnam, F. W. (1995). Traumatic stress and pathological dissociation. *Annals of the New York Academy of Sciences, 771,* 708–715.

Putnam, F. W. (1996a). Posttraumatic stress disorder in children and adolescents. In L. J. Dickstein, M. B. Riba, & J. M. Oldham (Eds.), *American Psychiatric Press review of psychiatry* (pp. 447–467). Washington, DC: American Psychiatric Press.

Putnam, F. W. (1996b). Special methods for trauma research with children. In E. B. Carlson (Ed.), *Trauma research methodology* (pp. 153–173). Lutherville, MD: Sidran Press.

Putnam, F. W. (1997). *Dissociation in children and adolescents: A developmental perspective.* New York: Guilford Press.

Putnam, F. W., & Carlson, E. B. (1997). Hypnosis, dissociation and trauma: Myths, metaphors, and mechanisms. In J. D. Bremner (Ed.), *Trauma, memory, and dissociation.* Washington, DC: American Psychiatric Press.

Putnam, F. W., Carlson, E. B., Ross, C. A., Anderson, G., Clark, P., Torem, M., Bowman, E., Coons, P., Chu, J. A., Dill, D. L., Loewenstein, R. J., & Braun, B. G. (1996). Patterns of dissociation in clinical and nonclinical samples. *Journal of Nervous and Mental Disease, 184,* 673–679.

Putnam, F. W., Guroff, J. J., Silberman, E. K., Barban, L., & Post, R. M. (1986). The clinical phenomenology of multiple personality disorder: Review of 100 recent cases. *Journal of Clinical Psychiatry, 47,* 285–293.

Putnam, F. W., Helmers, K., & Trickett, P. K. (1993). Development, reliability, and validity of a child dissociation scale. *Child Abuse and Neglect, 17,* 731–741.

Putnam, F. W., Hornstein, N. L., & Peterson, G. (1996). Clinical phenomenology of child and adolescent dissociative disorders: Gender and age effects. *Child and Adolescent Psychiatric Clinics of North America, 5,* 351–373.

Putnam, F. W., & Peterson, G. (1994). Further validation of the Child Dissociative Checklist. *Dissociation, 7,* 204–211.

Putnam, F. W., & Trickett, P. K. (1993). Child sexual abuse: A model of chronic trauma. *Psychiatry, 56,* 82–95.

Pynoos, R. S. (1993). Traumatic stress and developmental psychopathology in children and adolescents. In J. M. Oldham, M. B. Riba, & A. Tasman (Eds.), *Review of psychiatry* (pp. 205–238). Washington, DC: American Psychiatric Press.

Pynoos, R. S., & Nader, K. (1993). Issues in the treatment of posttraumatic stress in children and adolescents. In J. P. Wilson & B. Raphael (Eds.),

International handbook of traumatic stress syndromes (pp. 535–549). New York: Plenum Press.

Pynoos, R. S., Steinberg, A. M., & Goenjian, A. (1996). Traumatic stress in childhood and adolescence: Recent developments and current controversies. In B. A. van der Kolk, A. C. McFarlane, & L. Weisaeth (Eds.), *Traumatic stress: The effects of overwhelming experience on mind, body, and society* (pp. 331–358). New York: Guilford Press.

Quinn, K. M. (1995). Guidelines for the psychiatric examination of posttraumatic stress disorder in children and adolescents. In R. Simon (Ed.), *Posttraumatic stress disorder in litigation* (pp. 85–98). Washington, DC: American Psychiatric Press.

Raphael, B., & Martinek, N. (1996). Assessing traumatic bereavement and posttraumatic stress disorder. In J. Wilson & T. M. Keane (Eds.), *Assessing psychological trauma and PTSD* (pp. 373–395). New York: Guilford Press.

Raphael, B., Wilson, J., Meldrum, L., & McFarlane, A. (1996). Acute prevention interventions. In B. A. van der Kolk, A. C. McFarlane, & L. Weisaeth (Eds.), *Traumatic stress: The effects of overwhelming experience on mind, body, and society* (pp. 463–479). New York: Guilford Press.

Read, D., & Lindsay, S. (Eds.). (1997). *Recollections of trauma: Scientific research and clinical practice.* New York: Plenum Press.

Reed, L. D. (1996). Findings from research on children's suggestibility and implications for conducting child interviews. *Child Maltreatment, 1,* 105–120.

Renfrey, G., & Spates, R. C. (1994). Eye movement desensitization: A partial dismantling study. *Journal of Behavior Therapy and Experimental Psychiatry, 25,* 231–239.

Resick, P., & Schnicke, M. K. (1992). Cognitive processing therapy for sexual assault victims. *Journal of Consulting and Clinical Psychology, 60,* 748–756.

Resick, P., & Schnicke, M. K. (1993). *Cognitive processing therapy for rape victims.* Newbury Park, CA: Sage.

Resick, P. A. (1993). The psychological impact of rape. *Journal of Interpersonal Violence, 8,* 223–255.

Resnick, H. (1996a). Psychometric review of National Women's Study (NWS) Event History—PTSD Module. In B. H. Stamm (Ed.), *Measurement of stress, trauma, and adaptation* (pp. 214–217). Lutherville, MD: Sidran Press.

Resnick, H. (1996b). Psychometric review of Trauma Assessment for Adults (TAA). In B. H. Stamm (Ed.), *Measurement of stress, trauma, and adaptation* (pp. 362–365). Lutherville, MD: Sidran Press.

Resnick, H. S., Falsetti, S. A., Kilpatrick, D. G., & Freedy, J. R. (1996). Assessment of rape and other civilian trauma-related post-traumatic stress disorder: Emphasis on assessment of potentially traumatic events. In T. W. Miller (Ed.), *Stressful life events* (pp. 231–266). Madison, CT: International Universities Press.

Resnick, H. S., Kilpatrick, D. G., Dansky, B. S., Saunders, B. E., & Best, C. L. (1993). Prevalence of civilian trauma and posttraumatic stress disorder on a representative sample of women. *Journal of Consulting and Clinical Psychology, 61,* 984–991.

Resnick, H. S., & Newton, T. (1992). Assessment and treatment of post-traumatic stress disorder in adult survivors of sexual assault. In D. W. Foy (Ed.), *Treating PTSD: Cognitive-behavioral strategies* (pp. 99–126). New York: Guilford Press.

Resnick, P. J. (1995). Guidelines for the evaluation of malingering in posttraumatic stress disorder. In R. Simon (Ed.), *Posttraumatic stress disorder in litigation* (pp. 117–134). Washington, DC: American Psychiatric Press.

Ribbe, D. P., Lipovsky, J. A., & Freedy, J. R. (1995). Posttraumatic stress disorder. In A. R. Eisen, C. A. Kearney, & C. E. Schaefer (Eds.), *Clinical handbook of anxiety disorders in children and adolescents* (pp. 317–356). Northvale, NJ: Jason Aronson.

Riggs, D. S., Dancu, C. V., Gershuny, B. S., Greenberg, D., & Foa, E. B. (1992). Anger and posttraumatic stress disorder in female crime victims. *Journal of Traumatic Stress, 5,* 613–625.

Robin, R. W., Chester, B., & Goldman, D. (1996). Cumulative trauma and PTSD in American Indian communities. In A. J. Marsella, M. J. Friedman, E. T. Gerrity, & R. M. Scurfield (Eds.), *Ethnocultural aspects of posttraumatic stress disorder: Issues, research, and clinical applications* (pp. 239–253). Washington, DC: American Psychological Association.

Robins, L. N. (1988). Data gathering and data analysis for prospective and retrospective longitudinal studies. In M. Rutter (Ed.), *Studies of psychosocial risk: The power of longitudinal data* (pp. 315–324). London: Cambridge University Press.

Robins, L. N., Schoenberg, S. P., Holmes, S. J., Ratcliff, K. S., Benham, A., & Works, J. (1985). Early home environment and retrospective recall: A test for concordance between siblings with and without psychiatric disorders. *American Journal of Orthopsychiatry, 55,* 27–41.

Romans, S. E., Martin, J. L., Anderson, J. C., Herbison, G. P., & Mullen, P. E. (1995). Sexual abuse in childhood and deliberate self-harm. *American Journal of Psychiatry, 152,* 1336–1342.

Ross, C. A. (1997). *Dissociative Identity Disorder: Diagnosis, clinical features, and treatment of multiple personality* (2nd ed.). New York: Wiley.

Ross, C. A., Heber, S., Norton, G. R., Anderson, D., Anderson, G., & Barchet, P. (1989). The Dissociative Disorders Interview Schedule: A structured interview. *Dissociation, 2*(3), 169–189.

Rothbaum, B. O., & Foa, E. F. (1992). Cognitive–behavioral treatment of posttraumatic stress disorder. In P. A. Saigh (Ed.), *Posttraumatic stress disorder: Behavioral assessment and treatment* (pp. 85–110). Elmsford, NY: Maxwell Press.

Rothbaum, B. O., & Foa, E. F. (1996). Cognitive-behavioral therapy for posttraumatic stress disorder. In B. A. van der Kolk, A. C. McFarlane, & L. Weisaeth (Eds.), *Traumatic stress: The effects of overwhelming experience on mind, body, and society* (pp. 491–509). New York: Guilford Press.

Rowan, A. B., & Foy, D. W. (1993). Post-traumatic stress disorder in child sexual abuse survivors: A literature review. *Journal of Traumatic Stress, 6,* 3–20.

Ruch, L. O., Gartrell, J. W., Amedeo, S. R., & Coyne, B. J. (1991). The Sexual

Assault Symptom Scale: Measuring self-reported sexual assault trauma in the emergency room. *Psychological Assessment, 3,* 3–8.

Rudy, J. (1993). Contextual conditioning and auditory cue conditioning dissociate during development. *Behavioral Neuroscience, 107,* 887–891.

Ruskin, P. E., & Talbott, J. A. (1995). *Aging and posttraumatic stress disorder.* Washington, DC: American Psychiatric Press.

Rynearson, E. K., & McCreery, J. M. (1993). Bereavement after homicide: A synergism of trauma and loss. *American Journal of Psychiatry, 150,* 258–261.

Saigh, P. A. (1992). *Posttraumatic stress disorder: Behavioral assessment and treatment.* Elmsford, NY: Maxwell Press.

Saladin, M. E., Brady, K. T., Dansky, B. S., & Kilpatrick, D. G. (1995). Understanding comorbidity between PTSD and substance use disorders: Two preliminary investigations. *Addictive Behaviors, 20,* 643–655.

Sandberg, D. A., & Lynn, S. J. (1992). Dissociative experiences, psychopathology and adjustment, and child and adolescent maltreatment in female college students. *Journal of Abnormal Psychology, 101,* 717–723.

Saunders, B. E., Villeponteaux, L. A., Lipovsky, J. A., Kilpatrick, D. G., & Veronen, L. J. (1992). Child sexual assault as a risk factor for mental disorders among women. *Journal of Interpersonal Violence, 7,* 189–204.

Saywitz, K. J., Geiselman, R. E., & Bornstein, G. K. (1992). Effects of cognitive interviewing and practice on children's recall performance. *Journal of Abnormal Psychology, 101,* 744–755.

Saywitz, K. J., & Goodman, G. S. (1996). Interviewing children in and out of court. In J. Briere, L. Berliner, J. A. Bulkley, C. Jenny, & T. Reid (Eds.), *The APSAC handbook on child maltreatment* (pp. 297–318). Chicago: APSAC.

Saywitz, K. J., & Moan-Hardie, S. (1994). Reducing the potential for distortion of childhood memories. *Consciousness and Cognition, 3,* 408–425.

Saywitz, K. J., & Snyder, L. (in press). Narrative elaboration: Test of a new procedure for interviewing children. *Journal of Consulting and Clinical Psychology.*

Saywitz, K. J., Snyder, L., & Lamphear, V. (1996). Helping children tell what happened: A follow-up study of the narrative elaboration project. *Child Maltreatment, 1,* 200–212.

Scerbo, A. S., & Kolko, D. J. (1995). Child physical abuse and aggression: Preliminary findings on the role of internalizing problems. *Journal of the American Academy of Child and Adolescent Psychiatry, 34,* 1060–1066.

Schwab-Stone, M., Fallon, T., Brigs, M., & Crowther, B. (1994). Reliability of diagnostic reporting for children ages 6–11: A test–retest study of the Diagnostic Interview Schedule for Children—Revised. *American Journal of Psychiatry, 151,* 1048–1054.

Scott, M. J., & Stradling, S. G. (1994). Post-traumatic stress disorder without the stressor. *British Journal of Clinical Psychology, 33,* 71–74.

Scurfield, R. M. (1993a). Posttraumatic stress disorder in Vietnam veterans. In J. P. Wilson & B. Raphael (Eds.), *International handbook of traumatic stress syndromes* (pp. 285–295). New York: Plenum Press.

Scurfield, R. M. (1993b). Treatment of posttraumatic stress disorder among

Vietnam veterans. In J. P. Wilson & B. Raphael (Eds.), *International handbook of traumatic stress syndromes* (pp. 879–888). New York: Plenum Press.

Seligman, M. E. P. (1975). *Helplessness: On depression, development and death.* San Francisco: Freeman.

Shalev, A. Y. (1992). Posttraumatic stress disorder among injured survivors of a terrorist attack: Predictive value of early intrusion and avoidance symptoms. *Journal of Nervous and Mental Disease, 180,* 505–509.

Shalev, A. Y. (1996). Stress versus traumatic stress: From acute homeostatic reactions to chronic psychopathology. In B. A. van der Kolk, A. C. McFarlane, & L. Weisaeth (Eds.), *Traumatic stress: The effects of overwhelming experience on mind, body, and society* (pp. 77–101). New York: Guilford Press.

Shapiro, F. (1994). EMDR: In the eye of a paradigm shift. *Behavior Therapy, 25,* 153–156.

Shapiro, F. (1995). *Eye movement desensitization and reprocessing: Basic principles, protocols, and procedures.* New York: Guilford Press.

Shaunesey, K., Cohen, J. L., Plummer, B., & Berman, A. (1993). Suicidality in hospitalized adolescents: Relationship to prior abuse. *American Journal of Orthopsychiatry, 63*(1), 113–119.

Shilony, E., & Grossman, F. K. (1991). Depersonalization as a defense mechanism in survivors of trauma. *Journal of Traumatic Stress, 6,* 119–128.

Siegel, J. (1986). The Multidimensional Anger Inventory. *Journal of Personality and Social Psychology, 51,* 191–200.

Silverstein, R. (1994). Chronic identity diffusion in traumatized combat veterans. *Social Behavior and Personality, 22,* 69–80.

Simon, R. I. (1995). Toward the development of guidelines in the forensic psychiatric examination of posttraumatic stress disorder claimants. In R. Simon (Ed.), *Posttraumatic stress disorder in litigation* (pp. 31–84). Washington, DC: American Psychiatric Press.

Sipprelle, R. C. (1992). A vet center experience: Multievent trauma, delayed treatment type. In D. W. Foy (Ed.), *Treating PTSD: Cognitive-behavioral strategies* (pp. 13–38). New York: Guilford Press.

Smith, E. M., & North, C. S. (1993). Posttraumatic stress disorder in natural disasters and technological accidents. In J. P. Wilson & B. Raphael (Eds.), *International handbook of traumatic stress syndromes* (pp. 405–419). New York: Plenum Press.

Smucker, M. R., & Niederee, J. (1995). Treating incest-related PTSD and pathogenic schemas through imaginal exposure and rescripting. *Cognitive and behavioral practice, 2,* 63–93.

Solkoff, N., Gray, P., & Keill, S. (1986). Which Vietnam veterans develop posttraumatic stress disorders? *Journal of Clinical Psychology, 42,* 687–698.

Solomon, S., & Canino, G. (1990). Appropriateness of the DSM-III-R criteria for post-traumatic stress disorder. *Comprehensive Psychiatry, 31,* 227–237.

Solomon, S., Keane, T., Kaloupek, D., & Newman, E. (1996). Choosing self-report measures and structured interviews. In E. B. Carlson (Ed.), *Trauma research methodology* (pp. 56–81). Lutherville, MD: Sidran Press.

Solomon, S. D., Gerrity, E. T., & Muff, A. M. (1992). Efficacy of treatments for posttraumatic stress disorder. *Journal of the American Medical Association, 268,* 633–638.

Solomon, S. D., & Smith, E. M. (1994). Social support and perceived control as moderators of responses to dioxin and flood exposure. In R. J. Ursano, C. S. Fullerton, & B. G. McCaughey (Eds.), *Individual and community responses to trauma and disaster: The structure of human chaos* (pp. 179–200). Cambridge: Cambridge University Press.

Solomon, Z. (1989). PTSD and social functioning: A three year prospective study. *Social Psychiatry and Psychiatric Epidemiology, 24,* 127–133.

Solomon, Z., & Mikulincer, M. (1987). Combat stress reactions, posttraumatic stress disorder, and social adjustment: A study of Israeli veterans. *Journal of Nervous and Mental Disease, 175,* 277–285.

Solomon, Z., & Mikulincer, M. (1990). Life events and combat-related posttraumatic stress disorder: The intervening role of locus of control and social support. *Military Psychology, 2,* 241–256.

Solomon, Z., Mikulincer, M., & Hobfoll, S. E. (1987). Objective versus subjective measurement of stress and social support: Combat-related reactions. *Journal of Consulting and Clinical Psychology, 55,* 577–583.

Sonnenberg, S. M. (1988). Victims of violence and post-traumatic stress disorder. *Psychiatric Clinics of North America, 11,* 581–590.

Spurrell, M. T., & McFarlane, A. C. (1995). Life-events and psychiatric symptoms in a general psychiatry clinic: The role of intrusion and avoidance. *British Journal of Medical Psychology, 68,* 333–340.

Stamm, B. H. (Ed.). (1995). *Secondary traumatic stress.* Lutherville, MD: Sidran Press.

Stamm, B. H. (Ed.). (1996). *Measurement of stress, trauma, and adaptation.* Lutherville, MD: Sidran Press.

Steinberg, M. (1994). *Interviewer's guide to the Structured Clinical Interview for DSM-IV dissociative disorders—Revised (SCID-D).* Washington, DC: American Psychiatric Press.

Steinberg, M. (1995). *Handbook for the assessment of dissociation.* Washington, DC: American Psychiatric Press.

Steinberg, M. (1996). Diagnostic tools for assessing dissociation in children and adolescents. *Child and Adolescent Psychiatric Clinics of North America, 5,* 333–349.

Steinberg, M., Rounsaville, B., & Cicchetti, D. (1990). The Structured Clinical Interview for DSM-III-R Dissociative Disorders: Preliminary report on a new diagnostic instrument. *American Journal of Psychiatry, 147,* 76–82.

Steinberg, M., Rounsaville, B., & Cicchetti, D. (1991). Detection of dissociative disorders in psychiatric patients by a screening instrument and a structured diagnostic interview. *American Journal of Psychiatry, 148,* 1050–1054.

Steketee, G. S., & Foa, E. B. (1987). Rape victims: Post-traumatic stress responses and their treatment: A review of the literature. *Journal of Anxiety Disorders, 1,* 69–86.

Stine, S. M., & Kosten, T. R. (1995). Complications of chemical abuse and dependency. In M. J. Friedman, D. S. Charney, & A. Y. Deutch (Eds.), *Neurobiological and clinical consequences of stress: From normal adap-*

tation to *post-traumatic stress disorder* (pp. 447–464). Philadelphia: Lippincott-Raven.

Stone, A. M. (1992). The role of shame in post-traumatic stress disorder. *American Journal of Orthopsychiatry, 62,* 131–136.

Stone, N. M. (1993). Parental abuse as a precursor to childhood onset depression and suicidality. *Child Psychiatry and Human Development, 24,* 13–24.

Straus, M. A. (1979). Measuring intrafamily conflict and violence: The Conflict Tactics Scales. *Journal of Marriage and the Family, 41,* 75–88.

Surrey, J., Swett, C., Michaels, A., & Levin, S. (1990). Reported history of physical and sexual abuse and severity of symptomatology in women psychiatric patients. *American Journal of Orthopsychiatry, 60,* 412–417.

Sutker, P. B., Allain, J., Albert N., & Winstead, D. K. (1993). Psychopathology and psychiatric diagnoses of World War II Pacific theater prisoner of war survivors and combat veterans. *American Journal of Psychiatry, 150*(2), 240–245.

Tennant, C. C., Goulston, K., & Dent, O. (1993). Medical and psychiatric consequences of being a prisoner of war of the Japanese: An Australian follow-up study. In J. P. Wilson & B. Raphael (Eds.), *International handbook of traumatic stress syndromes* (pp. 231–239). New York: Plenum Press.

Terr, L. C. (1983). Chowchilla revisited: The effects of psychic trauma four years after a schoolbus kidnapping. *American Journal of Psychiatry, 140,* 1543–1550.

Terr, L. C. (1991). Childhood traumas: An outline and overview. *American Journal of Psychiatry, 148,* 10–20.

Tomb, D. A. (1994). The phenomenology of post-traumatic stress disorder. *Psychiatric Clinics of North America, 17,* 237–250.

Toth, S. L., Manly, J. T., & Cicchetti, D. (1992). Child maltreatment and vulnerability to depression. *Development and Psychopathology, 4,* 97–112.

True, W., Rice, J., Eisen, S. A., Heath, A. C., Goldberg, J., Lyons, M. J., & Nowak, J. (1993). A twin study of genetic and environmental contributions to the liability for posttraumatic stress symptoms. *Archives of General Psychiatry, 50,* 257–264.

Turnbull, G. J., & McFarlane, A. (1996). Acute treatments. In B. A. van der Kolk, A. C. McFarlane, & L. Weisaeth (Eds.), *Traumatic stress: The effects of overwhelming experience on mind, body, and society* (pp. 480–490). New York: Guilford Press.

Turner, S. W., McFarlane, A. C., & van der Kolk, B. (1996). The therapeutic environment and new explorations in the treatment of posttraumatic stress disorder. In B. A. van der Kolk, A. C. McFarlane, & L. Weisaeth (Eds.), *Traumatic stress: The effects of overwhelming experience on mind, body, and society* (pp. 537–558). New York: Guilford Press.

Ursano, R. J., Fullerton, C. S., & McCaughey, B. G. (1994). Trauma and disaster. In R. J. Ursano, C. S. Fullerton, & B. G. McCaughey (Eds.), *Individual and community responses to trauma and disaster: The structure of human chaos* (pp. 3–27). Cambridge: Cambridge University Press.

van der Kolk, B. A. (1987a). The psychobiology of the trauma response:

Hyperarousal, constriction, and addiction to traumatic reexposure. In B. A. van der Kolk (Ed.), *Psychological trauma* (pp. 63–87). Washington, DC: American Psychiatric Press.

van der Kolk, B. A. (1987b). The psychological consequences of overwhelming life experiences. In B. A. van der Kolk (Ed.), *Psychological trauma* (pp. 1–30). Washington, DC: American Psychiatric Press.

van der Kolk, B. A. (Ed.). (1987c). *Psychological trauma.* Washington, DC: American Psychiatric Press.

van der Kolk, B. A. (1987d). The role of the group in the origin and resolution of the trauma response. In B. van der Kolk (Ed.), *Psychological trauma* (pp. 153–171). Washington, DC: American Psychiatric Press.

van der Kolk, B. A. (1996a). The black hole of trauma. In B. A. van der Kolk, A. C. McFarlane, & L. Weisaeth (Eds.), *Traumatic stress: The effects of overwhelming experience on mind, body, and society* (pp. 5–23). New York: Guilford Press.

van der Kolk, B. A. (1996b). The body keeps the score: Approaches to the psychobiology of posttraumatic stress disorder. In B. A. van der Kolk, A. C. McFarlane, & L. Weisaeth (Eds.), *Traumatic stress: The effects of overwhelming experience on mind, body, and society* (pp. 214–241). New York: Guilford Press.

van der Kolk, B. A. (1996c). The complexity of adaptation to trauma: Self-regulation, stimulus discrimination, and characterological development. In B. A. van der Kolk, A. C. McFarlane, & L. Weisaeth (Eds.), *Traumatic stress: The effects of overwhelming experience on mind, body, and society* (pp. 182–213). New York: Guilford Press.

van der Kolk, B. A. (1996d). Trauma and memory. In B. A. van der Kolk, A. C. McFarlane, & L. Weisaeth (Eds.), *Traumatic stress: The effects of overwhelming experience on mind, body, and society* (pp. 279–302). New York: Guilford Press.

van der Kolk, B. A., Boyd, H., Krystal, J., & Greenberg, M. (1984). Post-traumatic stress disorder as a biologically based disorder: Implications of the animal model of inescapable shock. In B. A. van der Kolk (Ed.), *Post-traumatic stress disorder: Psychological and biological sequelae* (pp. 124–134). Washington DC: American Psychiatric Press.

van der Kolk, B. A., Greenberg, M. S., Orr, S. P., & Pitman, R. K. (1989). Endogenous opioids, stress induced analgesia, and posttraumatic stress disorder. *Psychopharmacology Bulletin, 25*, 417–421.

van der Kolk, B. A., & Kadish, W. (1987). Amnesia, dissociation, and the return of the repressed. In B. van der Kolk (Ed.), *Psychological trauma* (pp. 173–190). Washington, DC: American Psychiatric Press.

van der Kolk, B. A., McFarlane, A. C., & van der Hart, O. (1996). A general approach to treatment of posttraumatic stress disorder. In B. A. van der Kolk, A. C. McFarlane, & L. Weisaeth (Eds.), *Traumatic stress: The effects of overwhelming experience on mind, body, and society* (pp. 417–440). New York: Guilford Press.

van der Kolk, B. A., McFarlane, A. C., & Weisaeth, L. (Eds.). (1996). *Traumatic stress: The effects of overwhelming experience on mind, body, and society.* New York: Guilford Press.

van der Kolk, B. A., Perry, J. C., & Herman, J. L. (1991). Childhood origins of self-destructive behavior. *American Journal of Psychiatry, 148,* 1665–1671.

van der Kolk, B. A., van der Hart, O., & Marmar, C. R. (1996). Dissociation and information processing in posttraumatic stress disorder. In B. A. van der Kolk, A. C. McFarlane, & L. Weisaeth (Eds.), *Traumatic stress: The effects of overwhelming experience on mind, body, and society* (pp. 303–327). New York: Guilford Press.

Vaughan, K., Armstrong, M. S., Gold, R., O'Conner, N., Jenneke, W., & Tarrier, N. (1994). A trial of eye movement desensitization compared to image habituation training and applied muscle relaxation in posttraumatic stress disorder. *Journal of Behavior Therapy and Experimental Psychiatry, 25,* 283–291.

Vogel, J. M., & Vernberg, E. M. (1993). Children's psychological responses to disasters. *Journal of Clinical Child Psychology, 22,* 464–484.

Vreven, D., D., G., King, L., & King, D. (1995). The civilian version of the Mississippi PTSD Scale: A psychometric evaluation. *Journal of Traumatic Stress, 8,* 91–109.

Waldinger, R. J., Swett, C., Frank, A., & Miller, K. (1994). Levels of dissociation and histories of reported abuse among women outpatients. *Journal of Nervous and Mental Disease, 182,* 625–630.

Waller, N. G., Putnam, F. W., & Carlson, E. B. (1996). Types of dissociation and dissociative types: A taxometric analysis of dissociative experiences. *Psychological Methods, 1,* 300–321.

Weathers, F. W., Keane, T. M., King, L. A., & King, D. A. (1996). Psychometric theory in the development of posttraumatic stress disorder assessment tools. In J. Wilson & T. M. Keane (Eds.), *Assessing psychological trauma and PTSD* (pp. 98–135). New York: Guilford Press.

Webb, L. P., & Leehan, J. (1996). *Group treatment for adult survivors of abuse.* Thousand Oaks, CA: Sage.

Weisaeth, L. (1994). Psychological and psychiatric aspect of technological disasters. In R. J. Ursano, C. S. Fullerton, & B. G. McCaughey (Eds.), *Individual and community responses to trauma and disaster: The structure of human chaos* (pp. 72–102). Cambridge: Cambridge University Press.

Weiss, D. S. (1993). Structured clinical interview techniques. In J. P. Wilson & B. Raphael (Eds.), *International handbook of traumatic stress syndromes* (pp. 179–187). New York: Plenum Press.

Weiss, D. S. (1996). Structured clinical interview techniques. In J. Wilson & T. M. Keane (Eds.), *Assessing psychological trauma and PTSD* (pp. 493–511). New York: Guilford Press.

Weiss, D. S., & Marmar, C. R. (1993). Teaching time-limited dynamic psychotherapy for treating posttraumatic stress disorder and pathological grief. *Psychotherapy, 30,* 587–591.

Weiss, D. S., & Marmar, C. R. (1996). The Impact of Event Scale—Revised. In J. Wilson & T. M. Keane (Eds.), *Assessing psychological trauma and PTSD* (pp. 399–411). New York: Guilford Press.

Widom, C. S. (1989). Does violence beget violence? A critical examination of the literature. *Psychological Bulletin, 106,* 3–28.

Williams, L. M. (1994). Recall of childhood trauma: A prospective study of women's memories of child sexual abuse. *Journal of Consulting and Clinical Psychology, 62,* 1167–1176.

Williams, L. M. (1995). Recovered memories of abuse in women with documented child sexual victimization histories. *Journal of Traumatic Stress, 8,* 649–673.

Williams, M. B., & Sommer, J. F. (Eds.). (1994a). *Handbook of posttraumatic therapy.* Westport, CT: Greenwood Press.

Williams, M. B., & Sommer, J. F. (1994b). Toward the development of a generic model of PTSD treatment. In M. B. Williams & J. F. Sommer (Eds.), *Handbook of posttraumatic therapy* (pp. 551–563). Westport, CT: Greenwood Press.

Wilson, J., & Keane, T. M. (Eds.). (1996). *Assessing psychological trauma and PTSD.* New York: Guilford Press.

Wilson, J., Keane, T. M., & Smagola, J. (1996). *Trauma and the law: Assessing traumatic syndromes and PTSD in forensic contexts.* Unpublished manuscript.

Wilson, J. P. (1994a). The historical evolution of PTSD diagnostic criteria: From Freud to DSM-IV. *Journal of Traumatic Stress, 7,* 681–698.

Wilson, J. P. (1994b). The need for an integrative theory of post-traumatic stress disorder. In M. B. Williams & J. F. Sommer (Eds.), *Handbook of posttraumatic therapy* (pp. 3–17). Westport, CT: Greenwood Press.

Wilson, J. P., & Raphael, B. (Eds.). (1993). *International handbook of traumatic stress syndromes.* New York: Plenum Press.

Wilson, J. P., Smith, W. K., & Johnson, S. K. (1985). A comparative analysis of PTSD among various survivor groups. In C. Figley (Ed.), *Trauma and its wake* (pp. 142–172). New York: Brunner/Mazel.

Wilson, S. A., Becker, L. A., & Tinker, R. H. (1995). Eye movement desensitization and reprocessing (EMDR) treatment for psychologically traumatized individuals. *Journal of Consulting and Clinical Psychology, 63,* 928–937.

Wind, T. W., & Silvern, L. (1994). Parenting and family stress as mediators of the long-term effects of child abuse. *Child Abuse and Neglect, 18,* 439–453.

Wolfe, D., Sas, L., & Wekerle, C. (1994). Factors associated with the development of posttraumatic stress disorder among child victims of sexual abuse. *Child Abuse and Neglect, 18,* 37–50.

Wolfe, J., & Charney, D. (1991). Use of neuropsychological assessment in posttraumatic stress disorder. *Psychological Assessment, 3,* 573–580.

Wolfe, V. V., Gentile, C., & Wolfe, D. A. (1989). The impact of sexual abuse on children: A PTSD formulation. *Behavior Therapy, 20,* 215–228.

Wong, M. R., & Cook, D. (1992). Shame and its contribution to PTSD. *Journal of Traumatic Stress, 5,* 557–562.

Woodward, S. H. (1995). Neurobiological perspectives on sleep in post-traumatic stress disorder. In M. J. Friedman, D. S. Charney, & A. Y. Deutch (Eds.), *Neurobiological and clinical consequences of stress: From normal adaptation to post-traumatic stress disorder* (pp. 315–333). Philadelphia: Lippincott-Raven.

Yama, M. F., Fogas, B. S., Teegarden, L. A., & Hastings, B. (1993). Childhood sexual abuse and parental alcoholism: Interactive effects in adult women. *American Journal of Orthopsychiatry, 63,* 300–305.

Yama, M. F., Tovey, S. L., & Fogas, B. S. (1993). Childhood family environment and sexual abuse as predictors of anxiety and depression in adult women. *American Journal of Orthopsychiatry, 63,* 136–141.

Yehuda, R., Giller, E. L., & Mason, J. W. (1993). Psychoendocrine assessment of posttraumatic stress disorder: Current progress and new directions. *Progress in Neuro-Psychopharmacological and Biological Psychiatry, 17,* 541–550.

Yehuda, R., Giller, E. L., Southwick, S. M., Lowy, M. T., & Mason, J. W. (1991). Hypothalamic–pituitary–adrenal dysfunction in posttraumatic stress disorder. *Biological Psychiatry, 30,* 1031–1048.

Yehuda, R., Kahana, B., Southwick, S. M., & Giller, E. L. (1994). Depressive features in Holocaust survivors with post-traumatic stress disorder. *Journal of Traumatic Stress, 7,* 699–704.

Yehuda, R., & McFarlane, A. C. (1995). Conflict between current knowledge about posttraumatic stress disorder and its original conceptual basis. *American Journal of Psychiatry, 152,* 1705–1713.

Yehuda, R., Resnick, H., Kahana, B., & Giller, E. L. (1993). Long-lasting hormonal alterations to extreme stress in humans: Normative or maladaptive? *Psychosomatic Medicine, 55,* 287–297.

Young, M. B. (1988). Understanding identity disruption and intimacy: One aspect of post-traumatic stress. *Contemporary Family Therapy, 10,* 30–43.

Yule, W. (1994). Posttraumatic stress disorder. In T. H. Ollendick, N. J. King, & W. Yule (Eds.), *International handbook of phobic and anxiety disorders in children and adolescents* (pp. 223–240). New York: Plenum Press.

Index